Head Injury Recovery
in Real Life

Head Injury Recovery in Real Life

LARRY E. SCHUTZ
MICHAEL E. SCHUTZ

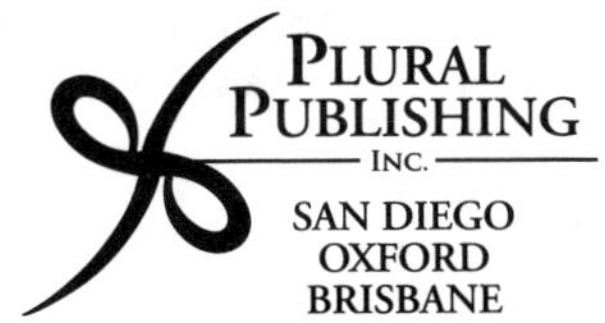

PLURAL PUBLISHING INC.

SAN DIEGO
OXFORD
BRISBANE

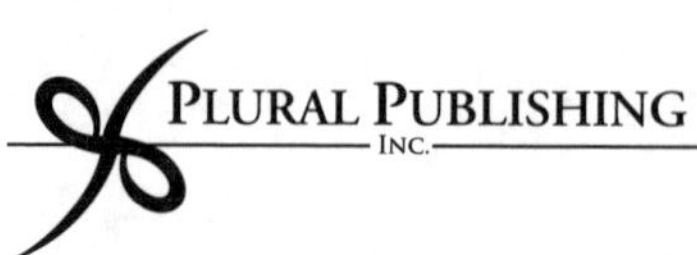

5521 Ruffin Road
San Diego, CA 92123

e-mail: info@pluralpublishing.com
Web site: http://www.pluralpublishing.com

49 Bath Street
Abingdon, Oxfordshire OX14 1EA
United Kingdom

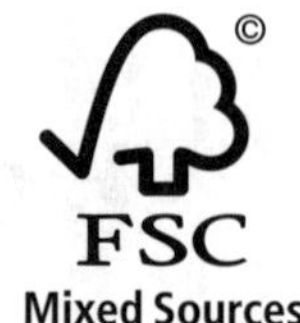

Library of Congress Cataloging-in-Publication Data:

Schutz, Larry E.
   Head injury recovery in real life / Larry E. Schutz and Michael E. Schutz.
         p. ; cm.
   Includes bibliographical references and index.
   ISBN-13: 978-1-59756-378-9 (alk. paper)
   ISBN-10: 1-59756-378-1 (alk. paper)
   1. Brain damage—Patients—Rehabilitation. I. Schutz, Michael E. II. Title.
   [DNLM: 1. Craniocerebral Trauma—rehabilitation—Personal Narratives.
2. Recovery of Function—Personal Narratives. WL 354 S396h 2010]
   RC387.5.S377 2010
   617.4'81044—dc22
                                                                2009040668

Contents

PART II. GREAT RECOVERIES AS INDIVIDUAL EFFORTS — 73

PART III. EXCEPTIONAL RECOVERIES AS PARTNERSHIPS WITH FAMILY — 187

PART IV. CONCLUSION — 253

Introduction

Some people may wonder why recovery from head injury needs to be the subject of a book. It is commonly assumed that an injury to the brain heals up; however, that idea is a myth (Swift & Wilson, 2001). Brain damage is permanent (Benton & Tranel, 2000). For many years, the National Head Injury Foundation (an organization of survivors and their families) issued its newsletter under this motto: "After head injury life is never the same." They felt it was important for members to understand that the healing process is less complete than most expect it to be.

Here is another common belief: "Permanent brain damage" makes victims so inept, crippled, stupid, and crazy that you can spot them at a glance (Nochi, 1998b). This is another myth (Hux, Schram, & Goeken, 2006). Most survivors look normal, hold up their end of a conversation, and accomplish most of the things they try to do. That is what makes traumatic brain injury (TBI) a "silent epidemic" (National Head Injury Foundation, 1982). You can't judge either the recovery needed or the recovery already achieved by appearances.

If the truth lies between these false extremes, then the crucial question is, "What recovers and what doesn't?" This is a question most people cannot answer, and even science has struggled to answer it. Severe head injuries were fatal until about 60 years ago. Research began to build a picture of recovery in the 1970s, but that only amounted to a few snapshots. Most studies looked at the earliest phases of recovery, at patients who were still in the hospital or spending a good part of the day at the outpatient clinic. The research, based on tests given by rehabilitation staff, measured recovery strictly in the terms of the "unreal" medical world. Even today, most published studies look at recovery through laboratory measurements. Very few look at real life, where recovery is different in some important ways (Ylvisaker & Gioia, 1998).

Although it has its limits, the research does tell a powerful story. Almost all survivors make great progress when they come out of coma.

They wake up terribly impaired and then their mental and physical skills stream back gradually (McKinlay & Watkiss, 1999). The early months bring huge gains because the injury has disrupted a great deal of living brain tissue, causing massive temporary effects (Katz & Black, 1999). However, by the second year this "natural" recovery is nearly done. At this point, the deficits that still remain are caused by the death of brain cells, and they will permanently interfere with the survivor's functioning (Jennett, 1997).

When they go home, survivors usually look and act normal in most ways (Roberts, 1979). Specialized tests reveal their long-term deficits in remembering newly learned information, exercising self-control, and handling difficult challenges (McCullagh & Feinstein, 2005). Under certain conditions these weakened cognitive (or thinking) skills cause emotional and behavioral problems (Marin & Chakravorty, 2005). Routine chores and tasks are usually not affected, but the out-of-the-ordinary challenges and interactions are a big problem. Important social relationships also become hard to handle—especially the reciprocal give-and-take that should occur with a spouse, friend, employer, coworker, or customer. Incidents keep happening, and eventually the roles and relationships can be ruined by the buildup of ill will—jobs and friendships lost, marriage emotionally estranged or broken (Wood, Liossi, & Wood, 2005).

The strangest part is that so many survivors respond to these difficulties passively: They make no effort to rescue the dying relationships or to replace the lost roles. They seem to learn nothing from the trial-and-error lessons of adaptation. People with other kinds of damage to the central nervous system, such as a spinal cord injury or blindness, also face permanent losses, but they make adjustments to get the lost parts of their lives back—that is called *functional recovery*. They develop new habits to work around their impairments (known as *adaptation to disability*). The most common cognitive deficits associated with TBI shut down this adaptation process. Many survivors fail to make *any* adjustments (Bergquist & Malec, 2005). The problem is so serious that TBI is sometimes called a disorder of adaptation (Craine, 1982; Reitan, 1988; Schutz, 2007b). Put simply, too many survivors just don't deal with their lasting symptoms.

Adaptation fails to take place when the effects of the injury are not recognized. The cognitive symptoms of TBI give the survivor an overpowering impression that the injury has not "changed me" in any major way, whereas companions are often struck by changes in personality (Prigatano, 1999b). How can survivors be different on the outside but the same on the inside? That is one of the reasons recovery is so complicated: A person who feels unchanged has no reason to adapt and every reason to go back to pre-injury life, doing things just as they were done before (Grosswasser & Stern, 1998). It is as if the person's sense of self and sense of the world were frozen at the moment the injury happened, making it impossible to deal with life as it is now or to prepare for what can and should be expected in the future (Damasio, 1994).

This research doesn't tell the whole story. In real life, TBI doesn't make adaptation to disability impossible; some people do adapt. A few articles tell the story of a survivor who went back to a responsible job or maintained important relationships (e.g., Evans, 2003; Howard, 2004; Lezak, 1995; Marin & Chakravorty, 2005; Newcombe, 1987; Nimgade & Costello, 2003; Oddy & Cogan, 2004; Paterson, 1980; Schutz, 1989; von Cramon & Matthes-von Cramon, 1994). We have also observed good functional recoveries achieved long after the discharge from the clinic (e.g., Lewis & Schutz, 1984). Thus, an open-minded review of all of the evidence finds that good recoveries are possible, even if they are uncommon outcomes.

The books and articles on TBI say nothing about *great* recoveries. A great recovery comes after an injury severe enough to compromise the essential skills for a full life. Moreover, a great recoverer adapts so well that these roadblocks are *completely* overcome. The recoverer not only resumes a full life, but also achieves excellence in competition against others with factory-fresh brains, day after day and year after year. Great recovery is about finding a way to do the hard things the injury *should* prevent doing, and then doing them at the highest level of quality and on a consistent basis. This level of recovery is so unexpected that it cannot be measured by the major TBI outcome scales (the Glasgow Outcome Scale and the Disability Rating Scale—see Wright, 2000). Some TBI experts even discount the possibility of a great recovery (Cope, 1996; Kraus, 1987; Marshall, 1987; Willer, Abosch, & Dahmer 1990). This book was written mainly to present 15 great recoveries, 12 of them in detail. These recoveries show that even severe TBI doesn't eliminate the ability to adapt at the highest level.

How did they do it? These recoveries can't be written off to good luck. Each one came at the cost of endless effort by the person, and in some cases, by the family. None of the 15 was a genius, a unique talent, or a wealthy person aided by a staff of helpers. Most of the families were supportive, and some even partnered in the recovery work, but others were no help at all. All of the survivors were treated in the same cognitive rehabilitation program, but the program clearly was not the magic ingredient because most of its graduates could not accomplish what these 15 did. Some of the great recoverers even underachieved when they were in therapy.

What they all did was to admit that the injury had changed them. They studied their mistakes and tried to avoid making them again. They stopped using their pre-injury ways of thinking and doing things and replaced them with new ways better suited to their damaged brains. They adopted a disciplined lifestyle of detailed schedules and plans and careful notes and reminders. They planned ahead to adjust for their impairments before their activities suffered any interference. They made it their business to do what they had been taught in the clinic, but they did not stop there. They redesigned and rebuilt the recovery strategies many times, custom-fitting them to meet the changing demands of their lives. They became passionate *self-therapists*, devoted to a life-long mission to reexamine their deficits and find ever-better ways to fix them.

The results they achieved were nothing short of spectacular. Some graduated from high school and college with top honors. Some went on to graduate school, passed licensing exams, and entered elite professions. Some worked in high-status jobs that demanded decision making and people handling, and earned top ratings and/or promotions. In the process, most led active social lives, and some met future spouses, got married, and started new families. Although they could no longer think in the way they did before the injury, they learned to get every important duty done at the same high level of quality as before. "It is exceptional to regain the premorbid (that is, pre-injury) level of functioning following a brain injury" (Hoegh, 1994). Most also gained a stronger sense of pride and purpose in life. Many were even grateful for the injury, because it gave them inspiration to become better people. Such remarkable accomplishments qualify these survivors as experts on the subject of recovery. For this reason, we asked them to tell their recovery stories in their own words. In addition, the stories are firsthand accounts of real life, mainly describing what happened after their final discharge from therapy. All but one have been back in real life full-time for between 5 and 16 years.

This book is written with three groups of readers in mind. The first one is survivors and their families. Each story includes a section of recovery advice the survivor offered them. Because the scientific and clinical facts about recovery are not explained in detail in books published for this group, we also wrote introductory chapters covering the history and science of recovery. Because most of these readers come from nonprofessional backgrounds, we wrote our explanations in plain English. If we felt we had to use a technical term, we explained it first. The senior author is a clinical neuropsychologist, a specialist in TBI rehabilitation for more than 25 years who designs and directs TBI programs; he usually writes in technical language. The junior author is a journalist whose job was to keep things simple (except for a small section at the end of each story written for neuropsychologists) and to choose the words that would paint a vivid picture of each issue and each recoverer. To the survivors and families: We want you to understand what can be done about TBI. We aren't promising that you can create one of these world-class recoveries for yourself, because they are, after all, exceptional. On the other hand, we won't tell you that you *can't* create one. Don't let anyone tell you that. It is never safe to bet against the recovery of a person determined to do everything that is necessary to succeed.

The second group is made up of cognitive rehabilitation professionals. In this specialty area, we have no tradition of publishing our most successful cases. Perhaps we should. Our main scientific tradition is based on the pursuit of general laws, focusing on the central tendencies of our research samples (Gigerenzer, 2000). TBI recovery is not adequately explained by central tendencies; the individual differences are so large that we need to learn from our extreme cases (Brooks, 1987). The best way to learn about unusual outcomes is from the subject's own narration (Bolles, 1988; Combs & Freedman, 1994; Nochi, 1998b). Self-descriptions of the best long-term recoveries define the upper limit for formulating "our goal . . . not so much to improve test scores as to improve the adaptation and success of patient's lives" (Eslinger, 2005, p. 6). They tell us how high we can "set the bar."

The third group is made up of neurorehabilitation students. Students often are taught to plan treatment to improve test scores, but a better objective is framed, "What could I do that would make the biggest difference in this person's future life?" The stories detail therapy events and recovery concepts that still impact these exceptional lives many years after their discharge—they point to the interventions that framed these successful futures. Some of these interventions can be used as described, and some of the recoverers' learning experiences can be recommended to your patients. These stories also remind us that great recovery is a human phenomenon, an achievement made not by lobes or by cognitive skills but by individuals. In the most effective treatment, the *person* receives the most attention (Prigatano, 1999a; Wood, 1990).

Think of recovery as a journey down a long, one-way road (Nochi, 1997): The survivor has changed forever and should not turn back to resume following his or her old path. But most survivors keep trying to double back, no matter how much oncoming traffic they encounter. The stories in this book were written by people who stopped trying to turn back and instead went forward to complete their journey successfully. In fact, they went farther down the road than almost anyone has gone. We should use their accounts as road maps—surely they know the way.

This book is dedicated to the memory of Betty Ann Schutz (1918–2005), our mother/grandmother. A professional from another era of health care, she felt a duty to try to understand all of her patients. Understanding often turned out to be a matter of taking the time to listen to what they had to say. It is also dedicated to Mae-Dell (Julie) Lacy and Henry Pfingstag, the teachers who changed our lives by stubbornly refusing to lower the bar under any circumstances.

Introduction

Chapter 1

How We Learned What We Know About Recovery

Traumatic brain injury (TBI) is a fact of life. The brain is highly vulnerable to damage in our world. Its consistency is mushy, like a bowl of warm oatmeal or gelatin salad (Sapolsky, 1996; Sohlberg & Mateer, 1989). Because it is not very durable, it is protected by being held fast inside a fluid-filled fabric bag (Walsh, 1978). There is a smooth, round skull in back and a rock-hard bone wall in front (Rose & Johnson, 1996). Unfortunately, this protection is incomplete, allowing damage to occur under certain conditions. A powerful push or a blow from in front spears the brain on the bony points inside the front wall (Jennett & Teasdale, 1981). Intense force applied to either side rakes it against the uneven sides of the skull (Lindgren, 1966). Glancing blows twist it on its stem, tearing the long nerve fibers in its stalk (Lezak, 1983). Enough blows, as in prizefighting, bruise and shrink it (Corsellis, Bruton, & Freeman-Browne, 1973; Roberts, 1969). In a hard fall, damage occurs when the head bounces on the ground and then the brain bounces off the inside of the skull (Reitan & Wolfson, 1986). An explosion or a bullet can destroy any part of it, so modern warfare is the ultimate breeding ground for brain damage (Boake, 1991; Luria, 1979). The destruction is permanent: Cells die and new ones are not born to replace them (Stein, Brailowski, & Will, 1995; Wade, 2005).

Though many dangerous activities risk brain damage, the modern epidemic of TBI (Bennett, Dittmar, & Ho, 1997; Uzzell & Stonnington, 1996b) arrived with the popularity of motor vehicles (Kraus & Chu,

2005). A crash at 35 miles per hour from hitting a tree on a neighborhood street or from a head-on collision in a parking lot damages the brain (Ommaya & Gennarelli, 1974). The faster the vehicle travels, the more force and damage an accident causes. Severe TBI became common when airplanes and cars became our main transportation (Long & Williams, 1988). Motor vehicle accidents are the main cause of TBI everywhere but the inner cities, where they are outpaced by violence against teens and young adults (Kraus, 1987).

In the late 19th century, science began studying the inner workings of the brain through the careful medical observation of strokes and penetrating brain wounds. Much of the work done between 1870 and 1970 involved mapping out "centers" for increasingly specific functions by classifying the effects of holes in different parts of the brain (Feinberg & Farah, 2003; Goldstein, 1942; Walsh & Darby, 1999). Most scientists felt certain that nothing could be done to repair brain damage. If brain cells in the control center for a skill were destroyed, that skill would always be impaired and the person's functioning would be forever limited, or so they assumed at that time (see Bach-y-Rita, 1989; Berrol, 1992; Rosenthal, 1999a; Stein, 1988).

In its first century, neurology had nothing to say about severe TBI because it was still a sure death sentence (Rose & Johnson, 1996). Trauma doctors learned how to keep these patients alive during World War II, after which ever-increasing numbers of injury victims were saved by improving technologies (Harti & Ghajar, 2005). The doctors saw patients getting better in the hospital, but had no idea what their future might hold until long-term outcome research results began to trickle in during the 1960s and 1970s (Clifton, 1989). The research showed that recovery stopped before they could resume normal lives, leaving them with serious adjustment problems (Bond, 1975, 1979; Gilchrist & Wilkinson, 1979; Levin, Grossman, Rose, & Teasdale, 1979; Lezak, 1978; Lishman, 1968; Rosenbaum & Najenson, 1976).

At the present time, with tens of millions of living survivors and almost as many pages of published scientific research on TBI, it is still hard to make sense of the recovery of a single survivor. The traditional methods of science are best suited to making statements about people in general (Gigerenzer, 2000), whereas they are difficult to apply to individuals (Brooks, 1987; Newcombe, 1987; Schutz, Rivers, & Ratusnik, 2009). The information in our first two chapters is based mainly on these general statements. We frequently use phrases like "most survivors" or "the typical survivor" to indicate that the principle comes from group-based research. Try to remember that the recovery of an individual could be an exception to almost any general rule.

Because there were no clinical services designed for TBI in the early 1970s, the therapies provided in the community were intended for another kind of disorder (Rosenthal, 1999b). Medications and medical treatments developed for mental health patients do not cure TBI (Cassidy, 1999; Lux, 1996; Pollack, 2005). Traditional psychotherapy for psychological disorders simply does not work (Goldstein & Ruthven, 1983; Horton, 1997; Malec, 1985; Morris & Bleiberg, 1986; Sbordone, 1990). Stroke therapy was designed to provide structured practice of impaired skills (Twitchell, 1951), but it does not have enough impact to restore the defective abilities (Burke, Guth, Guare, & Weslowski, 1999; Prigatano, Glisky, & Klonoff, 1996), and energetic, uncooperative TBI patients disrupted the orderly rehabilitation unit (Horn, 1992). Schools were equally unprepared, ill-equipped, and ineffective (Begali, 1992; Berko, Berko, & Thompson, 1970; Deaton, 1987a, 1987b; DePompei, Epps, Savage, Blosser, & Castelli, 1998; Telzrow, 1987). Poorly-recovered survivors got warehoused along with society's undesirables in jails (Finlayson & Garner, 1994; Hackler & Tobis, 1983) and psychiatric wards (Lishman, 1968). The community had no good answers for TBI (Jacobs, 1990; Stein et al., 1995).

America's first outpatient program for TBI was opened in 1968 at the Palo Alto V.A. Medical Center, Menlo Park Division, a vast mental hospital as big as a college campus. Nancy Cook, a clinical psychologist, gathered TBI patients living on all of the psychiatric wards into a day program called the Brain Injury Rehab Unit (BIRU) (Trexler, 1987). BIRU tried established psychological techniques with only limited success. In 1972, psychologists at Hawaii State (mental) Hospital set up their own, elaborate behavioral training program (Craine & Gudeman, 1981). These pioneers came to realize that new therapy methods specific for TBI were needed.

The whole picture changed in 1974 when Ben-Yishay and Diller, psychologists from NYU's Rusk Institute of Rehabilitation Medicine, developed cognitive rehabilitation for the Israeli Ministry of Defense (Boake, 1991; Christiansen & Caetano, 1999). The patients were combat veterans with TBI or penetrating head wounds. The program was a complex, "all-out" effort that included the education, skill training, counseling, and vocational therapy provided at centers for veterans of World War I with penetrating wounds (Goldstein, 1942; Poppelreuter, 1917). Psychologist/physician Poppelreuter (1917) had observed that his patients tended to withdraw from life as they recovered, and psychiatrist/neurologist Goldstein (1940/1963) explained that they withdrew to cope with the catastrophic anxiety and confusion they felt when confronted by situations they could not handle. Goldstein (1934/2000, 1952) advocated nesting the program in a customized, safe environment to encourage them to remain active. Ben-Yishay (1996) took his milieu in a different direction, framing the Israeli program in a type of high-intensity therapeutic community for insight training introduced in drug/alcohol rehabilitation. Finally, concepts and strategies of Russian psychologist/neurologist A. R. Luria (Ben-Yishay, 1996) were used in developing NYU's innovative brain therapy techniques for right brain disorders (Piasetsky, Ben-Yishay, Weinberg, & Diller, 1982) and carried over to the Israeli program. Luria's (1948/1963, 1966, 1973) basic idea (presaged by British neurologist John Hughlings Jackson—see Jackson, 1882/1998) was that the brain is more adaptable than early theories suggested because behavior is controlled by several intersecting networks rather than an individual control center (Churchland, 1998; Feinberg & Farah, 2003; Newcombe, 1987; Stein et al., 1995; Ylvisaker, 1998). When one network is damaged, the thought process can be rerouted through other, more intact networks to accomplish the objective (Luria, 1948/1963, 1979; Miller, 1984; Rosner, 1970). "Contemporary efforts at cognitive neuropsychological rehabilitation are based on Luria's approach" (Prigatano, 2005, p. 7). Unfortunately, Luria's ideas were not detailed enough to serve as a blueprint for TBI therapy (Piasetsky, 1982; Prigatano, 2005), but the Israeli group was able to develop its own blueprints (Ben-Yishay & Diller, 1983b; Gross, 1982), which have since been further modified on the basis of a generation of experience (Bleiberg, Cope, & Spector, 1989; Gross & Schutz, 1986; Schutz, 2007a, 2007b; Shallice, 2002; Shallice & Burgess, 1991; Stuss, Mateer, & Sohlberg, 1994). These psychosocial, rehabilitative, and neurocognitive concepts were combined in Israel into a year-long, full-time program of unprecedented complexity (Gordon & Hibbard, 2005).

The results were impressive: two to five times the ordinary recovery rate, with more than two thirds of discharged patients pursuing vocational activities, and half of them returning to stable, competitive jobs (Ben-Yishay & Prigatano, 1990). Later follow-ups found most of the former patients still working in competitive jobs more than a decade after their discharge (Hoofien, Gilboa, Vakil, & Donovick, 2001; Klonoff, Lamb, & Henderson, 2001). For the first time, a treatment procedure reliably corrected the major ability limitations of TBI in a lasting way (Rosenthal, 1983).

At about the same time, American hospitals were reinventing inpatient treatment for TBI. The Rehabilitation Act of 1973 created the Model Systems of Care program. In 1977, the first grant for TBI was issued to Santa Clara Valley Medical Center, a teaching hospital affiliated with Stanford University Medical School. Their program kept patients in treatment until they could function in the community. The length of stay averaged 4 months, with the most serious injuries taking as long as a year. Their outcome studies showed that a specialized, high-intensity program accelerates early recovery (Berrol, 1992; Cope, 1996).

The second Model Systems grant was awarded to Dr. Ben-Yishay, who returned to the United States to build an Israeli-type outpatient program at NYU in 1978. His program continues in operation today. New patients enter one "class" at a time for a 5-month cycle. Most who don't master recovery the first time through are asked back for another cycle. Today one cycle costs over $70,000, and many patients receive several cycles, remaining in therapy for as long as 3 years. As expensive as this therapy is, it continues to produce good outcomes.

Between 1977 and 1983, cutting-edge TBI programs were developed in eight more states (Illinois, Pennsylvania, New Jersey, Massachusetts, Florida, Oklahoma, Indiana, and Virginia). All of these programs provided fully specialized services including carefully crafted cognitive and psychological therapies. They employed dedicated treatment teams and applied their own outcome research results to improve the effectiveness of their interventions (Cope, 1996).

If the early 1980s established TBI as a distinctive, advanced professional specialty, the next decade was an era of misdirected program development:

> General acute care hospitals have opened new rehabilitation facilities over the last decade; these facilities serve as a new and supplemental revenue source. The result has been the proliferation of many new, small, relatively unskilled rehabilitation programs that provide more or less inappropriate treatments to complex catastrophic cases. This occurs because of the economic need to . . . generate revenue, rather than in response to balanced clinical judgment. (Cope, 1996, p. 297)

Within 10 years, more than 1000 self-proclaimed head trauma or cognitive programs were being advertised. The start-ups were often staffed by unqualified therapists (NIH, 1998). Many practiced the kind of old-fashioned physical rehabilitation that had proven to be ineffective for TBI in the past (Cope & Reynolds, 2005; Hoegh, 1994), with the addition of a few hours of so-called cognitive rehabilitation (often a conglomeration of testing tasks used as repetitive drills) (Schutz & Trainor, 2007; Ylvisaker, Hanks, & Johnson-Greene, 2002). New profit-oriented companies opened residential treatment centers, many of which were eventually closed for ethical violations (Banja, 1992). Barely a decade after its establishment, TBI rehabilitation had been saddled with an ugly reputation as shoddy, ill-conceived, unscientific, incompetent, and irresponsible (Bontke & Boake, 1991; Rosenthal, 1999a).

Even though TBI programs were opened in every major metropolitan area, specialized TBI rehabilitation never became the standard of care. Even in the boom years, only 5 to 15% of patients were admitted to TBI programs (Bontke, 1990; Gronwall, Wrightson, & Waddell, 1990; Kreutzer, Gordon, & Wehman, 1989; NIH, 1998). Most patients got no rehabilitation, some got technically limited care, and only a few got the kind of training that provided complete preparation for recovery.

In the present era, most TBI treatment is funded by medical insurance under managed care. This system has cut the funding and services for TBI dramatically (Sohlberg & Mateer, 2001). "All too often, the real needs of the individual with TBI are lost in the name of 'cost containment'" (Gordon, Hibbard, Brown, Flanagan, & Korves, 1999).

> Only a small number of private insurers include cognitive rehabilitation as a covered service . . . Many third-party payers as well as Medicare and Medicaid restrict scope, duration, timing and intensity of service and make no provision for cognitive treatment as life circumstances change. Some insurers disallow claims for cognitive rehabilitation while others have specifically excluded such treatment from their policies. (Katz, Ashley, O'Shanick, & Connors, 2006, p. ii)

Most TBI programs have closed, and of those that remain, few offer more than bare-bones services (Fordyce, 2003). The government funds 16 Model Systems of Care programs to operate with fewer restrictions, but they are too few and far between to help most newly injured patients. Thus, most patients "receive inadequate assistance" (Fordyce, 1994, p. 197), both among children (Greenspan & MacKenzie, 2000) and adults (Pickelsimer et al., 2007), while "the quality of life for survivors of traumatic brain injury . . . (remains) poor" (Berrol, 1992, p. xv).

In retrospect, it has become clear that TBI is unique among medical disorders and that only a fully specialized system of intensive treatment can provide the full benefits of recovery that our present technology allows. Under such ideal conditions, most patients with TBI are capable of making major progress toward recovery. If they are given less than comprehensive or fully specialized treatment, the quality of recovery usually suffers (Gowland & Gambarotto, 1994; Gronwall et al., 1990; Rotondi, Sinkule, Balzer, Harris, & Moldovan, 2007; Schootman & Fuortes, 1999). Thus, our society has at its disposal the methods to restore their lives, but "the need for services among people with TBI appears to greatly exceed the services delivered" (GAO, 1998). The current policy of withholding these services to most patients is illogical (Gordon et al., 1999): "When the benefit of a post-acute rehabilitation program is the salvage of a human life, it follows that any cost . . . is offset by the benefit" (Malec, Smigielski, DePompolo, & Thompson, 1993). It is also inhumane: "We are obligated to do everything possible to make their lives worth living" (Goldstein, 1942, p. 223).

Because most people are not offered the treatment they need to realize their full recovery potential, rehabilitation experts should at least share their knowledge of the principles of recovery with the untreated survivors, families, and community-based providers who are willing to help them. Most survivors and their families are people from ordinary backgrounds, with very little accurate knowledge about TBI. They do not understand what long-term TBI symptoms are like, and they fail to recognize those symptoms when they occur. They have no idea how to cope with the symptoms, and most efforts to recover are misguided and unsuccessful. Patients who make good recoveries through advanced rehabilitation receive a great deal of education about these matters, and they put that education to use in their daily life after they leave therapy. Thus people who have head injuries, and those who care for the survivors, have an absolute need for the specialized knowledge that is currently available only to TBI experts and discharged patients.

Much of the critically needed knowledge is published, but at present it is embedded in highly technical professional articles and textbooks. The principles of recovery do not have to be expressed in such a complicated fashion, but even if people received the information in plain language (Schutz, 2006a, 2006b), they would need to integrate the recovery disciplines into their daily life to make genuine progress on their own (Schutz, 2005c; Schutz & Schutz, 2005). The stories presented in this volume provide a promising starting point, by explaining some of the principles and by demonstrating how much progress a dedicated recoverer can make by following the expert guidelines.

Chapter 2

How Recovery Works— In the Clinic and in Real Life

TBI is common and costly enough to be a major public health problem.

The annual incidence of TBI in the United States has been variously estimated at 1.5 million (Centers for Disease Control, 1999; NIH, 1998), 2 million (National Health Interview Survey; see Kraus & McArthur, 1999), or more than 3 million cases (Silver, McAllister, & Yudofsky, 2005). Most (75–90%) are mild, requiring no more than brief hospital care (Bazarian et al., 2005; Bigler, 1990a; Kraus & Chu, 2005).

The most important statistic is the prevalence (frequency) of permanent ability limitations. Most studies assess physical abilities because they are easiest to measure. Permanent and total physical disability is the outcome for 10% of hospitalized cases (Kingston, 1985). There are 80,000 to 90,000 new cases per year (National Center for Injury Prevention and Control, 1999), or from 74 to 100 per 100,000 (Bryden, 1989; Willer, Abosch, & Dahmer, 1990). A study commissioned by the Centers for Disease Control estimates that 5.3 million Americans (or 2% of the population) cannot perform their daily living activities independently due to TBI (Langlois, Rutland-Brown, & Wald, 2006). However, it is not the physical abilities but cognitive and behavioral abilities whose loss produces the most serious and long-lasting problems after TBI (Gordon & Hibbard, 2005). The rate of cognitive/behavioral ability limitation is estimated at four to eight times the rate for physical abilities (Bigler, 1990a; Fisher, 1985), which means that many millions of survivors are affected. The annual cost of TBI to

American society in medical expenses and lost wages was estimated at $56 billion in 1995 (Thurman, 2001) and 60 billion in 2000 (Finkle-stein, Corso, & Miller, 2006). These facts identify TBI as a major public health problem (Katz, Ashley, O'Shanick, & Connors, 2006).

Recovery Depends on How Severe the Injury Is

The effects of a head injury are determined by a number of factors. The total amount of damage determines the kinds of challenges the survivor has to face. The amount of force applied to the brain determines how many brain cells die (diffuse damage), and that determines how long the person remains in coma as well as the size of the memory gap surrounding the accident. In turn, measures of the coma and memory gap predict every kind of long-term symptom and practical problem the injury causes. Some survivors also have areas of focal damage that are large enough to produce permanent losses of skills and abilities that depend on that part of the brain.

TBI damages lives in proportion to the severity level of the overall injury. The severity determines the length of convalescence, the extent of the permanent symptoms, the number of things that go wrong in life, the amount of coping that is needed, and the trouble that results from any failures to cope (Brooks, 1984a; Jennett & Teasdale, 1981; Levin, 1987; Lezak, 1983).

TBI is a combination of three kinds of injury (Alexander, 1987). The first, the destruction of a chunk or section of brain tissue, is called focal injury. A neurosurgeon creates a focal injury with a scalpel (more a tiny vacuum cleaner than a knife). Strokes cause focal injury by blocking blood flow to a section of brain until it dies, or by bursting a blood vessel, which kills most of the surrounding cells. Some tumors ruin every cell within their reach. A bullet, knife, or other object destroys cells all around its pathway (penetrating head wound) (Adams, Victor, & Ropper, 1997; Cooper, 1987). Focal damage occurs when the skull breaks and pieces of bone are driven into the brain (depressed skull fracture) (Adams et al., 1997; Harti & Ghajar, 2005). It also occurs when the impact force bursts a blood vessel inside the brain (intraparenchymal hemorrhage) (Dowling & Dacey, 1996). Large blood vessels can get torn where they enter the brain, flooding the top layer of brain cells with blood, which kills them on contact (subdural hematoma) (Becker, 1989; Jamieson & Yelland, 1972). A large blood clot puts brain cells beneath it under pressure, squeezing out enough of their blood supply to kill them, a problem in about half of the severe injuries (ischemic necrosis) (Andrews, 1992). When there is enough swelling on one side of the head, the bottom of the outside edge (temporal lobe) gets squeezed under the shelf of bone on which it normally sits. The bony ridge then cuts a groove into the brain, and the pressure kills the surrounding cells (transtentorial herniation) (Andrews & Pitts, 1991). The brain can get speared by the rough ridges or bony points on the inside of the skull (Holbourne, 1943), or at the point of impact when the skull is briefly bent inward by the blow (Gurdjian, 1975), producing bruised zones filled with tiny wedges of dead cells (contusions) (Ommaya & Gennarelli, 1974; Povlishock & Valadka, 1994). Most contusions occur in front and along the sides of the brain (Courville, 1945; Gurdjian, Webster, & Arnkoff, 1943; Ommaya, Grubb, & Naumann, 1970). The memory factories (hippocampi) are on the sides within a "box" made of bone, easily damaged by force, and torn cells spill out the harsh chemical (glutamate) they contain, which can kill surrounding cells (Bigler, 1990b, 2007; Sapolsky, 1996). Finally, rebounding off the skull damages the brain directly opposite the point of impact (countrecoup contusion) (Lindgren, 1966; Smith, 1974). In side impact, the rebound effect may be more damaging than the original blow (Courville, 1958; Dawson, Webster, & Gurdjian, 1951; Spatz, 1950). Impact in the front or back damages the front because the skull is rough there (Ommaya, Grubb, & Naumann, 1971). Areas of focal damage are usually surrounded by zones of swollen (edema) (Graham, 1999) or softened tissue (encephalomalacia) in which more cells have died (Plum & Posner, 1980).

Focal damage may (Alexander, 1987; Gennarelli, Spielman et al., 1982; Wilson, Hadley, Scott, & Harper, 1996) or may not have lasting effects (Gentry, 1991; Reitan & Wolfson, 1986). This seems to depend on the total number of cells killed (Chapman & Wolff, 1959; Goldstein, 1936; Lashley, 1938; Povlishock & Valadka, 1994). Small zones of damage often do not reach deep enough into the brain to produce permanent, significant symptoms (Alexander, 2003). In contrast, some war wounds from bullets and shell fragments cause symptoms that can still be measured after 20 years (Jarho, 1973; Lishman, 1968; Newcombe, 1969; Teuber, 1964).

Large areas of focal injury can destroy whole operating systems. In the frontal lobes, they leave behavior permanently out of control. In the back, they can destroy vision or balance. On the side, they often leave serious memory and/or emotion problems and sometimes language and/or perception disorders. Transtentorial herniation also has this kind of poor outcome (Giles & Clark-Wilson, 1993). Although rare, massive zones of focal damage can cause permanent and total dependence (Joseph, 1997; Kolb & Whishaw, 2003; Luria, 1966, 1973, 1980; Meier, Strauman, & Thompson, 1987; Roberts, 1979). We learn about the site and size of the damage from CT and MRI scans, which show them as 3-D pictures (Damasio & Damasio, 2003).

The second aspect of injury is called diffuse damage. The forces unleashed by a high-velocity impact destroy individual cells throughout the brain. The impact pulls and twists the brain out of shape, while waves of pressure sweep through it (Gilroy & Meyer, 1979; Graham, Adams, & Gennarelli, 1987; Katz & Mills, 1999). (You can make pressure waves by banging the side of a metal bowl of gelatin dessert.) The most serious damage is caused by an off-center blow, which produces a twisting force (Strich, 1961) that tears open the long, slender interconnecting "wires" running from the computing cells on the outer reaches to the energy wells deep in the brainstem (Andrews, 1992). The force also stretches interconnecting cells joining the computing stations, some to the breaking point (Adams, Mitchell, Graham, & Doyle, 1977). It rips open other connecting wires by raking them across the lumps of tissue located in the middle of the brain (Gennarelli, Thibault et al., 1982). Cells that are torn open bathe surrounding cells in harsh chemicals that can kill them (Katayama, Yoshino, Kawamoto, & Tsubokawa, 1996; Siesjo & Wieloch, 1985). Other destructive chemicals and immune system cells also pour in to attack healthy brain cells (Arnstein & Smith, 1999; Gennarelli & Graham, 2005). Damaged tissue swells, raising the pressure (Gentleman, Dearden, Midgley, & MacLean, 1993; Gennarelli & Graham, 2005) and temperature inside the skull (Dietrich, 1996), sometimes high enough to kill more cells (Seitelberger & Jellinger, 1971). Blood pressure fluctuates (Marion, Darby, & Yonas, 1991) and at both extremes more cells die (Bouma, Muizelaar, Choi, Newlon, & Young, 1991; Miller, Sweet, Narayan, & Becker, 1978). The filter that keeps harmful chemicals out of the brain's blood supply may start leaking (Partridge, 1985; Povlishock, Becker, Sullivan, & Miller, 1978). Accidents can also injure the brain indirectly via damage to the vital organs, which can malfunction badly enough to poison the relatively delicate brain (Epstein, Ward, & Becker, 1987; Gronwall, Wrightson, & Waddell, 1990; Povlishock & Valadka, 1994). In severe diffuse injury, every region loses some cells, whereas no structure is completely destroyed.

The third aspect is oxygen starvation (cerebral anoxia) (Ishige, Pitts, Hashimoto, Nishimura, & Bartkowski, 1987), which kills some cells in every TBI (Graham, Adams, & Doyle, 1979; Katayama et al., 1996) and can cause the worst symptoms when it is extreme (Price & Murray, 1972; Roberts, 1979). One study found significant anoxic damage in almost half of the patients (Adams, Graham, Scott, Parker, & Doyle, 1980). The most severe injuries cause all three kinds of damage (Adams, Graham, Gennarelli, & Maxwell, 1977; Graham et al., 1987).

Diffuse damage determines the lion's share of the long-term difficulties the survivor must face (Adams, Graham, Gennarelli, & Maxwell, 1991; Bigler, 1990b; Gennarelli, 1987; Jennett, 1990; Miller & Teasdale, 1985; Povlishock, 1989; Uzzell, 1986), although widespread (Blumbergs, Jones, & North, 1989; Pilz, 1983; Smith, 1996), diffuse lesions are usually too small to be seen on medical scans (Adams et al., 1989; Langfitt & Zimmerman, 1985). An indirect approach to measurement must be used. Two pioneering doctors in Glasgow, Scotland, Graham Teasdale and Bryan Jennett (1974), found that the severity of diffuse injury could be measured by the depth of the coma, and their method became an industry standard. Their Glasgow Coma Scale (GCS) assigns scores to basic reactions of eye opening, movement, and speech. The worse the injury is, the less a patient reacts, which results in a lower score. When examined by the admitting physician, "a comatose patient who is unable to open his or her eyes or follow commands and has a GCS score lower than 9 has a severe TBI by definition" (Harti & Ghajar, 2005). This examination usually occurs more than 1 and less than 2 hours post-onset.

Later research revealed that the length of coma was an even better measure than the depth of the coma (Katz & Mills, 1999). Coma duration is related to later recovery as measured by tests of intelligence, memory (Levin, Benton, & Grossman, 1982), and visual perception (Levin, Grossman, & Kelly, 1976, 1977). It also predicts the recovery of real-life abilities (Table 2–1).

Table 2–1. Describing Injury Severity Based on Coma Duration

Coma	*Recovery*
<24 hours	Almost all became fully independent (Carlsson, von Essen, & Lofgren, 1968)
>24 hours	75% fully independent, 2/3 regained normal social life (Pazzaglia, Frank, Frank, & Gaist, 1975)
	80% had measurable cognitive deficits 2 years later (Levin, 1987)
1–7 days	50% became fully independent (Carlsson et al., 1968)
1–7 days	49% had good overall recovery at 1 year post (Katz & Mills, 1999)
3 days+	Partial/total job disability 2–20 years later (Solch & Schyra, 1972)
7 days	>50% return to work within 6 months after holistic rehab (Schutz & Schutz, 1999)
7 day avg.	Unemployed 1–13 years later (no TBI rehabilitation) (Kinzel, in Roberts, 1979)
8 day avg.	Very few worked, most needed supervised living (Berrol et al., 1982)
	With TBI rehab, 65% worked, workshop or school (ChristensenCaetano, & Rasmussen, 1996)
9 day avg.	With TBI rehab, 50% held jobs (Schutz, Kleinschmidt, & Gorman, 1998)
<2 weeks	Associated with marked alterations of personality (Bond, 1984)
3 weeks+	Permanently disabling cognitive deficits (Levin, Benton, & Grossman, 1982)
3 weeks+	64% severely disabled at 1 year post (Katz & Mills, 1999)
4 weeks	Permanent neurological disabilities (Lambooy, vander Zwan, & Fossen, 1965)

Table 2–1. *continued*

Coma	*Recovery*
4 weeks	Unable to regain independence 1–10 years later (Carlsson et al., 1968)
1 month	93% less than good recovery (Multi-Society Task Force on PVS, 1994)
6 week avg.	Most needed physical care, supervised day activities (Berrol et al., 1982)
7 weeks	Supported employment led to working 2/3 of time (Wehman, 1996)
8 week avg.	Permanent severe disability (Lambooy et al., 1965)
8 week avg.	11% returned to work (Gilchrist & Wilkinson, 1979)
8 weeks+	Unable to hold competitive job (Schutz, Barry, Gross, & Tupper, 1984)

Injuries of low severity tend to have a better outcome, and recovery tends not to be blocked by medical or nonmedical complications. As the coma grows longer, it determines the long-term consequences to greater extent, making diffuse damage the main form (or prototype) of TBI (Bennett, Dittmar, & Ho, 1997; Bontke & Boake, 1991; Graham, 1999; Jennett, 1997; Morris & Marshall, 1998; Schutz, 2007a). In general, faster early recovery means more complete long-term recovery: the sooner coma ends and memory and other skills start to return, the better the ultimate outcome is likely to be (Berrol et al., 1982; Hagen, 1982; Lezak, 1976).

A severe injury is generally associated with permanent cognitive deficits and ability limitations (Schutz & Schutz, 2004). When coma duration is no more than 1 day, most survivors can regain independence and resume working at a competitive job (as opposed to a sheltered job), but their job security is not assured. With each added day of coma the odds of keeping the job drop. By 3 to 4 weeks of coma, the impairment is severe enough to undermine even independence in the home. When coma is measured in months, even the most intensive therapy usually does not restore full functioning in any area.

Coma duration is the most accepted measure of the severity of injury in the United States, but other measures are also used (Brink, Garrett, Hale, Nickel, & Woo-Sam, 1970; Ewing-Cobbs, Levin, & Fletcher, 1998; Heiskanen & Kaste, 1974; Nelson, 1992). In Europe, post-traumatic amnesia (PTA) is the preferred measure (Russell & Nathan, 1946; Table 2–2). PTA is measured in two ways: the memory gap *after* the injury, and the total gap *surrounding* the injury, both approaches being consistent with the definition advanced by Russell and Smith (1961). PTA predicts future test scores better than coma (Brooks, 1972, 1984a; Brooks, Aughton, Bond, Jones, & Risvi, 1980), and remains the best predictor of occupational status and psychosocial symptoms 10 years later (Draper, Ponsford, & Schonberger, 2007).

The most extreme injuries inflict so much permanent damage that they impair basic eye and posture reflexes, cause multiple months of coma and post-traumatic amnesia, and rarely permit a good recovery (Alexandre, Colombo, Nertempi, & Benedetti, 1983; Boller, Albert, LeMay, & Kertesz, 1972; Brink et al., 1970; Eisenberg & Weiner, 1987; Giannotta, Weiner, & Karnaze, 1987; Levin, 1987; Miller & Teasdale, 1985; Overgaard et al., 1973; Pagni, 1973; Vapalahti & Troupp, 1971). Recovery from these injuries, qualitatively different from that of most severe injuries (Eames & Wood, 1989; Roberts, 1979), will not be discussed at length here.

Table 2–2. Describing Injury Severity Based on PTA Duration

PTA	*Significance*
<1 day	Probable rapid and complete recovery (McKinlay & Watkiss, 1999)
1 day	Conventional cutoff point for severe injury (Jennett & Teasdale, 1981)
1 day+	Transient cognitive impairments (children) (Oddy, 1993)
1 day+	Permanent cognitive impairments (Corkin, Hurt, Twitchell, Franklin, & Yin, 1987)

Table 2–2. *continued*

PTA	Significance
1–6 days	Probable recovery in weeks to months (McKinlay & Watkiss, 1999)
<8 days	90% good recovery (Jennett, Snoek, Bond, & Brooks, 1981)
7–14 days	Probable recovery in months with residual problems (McKinlay & Watkiss, 1999)
8–14 days	80% good recovery (Jennett et al., 1981)
<13 days	Fewer permanent deficits, better vocational prognosis (van Zomeren & vanden Burg, 1985)
<14 days	At 1 year, 76% good recovery (Katz & Mills, 1999)
>13 days	More permanent deficits, worse vocational prognosis (van Zomeren & vanden Burg, 1985)
>13 days	Likely to have persistent cognitive deficits (Brooks, Campsie, Symington, & Beattie, 1987)
14–28 days	Recovery across 1 year+, permanent limitations (McKinlay & Watkiss, 1999)
15–28 days	66% good recovery (Jennett et al., 1981)
3 weeks+	Permanent measurable impairment is likely (Jennett, 1997)
3 weeks+	Permanent cognitive impairment (children) (Oddy, 1984)
28 days+	Long-term disability expected (McKinlay & Watkiss, 1999)
28 days+	73% less than good recovery (Jennett et al., 1981)
28 days+	Severe disability is the most likely outcome (Levin, 1987)
56–84 days	At 1 year, 75% with moderate disability (Katz & Mills, 1999)
84 days+	At 1 year, 100% with severe disability (Katz & Mills, 1999)

Recovery Depends on What Kind of Person Got the Injury

> The extent of recovery and the amount of long-term disability also depend on what the person was like before the injury. The more assets and resources (intelligence, education, wealth, mental health, self-control, character, stability, family support) the person had before the injury, the better he or she is likely to do after the injury. Younger people also have better physical recoveries.

Recovery is not just a matter of how much the brain was damaged, but of how the survivor is able to deal with the damage. Symonds (1970) pointed out that recovery depends not only on the kind of injury that the head got, but the kind of head that got the injury (Symonds, 1970). In other words, many personal characteristics affect recovery potential.

The more sound and healthy the brain was at the time of the accident, the better it should recover (Gennarelli & Graham, 2005). Thus, if the brain was damaged by a previous injury or some other brain disorder, recovery potential may be reduced; if the preexisting condition was serious, it may be reduced quite a bit (Jennett, 1997). Aging "damages" the brain enough by age 35 to 40 to have a small measurable impact on cognitive recovery (Eisenberg & Weiner, 1987; Roberts, 1979), and the effect increases into old age (Goodman & Englander, 1992), due in part to problems with general health (Giannotta et al., 1987; Meier et al., 1987). It should be noted that maturity may also allow older persons to benefit more from their therapy (Thomsen, 1989).

There is a major age advantage in physical recovery beginning in childhood (Miller & Teasdale, 1985; Teuber, 1975; Uzzell & Stonnington, 1996a), the Kennard (1940) principle. However, young children are also disadvantaged by interference with normal development of their social and other complex skills (Chapman, 2007; Donders & Waurschausky, 2007).

Chronic use of alcohol damages the brain, and TBI patients with a history of abuse tend to have a poorer outcome (Brooks et al., 1989; Jurkovich et al., 1993; Ruff et al., 1990; Sparedo & Gill, 1989; Tarter &

Edwards, 1985). The combination of alcoholism and aging has even stronger effects on recovery potential (Orosz, 1979). Alcohol is present in more than half of emergency room admissions for TBI (Kraus & Chu, 2005). Up to two thirds of survivors have a history of alcohol/drug problems (Corrigan, 1996). Abstinence from all substances is recommended for best recovery (Kreutzer, Leininger, & Harris, 1990; Schutz, 2006a).

If recovery is about rebuilding a life through the use of a damaged brain, then access to other resources for reconstruction should also affect recovery, and it does. Psychological assets including mental health, good character, intelligence, social status, family stability, coping skills, and good work history are associated with better recovery (Alfano, Paniak, & Finlayson, 1991; Dikmen & Reitan, 1977, 1978; Fordyce, Roueche, & Prigatano, 1983; Kozol, 1946; Lishman, 1978; Long & Williams, 1988; Lynch, 1982a; Max, 2005; Najenson, Grosswasser, Mendelson, & Hackett, 1989; Rusk, Block, & Lowman, 1969), as is the help of concerned and well-adjusted family members (Farmer & Stucky-Ropp, 1996; Klonoff, 1971). A high level of education also predicts a better outcome (Gilchrist & Wilkinson, 1979; Levin, O'Donnell, & Grossman, 1979). A history of preinjury mental health is associated with resistance to depression after the injury as well as successful recovery (Malec, Testa, Rush, Brown, & Moessner, 2007). A history of good school adjustment predicts better recovery (Fahy, Irving, & Millac, 1967; Fuld & Fisher, 1977; Haas, Cope, & Hall, 1987). Well-adjusted survivors can handle more damage than those who barely managed before the injury (Bennett et al., 1997; Binder, 1986; Prigatano, 1999a).

Personality can also be either an asset or an obstacle to recovery. Patients who are more agreeable, conscientious, and outgoing before injury tend to have better vocational recoveries (Schutz & Micucci, 1984; Schutz & Wanlass, 1986): The better a person got along with others before the injury, the fewer social problems the injury is likely to cause. Higher preinjury self-esteem also goes with fewer postinjury difficulties in dealing with other people (Johnson & Newton, 1987). TBI can improve personality in some cases (Bennett et al., 1997). Headstrong or difficult people temporarily become cooperative in the first few weeks or months after coming out of coma (Gronwall et al., 1990). Those with disabling shyness before injury may be brought out of their "shells" and remain more sociable over the long term, which may be seen as a personality upgrade by all concerned (Eames, 1990; Lynch, 1982a; Thomsen, 1990). Personalities high in risk-taking are especially likely to sustain TBI (Fahy et al., 1967; Fuld & Fisher, 1977; Jamieson & Kelly, 1973; Rose, 1988), and tend to have less successful recoveries (Humphrey & Oddy, 1981; Levin & Grossman, 1978; Schutz & Micucci, 1984).

The Mental Functions That Recover Over Time

People waking up from coma are terribly impaired in all areas, but most quickly improve in many ways. The improvement happens as the disrupted brain functions improve, and some even return to normal. Within about 6 months, much of this "natural recovery" is completed. Some of the things that usually improve include talking, walking, using well-learned skills, remembering knowledge learned before the injury, and paying attention to one thing at a time. Thanks to natural recovery, most survivors reach the point where they can be left alone at home. They also give the appearance of being normal in most situations.

Brain symptoms begin improving when coma lifts. The brain of a coma patient is not just damaged, but also disorganized in many ways. Major temporary effects occur because trauma disrupts the many, closely regulated physical and chemical processes that support brain function. For example, thinking continues only if a steady supply of brain chemicals (neurotransmitters) and a rich supply of blood arrive as soon as the thinking starts (Goldberg, 2001). If these supplies are delayed, thinking deteriorates (Envoldsen & Jensen, 1978; Lewelt, Jenkins, & Miller, 1980). Some brain cells are swollen, stretched, or partly torn, needing months to heal up enough to go back on-line (Finger & Stein, 1982; Thomas & Trexler, 1982; Uzzell, Dolinskas, Wiser, & Langfitt, 1987). The recovery of these disrupted systems takes no special effort. It is natural or "spontaneous" recovery that occurs with time (Kolb & Gibb, 1999).

Early natural recovery gains are dramatic (McKinlay & Watkiss, 1999). A patient fresh out of coma can do very little, say very little, and understand very little because the whole brain is malfunctioning in so many ways (Lezak, 1983). The person usually does not know where he or she is, the date and the time of day, the fact that this strange place is a hospital, or why he or she is staying there (Levin, Benton, & Grossman, 1982). There is no ability to care for self, even to use the bathroom. Nothing can be learned yet, so there is no point in explaining anything (Hagen, 1982). These problems improve from one day to the next. A parent or spouse may go home at night and the next day find that the loved one has started eating, dressing, or learning again. This "miracle" goes on day after day, but gradually the rate of improvement slows down (Deaton, 1987b).

The recovery of mental and physical abilities is predictable. Simple skills come back first, including basic mental abilities like counting, naming things, and holding information in mind for a few seconds (*focal attention* and *working memory*), along with routine practical skills like self-feeding and brushing teeth. Later, more complex skills improve: explaining, searching and finding, doing mental calculations, tying shoes, shaving, applying makeup, walking across uneven surfaces and up staircases. The highest skills come back last, if at all. If the injury is mild, the sequence goes quickly, whereas if it is severe, everything comes back more slowly: the bigger the injury, the more gradual the "recovery slope" (Arlinghaus, Shoaib, & Price, 2005; Berrol et al., 1982). Physical abilities return over the first half-year, supporting the return of self-care and other daily living skills (Brooks, Campsie, Symington, Beattie, & McKinlay, 1986; McLean, Dikmen, Temkin, Wyler, & Gale, 1984; Panikoff, 1983); these areas usually have no serious, permanent deficits (Burke, Guth, Guare, & Weslowski, 1999; Fahy et al., 1967; Levin, 1987; Miller, Benson, & Johnson, 2003; Ponsford, Olver, & Curran, 1996; Solch & Schyra, 1972).

Some thinking skills also tend to come back strong. Often by mid-year, all but the most extremely impaired patients can keep a normal amount of information in mind for short periods of time (Dye, Milby, & Saxon, 1979; Gronwall & Sampson, 1974; Reitan & Wolfson, 1986; Vigoroux et al., 1971). At this point, survivors complete routine activities and participate in conversations without losing track of what is being said. Scores on intelligence tests tend to return to the normal range (or near normal) soon after (Mandleberg & Brooks, 1975). Conversational speech usually also comes back well (Levin, Grossman et al., 1979), although problems with expressing and comprehending the most complicated statements persist (Coelho, Liles, & Duffy, 2006; Hagen, 1982). These gains restore a normal appearance (Gouvier, 1986; Gordon et al., 1998; Halligan & Wade, 2005; Hux,

Schram, & Goeken, 2006): Four out of five survivors no longer "look head-injured" by the end of the first year of recovery (Roberts, 1979).

Natural recovery also brings back access to the mental library of preinjury knowledge, although access may be inconsistent because the search process can get disorganized easily (Bennett et al., 1997; Burke et al., 1999; Goldstein & Levin, 1991; Kiefer, Ahlegian, & Spitzer, 2005; Maestu et al., 2005). Along with facts and figures, the knowledge of how to do things (remote procedural memory) usually comes back strong (Schmitter-Edgecombe, 2006; Sohlberg & Mateer, 2001). Thus, most patients remember how to perform their developed skills, from using language, reading, and doing math to driving a car, operating a computer, doing hobbies, crafts, sports, job routines, and all other special skills. Any abilities learned and used in the years before the injury are likely to come back (Burgess & Wood, 1990).

In adults, enough natural recovery is completed to estimate long-term functioning after 6 to 12 months (Dikmen, Reitan, & Temkin, 1983; Mandleberg, 1975). Deficits present at 2 years post-injury are usually permanent (Corrigan, Smith-Knapp, & Granger, 1998; Olver, Ponsford, & Curtin, 1996): "It is unrealistic to expect significant improvement in physical deficits, cognitive functions, behavior or personality problems after two years" (Jennett, 1997, p. 443). However, in some cases individual test scores can improve beyond 2 years (Millis et al., 2001), and children sometimes make substantial late recoveries (Lehr, 1990). There is no time limit on self-created recovery through the use of compensation strategies (Gronwall, Wrightson, & Waddell, 1998).

The Mental Functions That Do Not Recover: The Lasting Deficits

TBI that produces coma always destroys part of the brain, and that loss always causes some lasting deficits. The most extreme injuries permanently impair all cognitive skills, but most injuries do not eliminate skills. Instead, the injury makes the skills inconsistent, prone to breaking down under certain circumstances. Unfortunately, some of the resulting defects, particularly those affecting new learning and the executive functions, have serious consequences.

As natural recovery slows down in the months after the injury, it becomes apparent that the most serious symptoms are not going back to normal. These islands of cognitive defect grow more and more sharply defined as the last temporary effects clear up (Bond, 1979; Bond & Brooks, 1976; Katz & Mills, 1999). The World Health Organization (WHO, 1980) classified symptoms into three categories. The first level is called *impairment*, the loss of basic physical or mental skills. Impairments undermine the cognitive processes that produce effective behavior. The other two levels, *disability* and *handicap*, will be explained in the next two sections.

Forgetfulness is the most common TBI symptom (Brooks, 1984a). In one study, memory problems were reported for 87% of severely injured survivors (McKinley & Watkiss, 1999). At 5 years post-onset, two thirds of the survivors in another study complained of memory problems (Jennett, 1997). However, there are many kinds of memory (Baddeley, 1990), and after TBI memory works fine for some purposes but not for others (Evans & Preston, 1990). There is a tendency to forget new learning, although information that seems important can often be recalled if attention is devoted to learning it (Mateer & Raskin, 1999). On the other hand, when a lot of information is presented at one time, it is not possible to think about all of it, and much or most may be forgotten, particularly the parts that do not seem important or interesting.

In practical terms, recall from conversations, phone calls, books, newspapers, magazines, and professional consultations is seldom complete and reliable (Bontke, Brockman, Clio, Robert, & Worthington, 1998; Filley, 2001; Goldstein, 1942; Gronwall & Wrightson, 1981; Lezak, 1987b). Learning the curriculum in high school or college tends to be strongly affected (Blosser & DePompei, 2003; Ewing-Cobbs et al., 1998; Holmes, 1988). Survivors also tend to forget the sequence and details of the events of their day (episodic memory) as well as their commitments to do something at a certain future time (prospective memory) (Sohlberg & Mateer, 2001). Even these problems can be prevented when time is taken to focus on the information and its importance (Geschwind, 1982), but such intense study is not always practical (Cermak, Verfaillie, & Lanzone, 1999). Most injuries cause enough focal damage to the memory-making centers to produce lifelong difficulties with these advanced memory skills (Bigler, 2007; Goldstein & Levin, 1991).

Attention is another area of long-lasting difficulty caused by TBI (e.g., Benton, 1987; Levine et al., 2002; Lezak, 1987b), reported to affect 33 to 62% of survivors at 1 to 2 years post-onset (McKinley & Watkiss, 1999). Just as with memory, there are many kinds of attention, and all are not equally affected (van Zomeren & Brouwer, 1994). As with memory, even the most strongly affected functions are not consistently defective. Manly (2003) points out that

> variability is a central, if not definitive, feature of "attention" deficits. The fact that performance on a task may, at one time, be adequate and, at another, quite deficient suggests that many of the basic components required for performance . . . are present but for some reason are unreliably orchestrated to produce the desired results. (p. 43)

Cognitive fluctuation or inconsistent attention is a trademark of TBI (Salthouse, 2007; Sbordone, 1997; Schutz, 2005d; Stuss, Murphy, Binns, & Alexander, 2003), seen in every kind of task and situation (O'Shanick & O'Shanick, 2005; Wood, 1990). More consistent and serious breakdowns of attention are reserved for the most difficult tasks. For example, when rapid choices among many alternatives must be made, the survivor often makes poor decisions (van Zomeren, Brouwer, & Deelman, 1984). As the speed at which the information is presented increases, decision making breaks down even more frequently (Adams, Graham, Murray, & Scott, 1982; Brouwer & van Wolffelaar, 1985). This relationship between task difficulty and attention errors holds true for everyone (Broadbent, 1971; Kahneman, 1973; Reason, 1990), but task difficulty has a much greater effect on a damaged brain than on an undamaged one (Gronwall, 1987).

In cognitive impairment, the lower levels of the skill often work well; deficit appears selectively at the higher levels (Goldstein, 1942; Poppelreuter, 1917). For this reason, skills are most prone to fail when used to do something unusually difficult (Thomas & Trexler, 1982), or, in other words, when high levels of mental and physical effort are employed (Jennett, 1997; Schutz, 2005b; Wood, 1987). This selective loss of function at the highest levels of difficulty is observed for both memory and attention skills (Dell'acqua, Sessa, & Pashler, 2006; Goldstein & Levin, 1991; Hein, Schubert, & von Cramon, 2005; Park, Moscovitch, & Robertson, 1999).

The third and by far the most important long-lasting deficit concerns the executive functions (Lezak, 1987a; Worthington & Walker, 2008). The phrase *executive functions* is unfamiliar to most people outside of neuroscience. It was coined by Hans-Lukas Teuber (1964) to refer to a special set of advanced cognitive functions impaired by penetrating wounds of the frontal lobes. The term was chosen because these functions (initiation, response suppression, impulse control, mental flexibility, error-checking, and problem-solving by planning and anticipation) are all used in *executing* any behaviors that must be thought through (Lezak, 1987; Luria, 1966).

At the heart of Teuber's (1964) executive, as elaborated by Luria (1973), is a complex (metacognitive) self-management system (SMS) that orchestrates the brain's highest level thought processes (Bennett et al., 1997; Calvin, 1996; Goldberg, 2001). These processes include keeping an accurate account of what the self can and cannot do (Bleiberg, Cope, & Spector, 1989; Carver & Scheier, 2001; Kelly, 1955; Markus, 1977; Stuss, Mateer, & Sohlberg, 1994). Environmental opportunities and hazards are carefully scanned (Pribram, 1960, 1973, 1986) and attention is allocated to deal with those that are adaptively important (Norman & Shallice, 1986; Picton, Alain, & McIntosh, 2002; Posner & Petersen, 1990; Shiffrin & Schneider, 1977). Such events trigger an executive routine for testing and selecting goals, plans (Calvin, 1989; Duncan, 1996; Grafman, 2002; Miller, Galanter, & Pribram, 1960; Walter, 1953), strategies, and intentions to act (Bernstein, 1967; Gollwitzer, Fujita, & Oettingen, 2004; Locke & Latham, 2002; Schmidt & Lee, 1999; Shallice & Burgess, 1991). Quality control is maintained by allocating enough brain circuitry to provide the right amount of mental effort (Duncan & Miller, 2002; Edelman & Tononi, 2000; Goldberg, 1985) to properly control the pace and quality of the thinking and action (Fuster, 2005; Locke & Latham, 2002). Planned acts are initiated at the right time (Mesulam, 2002; Stuss & Benson, 1986). Finally, errors in following the plan are monitored and fixed (Bernstein, 1967; Gross, 1982; Kosslyn & Koenig, 1992; Luria, 1973; Miller et al., 1960; Shallice, 1972; Shallice & Burgess, 1996) and self-corrective lessons learned from the outcome (Damasio, 1994; Goldberg, 2001; Stuss, 1991).

Unlike other major brain systems (Burgess & Wood, 1990; Luria, 1973), the SMS spends most of the time off-line (Passingham, 1995; Shiffrin & Schneider, 1977). Most behavior runs "on automatic pilot" via prefabricated plans (Gazzaniga, 1998; Rabbitt, 1998; Shiffrin & Schneider, 1977) that bypass the SMS (Stuss, 1991). The SMS monitors events via a problem-solving network (the central executive—see Mesulam, 2002) that remains on standby (Miller et al., 1960) until a signal indicating trouble is detected (Bechara, Damasio, Damasio, & Lee, 1999; Gray & McNaughton, 2003; Heilman, Bowers, & Valenstein, 1993; Jahanshahi & Frith, 1998; Posner & DiGirolamo, 1998). This network then runs a series of cycles (or feedback loops) to calculate the risk of harm and loss (Norman & Shallice, 1986; Shallice, 1982, 1988).

If the stakes are high enough, the SMS is activated and takes control to plan a better solution (Mesulam, 2002; Miller et al., 1960; Schutz, 2005a) through additional cycles of high-level thinking (Baddeley & Hitch, 1974; Neisser, 1967; Shallice, 1972; Shiffrin & Schneider, 1977; Sigman & Dehaene, 2006; Turk et al., 2004). As such, operation of the SMS

> . . . is context-dependent rather than categorical. The manifestations . . . become particularly prominent when the environment contains distractors, when ambiguity and conflict are high, when appearance and significance are at odds, when events must be interpreted in light of contextual peculiarities, when prepotent response tendencies must be restrained for some long-term purpose, when decision trees have multiple branches, and when the egocentric view must be transcended. (Mesulam, 2002, p. 24)

So when a solution is neither obvious nor easy the SMS is activated. For example, the SMS needs to take charge in unfamiliar situations because there is no solution on file (Burgess, 1998).

TBI essentially closes down the SMS (Bleiberg et al., 1989; Braunling-McMorrow, 1998; Kennedy & Coelho, 2006), causing a set of problems in directing attention, organizing action, and noticing errors called the *dysexecutive syndrome* (Baddeley & Wilson, 1988). These are TBI's most prominent symptoms (Stuss & Gow, 1992), causing the most serious and disruptive limitations of real-life activities (Crawford & Henry, 2005; Pelham & Lovell, 2005).

Early accounts attributed the dysexecutive syndrome of TBI to frontal-lobe contusions, following the older tradition of localizing damage to control centers (Churchland, 1998; Newcombe, 1987; Stein, Brailowski, & Will, 1995). This explanation works for large, deep frontal contusions (Luria, 1973), but TBI often does not cause this kind of damage (Harti & Ghajar, 2005), so another explanation is needed (Schutz, 2007a). Dysexecutive syndrome can also be attributed to diffuse damage to the networks that connect to the frontal lobes (Cicerone, Levin, Malec, Stuss, & Whyte, 2006; Stuss & Benson, 1986). By this account, TBI causes the executive symptoms by

> "unplugging" neural networks from one another. . . . These changes create "networking" lapses for the individual during functional activities. Lapses may vary from transient problems with . . . problem solving to more overt problems with stopping ongoing behaviors. (O'Shanick & O'Shanick, 2005, p. 246)

When traumatic force is applied to the brain, the resulting pressure waves selectively tear the long, thick fibers linking the far ends of the central executive network (Bigler, 2005; Geschwind, 1965; Povlishock, Kontos, & Ellis, 1989; Schutz, 2007a). After the injury, messages get more garbled with each cycle, quickly "crashing" this network (Bisiach & Geminiani, 1991; Gross, 1982; Gross & Schutz, 1984; Quartz & Sejnowski, 2002; Schutz, 2007a) and locking the executive system into standby mode (Cooper & Shallice, 2000; Gross & Schutz, 1986; Schutz, 2007b; Stuss, Mateer, & Sohlberg, 1994). The shut-down routine sounds an "all clear" signal that everything is working perfectly, preventing awareness or suspicion that there was a problem (Heilman, 1991).

"In the absence of an executive system, information is processed automatically" (Fernandez-Duque, Baird, & Posner, 2000, p. 289). Urges are put into action with no thought (Benton, 1968; Brown, 1987; Cole, 1998; Gazzaniga, 1998; G. Goldberg, 1985; Shallice & Evans, 1978). Objects of temptation "capture" behavior (L'Hermitte, 1986; Norman, 1988) as other goals, including those of the highest priority, are instantly abandoned (Duncan, Emslie, Williams, Johnson, & Freer, 1996; Wood & Liossi, 2006). No effort is made to anticipate how other people might react to or be affected by actions (Lezak, 1987a). If an error is made, it is likely to escape notice (Hart, Giovannetti, Montgomery, & Schwartz, 1998; McGlynn & Schacter, 1989; Zaidel, 1987) and regret (Bechara, Damasio, Damasio, & Anderson, 1994; Elliott, Dolan, & Frith, 2000; Shallice & Burgess, 1991), so the same wrong moves get made again and again (Berko, Berko, & Thompson, 1970; Brooks, 1990; Deutsch, 1998). Things are now done in the "quick and dirty way" even when there are compelling reasons to be careful and thoughtful (Archibald, Mateer, & Kerns, 2001; Buchtel, 1987; Stuss & Buckle, 1992; Varney & Menefee, 1993). Although well-known, familiar risks and hazards may be avoided most of the time (Giles & Clark-Wilson, 1993; Levin, Goldstein, High, & Williams, 1988), no attention is paid to unfamiliar ones, no matter how obvious they may be to everyone else (Mazziotta & Phelps, 1986; Stuss, 1987). All of these faulty actions are forms of impulsive behavior (Votruba et al., 2008), which is often described as the main behavioral symptom of TBI (Bleiberg et al., 1989; Fryer & Fralish, 1998; Schutz, 2007a; Wood, 1987). This impulsivity is also seen in preadolescence, before the executive system has matured enough to assume control of behavior (Diamond, 2002; Jennett, 1997). Moreover, behavior is inflexible: Things are always done in exactly the usual way, even when that way obviously does not fit the situation (Fernandez-Duque et al., 2000; Stuss & Gow, 1992; van Zomeren & Spikman, 2005).

The central executive network is also the primary gateway for activating other, advanced brain systems, so when it shuts down, other critical thinking functions also go off-line. The network that uses the lessons of past experience to guide present-day behavior and inspires emotional effort to overcome special obstacles (Gray & McNaughton, 2003; Pribram & McGuinness, 1975) is wired through the central executive, so they shut down together (Mesulam, 2000, 2002). In addition, "neuroimaging findings have shown activation of frontal areas associated with paying attention in the context of strong mental effort. . . . The alert state is critical for optimal performance in tasks involving higher cognitive functions" (Raz, 2004, p. 27; see also Posner & Petersen, 1990; Szamietat, Schubert, Muller, & Von Cramon, 2002). This frontal attention network focuses the mind with extra effort to respond more effectively to adaptive challenges (Bushara, Grafman, & Hallett, 2001; Duncan & Miller, 2002; Raizata & Poldrack, 2006). After TBI, this added effort is not recruited when responses are readied (Marshall, 1987; Posner & Fan, 2008; Prigatano, 1987; Seignourel et al., 2005; Stuss et al., 2003; Wood, 1987). Finally, executive error processing stops updating the self-image (Kennedy & Coelho, 2006), promoting a false certainty that old methods, goals, and dreams still remain valid (Grosswasser & Stern, 1998).

Head trauma also reduces the brain's extra, "reserve" capacity (Lezak, 1983). Quality control deteriorates when body and brain are taxed by overload from excessive demands, a situational effect (Brooks, 1990). Some partially damaged brain cells now work properly only under perfect conditions (Becker, 1989). They leak excess acid, shut down nearby cells (Kaila & Ransom, 1998; Kauppinen & Williams, 1998), and cause cognitive interference after too much continuous use (Gronwall & Wrightson, 1974; Janus, 1996; Kowalske, Plenger, Lusby, & Hayden, 2000; McKinlay & Watkiss, 1999; Sbordone, 1991; Stuss et al., 1989), stress (Campbell & Dollaghan, 1990; Chapman & Wolff, 1959; Clark, 1968; Guercio & Fralish, 1998; Prigatano, 1987; Russell & Sharratt, 1992), or stimulation (Blanton, Porter, Smith, & Wolf, 1999; Hartley, Morrison, & Arnold, 1989; Wood, 1990) from high levels of arousal (Filley, Cranberg, Alexander, & Hart, 1987; Gronwall, 1987; Trexler, 1982), novelty (Goldstein, 1942), anxiety (Bender, 1949; Feinstein, 1999; Gronwall et al., 1990; Martinelli, Zasler, & Tiernan,

2005; Nimgade & Costello, 2003), depression (Uomoto, 1992), frustration (Deaton, 1991; Miller et al., 1960), or other emotionality (Ben-Yishay & Prigatano, 1990; Braunling-McMorrow, 1998; Cole, 1998; Cooley, Glang, & Voss, 1997; Sherr & Langenbahn, 1992; Simon, 2001). The overload causes confusion and makes behavior even more impulsive (Brown, 1977; Burgess & Wood, 1990; Eames, 1990; Goldstein, 1942; Pashler, 1998). If it continues, it can interrupt the train of thought and can even blank out the mind entirely (Bennett et al., 1997; Goldstein, 1934/2000, 1952; Prigatano, 1999a). After the overload ends, effective functioning usually resumes.

The executive is not "broken" in the sense that every situation produces dysexecutive symptoms (Wood, 1987; Ylvisaker & Gioia, 1998). "Generally it is not the case that patients . . . cannot perform an action at all; rather, they do not independently initiate the action at a particular time or place" (Stuss et al., 1994, pp. 223–224). Instead, symptoms are context-specific (Luria, 1979; Trexler, 1982), not so much a problem in *what* the brain is capable of doing as it is in *when* it fails to function properly (Burgess, 1998; Evans, 2005; Rabbitt, 1998). The executive system is called into operation for tasks of high difficulty (Hasher & Zacks, 1979; Hockey, 1993; Raizata & Poldrack, 2006; Thomas & Trexler, 1982), so much so that the terms executive and effortful have been treated as synonymous (Sigman & Dehaene, 2006). Dysexecutive symptoms are rare when doing familiar things with familiar people, the lifestyle toward which long-term survivors are inclined (Goldstein, 1934/2000; Trexler & Fordyce, 1996). Consequently, they may underestimate the dysexecutive syndrome because their lifestyle prevents them from experiencing it (Gronwall, Wrightson, & Waddell, 1998; Lehr, 1990). Clinical tests, and the research based on them, also underestimate dysexecutive symptoms (Anderson, Damasio, Tranel, & Damasio, 2000; Coelho, Ylvisaker, & Turkstra, 2005; Johnstone & Callahan, 1996; Manchester, Priestly, & Jackson, 2004; Stuss & Levine, 2002).

Despite these technical limitations, executive as well as memory and attention deficits detected at 10 years post-onset (Draper & Ponsford, 2008) are still related to the overall severity of the injury (as measured by post-traumatic amnesia). Moreover, the participants in this study had completed intensive therapy, indicating that the therapy did not remove the deficits. Because they do not appear to go away and are not cured, they must be coped with in some way.

Functioning in Real Life: The Lasting Ability Limitations

Severe TBI can interfere with the important tasks of life. Many survivors get their old jobs back or get hired for new jobs in the same field, but these jobs may be lost later on due to problem behaviors in the workplace. Serious social errors can drive friends away and prevent making new ones. Spouses can become so burdened and frustrated by high-maintenance behaviors and limited help and support from the survivor that the marriage is ruined. Children may have difficulty in getting along with parents who have head injuries for the same reasons. The more the chosen lifestyle demands from the survivor, the more problems the long-lasting deficits tend to cause in trying to meet those expectations.

The second category of post-injury problems in the WHO (1980) classification is called *disability*. Whereas impairment concerns problems measured in the clinic, disability is about problems that occur in real life when trying to perform goal-directed activities. These concepts have a cause-effect relationship: Disorder causes impairment, which causes disability. However, impairment does not always have to produce disability, depending on how the individual, the family, and the person's social world respond to the impairment (Diller, 1987).

In 2001, WHO revised its classification scheme, replacing the negative word *disability* with its opposite, *ability*. This change was motivated by concern about the subtle discrimination that comes from defining survivors in terms of what is wrong with them, and thus underemphasizing their strengths and assets (Nochi, 1998b; Wade, 2005). In some cases, reference to the word disability cannot be avoided without changing the meaning of a concept or study, but we have tried to use the new terminology wherever possible in this book.

Most of the research on abilities focuses on general categories of functioning, including working, attending school, driving, interacting socially, and performing the "activities of daily living." The last category is a more specific list of universal, practical tasks that usually includes shopping in the community, managing financial affairs, home management, meeting health care needs, meal preparation, dressing, grooming, toileting, and ambulation or personal mobility. Some studies also measure the length of time survivors can go without supervision at home.

As we discussed earlier, all abilities are generally affected by the overall severity of the injury (Alexander, 1987, Brooks, 1987); however, measures of function are only modestly related to measures of severity. This weak relationship exists because the most massive injuries usually compromise all abilities and the mildest ones usually spare all abilities, but in between the two extremes outcome is influenced by the person's choices and resources (Long, 1998; McKinlay & Watkiss, 1999; Sbordone, 1998). Some survivors with intermediate injuries can pull together their resources and function at an adequate level of ability (Diller & Ben-Yishay, 1987), whereas in other cases personal weaknesses magnify the ability limitations from a deficit (Alexander, 1995; Binder, 1986; Raskin & Mateer, 2000). For example, motivation tends to have major effects on abilities after TBI (Prigatano, 1999b). The ways in which the survivor tries to cope with the deficits can either improve or reduce abilities (Goldstein, 1934/2000, 1952). In addition, various features of the physical and/or social environment can either help or hinder the use of abilities (Gross & Schutz, 1986; Hart & Hayden, 1986; Wilson, 2003). These situational influences on functional recovery can be strong (Brooks, 1987). For example, some individuals live preinjury lifestyles that are so taxing that they can barely be managed prior to the injury, and these are likely to become unmanageable after the injury. The possibility of recovering from a severe injury with no ability limitations of any kind is so remote that it is dismissed as unrealistic (Cope, 1996; Kraus, 1987; Marshall, 1987; Willer et al., 1990).

Friendships and Other Social Relationships

Social functioning is affected by personality changes and behavior problems, which are found after 67 to 90% of severe injuries (Crosson, 1987; Grant & Alves, 1987; Jacobs, 1987; Jennett, Snoek, Bond, & Brooks, 1981; Lishman, 1968; Thomsen, 1974; Timming, Orrison, & Mikula, 1982; Weddell, Oddy, & Jenkins, 1980). Out-of-control, impulsive, or aggressive public behavior is usually the most upsetting symptom for social partners (Cassidy, 1990; Eames, 1990; McKinlay, Brooks, Bond, Martinage, & Marshall, 1981; Oddy, Humphrey, & Utley, 1978a;

1978b). Survivors may be unable to banter or chat, with uncomfortable pauses in which the survivor has nothing to say. Friends get distressed by hearing the same stories over again. Often there are fewer shared activities around which to maintain the friendship, as survivors may be prohibited from some preinjury leisure activities and the common ground may be reduced when the friends go off to college, marry, and develop careers (Lehr, 1990).

Social behavior is more affected by the dysexecutive syndrome than by any other deficit (Burgess & Wood, 1990; Coelho, Liles, & Duffy, 1992; Jacobs, 1989; Kozloff, 1987; Rosenthal & Bond, 1990; Tyerman, 1996). The SMS dictates how to treat friends, by keeping behavior in line with the social rules that fit the context (Luria, 1979; Picton et al., 2002; Pribram, 1973, 1986; Schulkin, 2000). Survivors' social behavior is often inappropriate to the context, ignoring the friend's needs, concerns, and expectations (Burgess & Wood, 1990; Grafman, 2002; Jacobs, 1990; Sohlberg & Mateer, 1989). When survivors lose sight of these needs, the things they do and say are seen as insensitive, hurtful, or selfish (Eisele, Lust, & Aram, 1998; Hagen, 1982; Scheff, 1990). For example, a survivor might use crude or offensive language in the presence of a friend's elderly parent or young child (Goldstein, 1934/ 2000; Head, 1926) because the survivor gave no thought to how the friend would be affected (Craik & Lockhart, 1972; Miller et al., 1960). Failures to show appropriate consideration (polite conduct, inquiring about others, expressing sympathy after personal tragedies, recognizing special events, giving thanks for help received, and so on) lead friends to feel unappreciated or disrespected (Fralish, 1998; Levin, 1985; Livingston, 1990; Prigatano, 1987; Ylvisaker & Szekeres, 1998). When repeated, such behaviors may be taken as offensive personal insults (Coelho et al., 1992; Eames, 1990; Sohlberg & Mateer, 1989; Uomoto, 1992; Ylvisaker & Urbanczyk, 1994) because they make the partner feel devalued (Scheff, 1990). If this behavior continues, it can lead to bitter social rejection (Burgess & Simons, 2005; Nochi, 1998a).

Many survivors even have difficulty in meeting expectations for basic friendship maintenance behaviors, such as issuing invitations, keeping up contact between visits with letters or phone calls, playing the considerate host, or giving thanks (Elsass & Kinsella, 1987; Tyerman, 1996; Wood, Liossi, & Wood, 2005). In many instances, family members make all of the social arrangements and responses for the survivor (Lezak & O'Brien, 1990; Thomsen, 1990).

When survivors try to meet new friends or get dates on their own, they often mishandle the early "feeling-out" process. Whereas most people approach new contacts slowly, waiting for signals that the other person is interested, survivors tend to get carried away by the desire for closeness and make more abrupt advances, which unsettles the target person and often leads to a rejection. Defects in these interaction-management skills, and the survivor's general difficulties in dealing with everything new or unfamiliar (Burgess, 1998), help to explain why new friendships tend to be so rare (Schutz, Kleinschmidt, & Gorman, 1998).

Although the research says little about successful social recoveries, we have seen some survivors maintain strong social networks and initiate many new friendships. These successful individuals invest extra effort and care in their friendships. Often, they are outgoing personalities for whom interaction is motivating and rejection is intolerable (Schutz & Wanlass, 1986). Those who make new friends also tend to be flexible in pursuing and accepting friendship opportunities with less prestigious people. Many survivors have lost some of their preinjury social status, making friendship possible only with other people who are also lower in status. Survivors who fail to adjust to this change in their social "market value" may fail to make any new friends.

Working

The best-researched ability domain is vocational (Newcombe, 1987). The vocational effects of TBI are complex. Return-to-work rates that range from 20 to 80% "probably reflect differential tolerance of employers, different degrees of severity of injuries in the samples reported, different durations of follow up, different criteria for judging return to work, etc." (Brooks, 1987, p. 67; see also Crepeau & Scherzer, 1993; Gordon, Zafonte, et al., 2006; Jacobs, 1989). Most published studies examine work status within the first 1 or 2 years-post onset. Most survivors reenter the work force by returning to the preinjury job (Najenson et al., 1974) unless physical disabilities prevent it (Brooks, 1987). Although they usually remember how to do the job, their success tends to be only temporary because of critical changes in workplace behavior (Ben-Yishay, Silver, Piasetsky, & Rattok, 1987; Brooks, 1987; Diller, 1987; McKinlay & Watkiss, 1999) and social skills (Jacobs,

1989; Najenson et al., 1974), especially in the presence of the dysexecutive syndrome (Arlinghaus et al., 2005). Even though the behavior problems may occur only some of the time, a growing track record of "uncouth" or "irresponsible" behavior is taken as evidence of a bad attitude or abandoned personal commitment to the job (Boll, 1982; Goldberg, 2001; Nochi, 1998b). At some point, such behaviors are no longer excused and job security begins to deteriorate. As the workplace interpersonal climate becomes more unpleasant, the survivor may feel mistreated and quit or the employer may terminate the job. Several instances of this pattern are reviewed in the sketches of unsuccessful recoveries presented in Chapter Three.

When the injury takes place in childhood or adolescence, there may be no preexisting set of workplace social habits. Under these conditions, the default, impulsive behaviors may break even the most basic rules of vocational conduct (Deaton, 1990). For example, on her first day working in retail sales, a former college student was assigned to stock the shelves of the small clothing store after business hours. Her supervisor, shocked to see how little she accomplished in 3 hours of stocking, gave her a verbal dressing-down. Unaccustomed to being accused of lethargy, the survivor made some accusations of her own and was fired on the spot. Another young lady, fresh out of high school, was hired for a long string of brief, entry level jobs, and then fired for being late to work, late returning from breaks, failing to carry out orders, showing up for work reeking of marijuana, and requesting extended vacation time starting in her first week on the job. Several instances of this pattern are also reviewed in Chapter Three.

In other cases, the injury has damaged a vocational skill that is essential to the survivor's preinjury occupation, and this disqualifies the survivor. For example, we have seen patients with experience as food servers in upscale establishments who were unable to resume those jobs because they could not learn customers' names or remember their meal orders. Court reporters, air traffic controllers, and paramedics are expected to make very quick decisions and responses, and we have examined survivors who cannot respond quickly enough. Assembly line jobs and retail sales in a busy store may become impractical for the same reason. Manual laborers with permanent physical impairments may be unable to return to their former jobs (Brooks, 1984b). Many survivors lose jobs that require on-line problem solving and good judgment, especially in sensitive handling of customer issues (Schutz & Wanlass, 1986).

Sometimes, the vocational outcome results less from the suitability of the job than from the standards of the particular company or supervisor (Oddy, 1984). Some companies do not tolerate any loss of consistency of performance in a critical position. Others find sheltered niches that do not require working at full capacity, a courtesy often reserved for high-level employees or family members (Brooks, 1987). For example, we have seen large companies create essentially sheltered jobs for functionally limited executive engineers. Some individuals can counterbalance their deficiencies by being attractive or personable, or by making extra efforts to be indispensable in some capacity. Job retention is higher in survivors with high intelligence (Newcombe, 1987) and/or greater insight (Diller, 1994; Ezrachi, Ben-Yishay, Kay, Diller, & Rattok, 1991; Sherer et al., 1998), presumably because they offer more assets.

Finally, vocational functioning can be influenced by the availability of disability benefits (Lishman, 1987). When patients receive a living wage in the form of disability payments or pension, they may refrain from trying to return to work as long as the benefits are available. We have known many survivors (including Tom—see Chapter Thirteen) who are careful not to jeopardize their disability benefits by taking a chance on starting a new career.

Going to School

TBI also has devastating, delayed effects on the educational process (Lehr & Savage, 1990). Most returning students look so normal that they are placed back in their preinjury classroom without hesitation, but impaired learning and adaptation prevent them from making normal progress after their return (Chapman, 2007; Savage & Woolcott, 1994; Ylvisaker et al., 2001). They may continue to function in the normal range for months or years depending on their preinjury level and help from family and teachers, but a decline into failure is hard to escape if they remain in the educational system long enough (Ewing-Cobbs et al., 1998; Taylor et al., 2002). They also tend to become behaviorally and socially maladjusted because the classroom and the schoolyard are not structured enough to restrain their impulsive behavior or teach them to follow the social rules that grow more complex as they mature (Max, 2005).

Unfortunately, the presence of the TBI is almost never recognized, in spite of a federal law requiring classification of students with

TBI (Glang, Todis, Sohlberg, & Reed, 1996; Slomine et al., 2006; Walker, 1997). If unidentified, they are left at risk for frustration, failure, social rejection, and retention or placement in special education for disorders other than TBI (Deaton, 1990; Telzrow, 1990). Many students injured in late high school struggle with more problems in college, where the levels of special services and TBI awareness are even lower (Holmes, 1988; Rivers, Schutz, & Lobato, 2007; Triplett, Hill, Freeman, Rajan, & Templer, 1996). These problems with new learning are not limited to students. Survivors have problems in job training programs, and in learning complex instruction sets like those of computer programs.

TBI does not make it impossible to function in school (Deaton, 1990). A carefully designed special education or rehabilitation program can teach adolescents the compensatory techniques that boost the learning and self-organization capabilities they need for success in school or college (Chan, McDermott, & Roediger, 2006; Schutz, 1989, 2005f; Schutz & Schutz, 2000). Promising educational rehabilitation programs developed for younger students (Blosser & DePompei, 2003; Ylvisaker & Szekeres, 1996) need to be examined by outcome research.

Driving

Safe driving requires rapid reactions, consistent vigilance, and the periodic use of the SMS to avoid unexpected traffic hazards and deal with other assorted vehicular problems. Thus the deficits of severe TBI are fundamentally incompatible with driving safety (van Zomeren, Brouwer, & Minderhoud, 1987). Although this analysis is beyond dispute, we have been amazed that many severely injured patients were cleared to drive by scrupulous testing and maintained superior safe-driving records for years afterward (Schutz , 2007a; Schutz & Gorman, 1996). A scientific explanation for this phenomenon has not been offered, and the research on driving is quite limited (van Zomeren, Brouwer, & Deelman, 1984). However, we can offer at least a speculation. We believe that most people understand the dangers of driving better than they understand other risks and hazards, which helps to mobilize the mental effort needed to optimize their driving performance. We required the members of our treatment program to demonstrate their ability to sustain a high level of self-regulation before releasing them to drive. Those who failed to prove this capability in therapy (and resumed driving without consent) had a much poorer driving safety record, often with frequent accidents (Schutz & Gorman, 1996).

Independence in the Home and Community

When they reach the post-acute level, most survivors of severe injuries perform basic self-care tasks and activities of daily living without supervision (Hall et al., 1996; Panikoff, 1983; Wood, 1987). However, they may be less than perfectly consistent or may execute the tasks at below the highest level of quality control (Porch, Collins, & Wertz, 1974), particularly in the presence of dysexecutive syndrome (Schutz & Tercero, 1985). Individual differences in personality and substance use also contribute to the persistence of safety problems (Corrigan, 1996). Long-lasting safety and judgment problems are also associated with right posterior focal damage (Jongbloed, 1986; Schutz, 2005a) or extensive damage to both frontal lobes (Goldberg, 2001; Luria, 1973). For example, an elderly, somewhat frail woman with bifrontal and right parietal traumatic contusions lived alone and invited homeless strangers from a nearby public park to have dinner in her home. On some occasions she was not immediately able to convince her dinner guests to leave after the meal. Although her relatives, friends, and attorney urgently warned her against the practice, she saw nothing wrong with it and planned to continue.

Marriage and Family Roles

The typical survivor must be supervised and managed to minimize behavior problems (Brooks & McKinlay, 1983; Brooks, Campsie, Symington, & Beattie, 1987; Jennett et al., 1981; Mauss-Clum & Ryan, 1981; Thomsen, 1984, 1990). Brooks (1984b) found 65% of spouses feeling burdened by care requirements at 12 months post-onset. This level increased over time, with 89% reporting moderate to severe burden at 5 years post-onset (Brooks et al., 1986).

The problem behaviors and personality change are also taxing for many spouses (Peters, Stambrook, Moore, & Esses, 1990), including apathy, irritability, rapid frustration, impatience, emotional outbursts, immaturity, self-centeredness, restlessness, and lack of self-control (Bond, 1975; Kay & Cavallo, 1994; Lezak, 1988; Oddy et al., 1978b; Rosenbaum & Najenson, 1976; Urbach & Culbert, 1991). Conversation may be empty or egocentric, conduct may be insensitive to the partner's needs, reasonable give-and-take may be lacking, the survivor may be untrustworthy in handling responsibilities, and the sexual relationship, if one continues, may be less frequent and less satisfying (Kay & Cavallo, 1994; Tyerman, 1996). Parenting can be quite difficult for survivors, especially because of the inflexibility (Uomoto & Uomoto, 1999).

The Opportunity to Participate in a Normal Life

> Eventually, most survivors lead abnormal lives, with few friends, few major responsibilities, and no productive activity. Students tend to drop out of mainstream education into special classes and vocational training, and/or to be exiled from higher education.

The third category in the original WHO (1980) scheme is called *handicap*. Handicap occurs when normal roles, activities, and opportunities are withheld from a person with a disability (Finlayson & Garner, 1994). The revised scheme (WHO, 2001) eliminates the negative term of handicap and replaces it with its essential opposite, *participation*. Participation rights are usually preserved in TBI because of survivors' normal appearance (Truelle & Robert-Pariset, 1990). The barriers to participation arise as a delayed consequence of how the restored opportunities are handled. Because survivors seem normal, they are held to normal standards of performance and conduct (Boll, 1982; Condeluci, 1998) and denied the special help and tolerance reserved for "the handicapped" (Nochi, 1998a; Slomine et al., 2006). Their permanent cognitive deficits usually render them unable to meet these standards without accommodations or help. Repeated failures to meet the standards are usually judged as reflecting personal qualities of inadequacy, laziness, bad attitude, or if problem behaviors are prominent, psychological disorder (Goldberg, 2001; McKinlay & Watkiss, 1999; Nochi, 1998b). If failures continue, the judgment often becomes moral, as a "bad" spouse, friend, or worker, and that role may be taken away by divorce, estrangement, or dismissal. If the survivor should attempt to find another spouse, friend, or job based on the same, normal expectations, the pattern tends to repeat itself. Eventually, survivors often give up on participation in these roles and live out a limited life instead (Goldstein, 1934/2000, 1942; Jacobs, 1989, 1990). This participation effect usually appears only after a period of delay (Burgess & Simons, 2005), which makes it unlikely that either the survivor or the associates will connect the problems with the injury (Boll, 1982; Gordon et al., 1998; Hux et al., 2006; Max, 2005; Swift & Wilson, 2001).

Social deficits can destroy enough friendships to produce social isolation (Kozloff, 1987; Thomsen, 1984). During the first decade, the prevalence of social isolation is estimated at 21 to 38% (Jacobs, 1989). Severe long-term limitations in social function may affect as many as 90% (Dawson & Chapman, 1995). Social losses tend to be greatest from injuries early in life: After severe TBI, children appear to be unable to build adult-level social repertoires (Deaton, 1987b; Lehr, 1990; Prigatano, O'Brien, & Klonoff, 1993).

Panting and Merry (1972) reported that 30% of their subjects divorced. Brooks (1987) reported a 12% rate of separation or divorce across the first 5 years post-onset. Thomsen (1984) reported that injured men were more likely to remain married, whereas injured women were more likely to be divorced. Some marriages end abruptly because of physical violence (Wood & Liossi, 2006). Although many marriages remain intact, the quality of the marital relationship is often badly damaged (Mauss-Clum & Ryan, 1981) as the survivor has "changed from being a companion and a confidant to being someone who needs to be watched and managed" (McKinlay & Watkiss, 1999, p. 82). When responsibilities are gradually taken away because of unacceptable errors, the role of a marital partner and parent can be almost completely replaced by one that more closely resembles that of a preadolescent child, a result that tends to be equally frustrating and dissatisfying for the family and the survivor (Kreutzer, Zasler, Camplair, & Leininger, 1990; Lezak, 1988; Rosenbaum & Najenson, 1976; Rosenthal, 1989).

Once again, although the research reveals that the most common outcome is starkly restricted social and familial participation, we have seen positive exceptions to this pattern. Some survivors never stop being deeply loved by their spouses and/or their friends. It is our impression that this positive result occurs when survivors of unusually good character have close and intimate relationships with partners of unusually good character. One clear example is provided by a retired couple who had enjoyed spending all day together. After she suffered a grossly dementing injury, she followed his lead in everything they did. As a result, she maintained nearly full participation, and both found the relationship rewarding. It is interesting that such closely connected partners seldom perceive a personality change. It seems that they continue to perceive the "person inside" and dismiss the overt behavior changes as nonessential.

For single survivors, and for those who lose their partner or spouse after the injury, the participation barrier can be extremely steep because of the previously-discussed defects in the strongly executive-based ability to form a new relationship. Oddy et al. (1978b) report that 60% of a group of younger long-term survivors had no romantic partner, a major area of personal dissatisfaction. We have known many survivors who wanted but could not get a date for 10 years or longer. Some who have been able to temporarily control their impulses of attraction can get dates but cannot negotiate the extended courtship ritual that leads to a relationship.

Severe behavior problems, from violent or antisocial acts, can lead to exile from the family, the workplace, and even the community as a whole (Lishman, 1973). One study reports that at 5 years post-onset, 54% of a group of severely injured survivors threatened violence and 20% had assaulted a family member (Brooks et al., 1986). Mood swings (Levin, Benton, & Grossman, 1982) also trouble family members and drive away friends and peers. Studies find up to 77% of severely injured survivors to be depressed, and almost as many to suffer from severe anxiety symptoms (Kim et al., 2007; Malec et al., 2007). A number of other studies find half of their samples showing sufficient symptoms to earn a psychiatric diagnosis (Lezak, 1987a). These symptoms can lead to confinement in a mental hospital, particularly when there is suicidal behavior or loss of reality contact (Davison & Bagley, 1969; Lishman, 1987). A recent Canadian study of the first 10 years post-onset found the incidence of psychiatric hospitalization to be three times as great after the injury as it had been prior to injury (Cameron, Purdie, Kliewer, & McClure, 2008). Another study found suicide more likely after TBI. The suicide rate varied with the severity of the injury, but it did not reach 1% in any group (Teasdale & Engberg, 2001).

Survivors who lived marginal preinjury lifestyles are particularly likely to cross legal boundaries and face participation-limiting penalties (Jacobs, 1990). For example, one survivor indulging in a cocaine binge turned his middle-class home into a "crack house," with unsavory associates coming and going at all hours and the front door left ajar for extended periods. Eventually, this flagrant conduct led a term of imprisonment and a marital separation. Another survivor who had just completed rehabilitation, still resentful because he was not released to drive, drank a six-pack of beer, stole his sister's car, and went on a 100 mile per hour dash to the state border, which also ended in a prison term.

Most survivors leave the work force before reaching retirement age (Malec, 2005). For those who fail to get hired or to keep a job of the kind held before the injury, there are always jobs with lower expectations and standards that they could get and probably keep (Weddell et al., 1980; Wehman, 1991), but these tend to be lower in prestige and pay and most survivors refuse to seek or accept them (Cope, Cole, Hall, & Barkans, 1991; Dresser, 1973; Jacobs, 1989; McMordie, Barker, & Paolo, 1990; Rosenthal, 1989; Wehman, Kreutzer, Sale, & West, 1989), even when it is their only viable alternative (Grosswasser & Stern, 1998; Najenson et al., 1974) to severe financial hardship (Schutz, 2007a). Extreme examples include a world-class race car driver with a profound head injury sustained in competition who reconciled himself to the loss of his racing career only after several years in a wheelchair. A drag racer with a brainstem injury still expected to resume her racing career after 5 years in a wheelchair. The most common recovery pattern is the unsuccessful pursuit of the old career at the former level of status, followed by a total withdrawal from any vocational activity. The 5-year employment rate has been estimated at 27%, though flaws in this research may significantly overestimate the true rate (Hart et al., 2006). As the years pass, the percentage remaining in the work force appears to dwindle. Productive employment at and beyond the second decade post-onset is estimated at less than 10% (Prigatano, 1999a; Prigatano & Ben-Yishay, 1999). For those who maintain employment, it is not clear what percentage have adjusted to employer expectations as opposed to being maintained in a position supported by relaxed or sheltered standards (Oddy, 1984).

Students with TBI also encounter slowly developing participation barriers. The research in this area is limited to anecdotal examples and short-term follow-up studies, but both indicate that continuing failure experiences discourage and eventually disenfranchise students, as they either drop out of school or are relegated to subacademic courses of study (Ewing-Cobbs et al., 1998; Johnson, Thomas-Stonell, Rumney, & Oddson, 2006; Max, 2005; Slomine et al., 1996; Taylor et al., 2002; Telzrow, 1987; Ylvisaker & Szerkes, 1996). There are some exceptions to this pattern: Some students earn passing grades in college after TBI, but "extraordinary effort," determination, and work ethic are required for this success (Todis & Glang, 2008).

In summary, most survivors get to resume a normal life but cannot maintain it. Those judged and excluded because they could not meet minimal expectations for behavior or performance are even denied the grace of attributing their failure to the injury. These consequences underscore the critical need to adapt to deficits, without which long-term prospects may be foreclosed. Of those survivors who have maintained long-term participation, it is not clear how many did so through adaptation, and how many were given special accommodations. It should be noted that research on long-term participation is so limited (Cicerone, 2004; Diller, 1994) that these conclusions can be only tentative and not definite; there may be pathways to continued participation that have not yet been investigated.

Adaptation to the Injury

It is generally believed that survivors do not adapt to their ability limitations because they do not immediately recognize and understand their deficits. Although this short-term blindness to deficit is a common symptom of damage to the executive system, it is also not the whole story. It is possible to gain a partial recognition of deficits. In addition, survivors can learn to cope emotionally by developing healthier attitudes toward their present life. It also seems likely that survivors can start the process of adaptation whenever they recognize a need to do so, even after many years.

The deficits and serious consequences of TBI become permanent limitations on life *unless* the survivor adapts to them. Survivors who gain no insight achieve no adaptation and end up living with the injury's worst consequences (Bergquist & Malec, 2002; Bogod, Mateer, &

MacDonald, 2003; Burgess, Alderman, Evans, Emslie, & Wilson, 1998; Lengfelder & Gollwitzer, 2001; Ownsworth & Fleming, 2005; Toglia & Kirk, 2000):

> When (the survivor) lacks insight, he cannot appreciate the way in which other people react to what he does, and because of this he does not see the need to alter how he acts. (Lacking the) ability to judge the effect of what we say and do on other people, and use this knowledge to modify our behavior, . . . the person may genuinely believe that there is nothing wrong with him, or he may focus on a minor consequence of the accident, such as a stiff knee, and deny he has any other problems. Of course, as long as he doesn't see that there is any need for it he will be unlikely to make much progress. . . . It will be hard to convince him that he should work on overcoming a concentration problem, for example, if he is sure that his concentration is as good as it ever was. (Gronwall et al., 1990, pp. 56–57)

Adaptation requires realization that the self can cope with the deficits (also called self-efficacy) (Diller, 1994; Smith, Jostmann, Galinsky, & van Dijk, 2008) and an attitude of self-responsibility to do something about them (self-accountability) (Dumont, Gervins, Fougeyrollas, & Bertrand, 2004; Lazarus & Folkman, 1984; Schutz, Barry, Gross, & Tupper, 1984; Trexler & Fordyce, 1996). Without adaptation to disability, survivors cannot effectively manage their own lives (Ben-Yishay & Prigatano, 1990; Braunling-McMorrow, 1998; Burke et al., 1999; Levin, 1991; Liu, Chan, Lee, Li, & Hui-Chan, 2002; McMahon & Frasier, 1998). If they were to begin adapting, they could start a recovery process and regain some control over life. For this reason, the adaptive deficit can be considered the most serious problem caused by TBI, because it traps them in a state of permanent impairment, ability limitation, and unprotected participation.

By presuming survivors to be totally incompetent at adaptation, researchers have prejudged them as unable to create positive recovery experiences (McGrath, 2004). The "old school" research reveals nothing but difficulties and losses (Jacobs, 1987, 1988, 1989, 1990; Thomsen, 1984, 1990), but this may be because it looks only for negative outcomes (Gordon, Hibbard, Brown, Flanagan, & Korves, 1999). A new understanding of survivors' positive adaptive capabilities is emerging.

Human adaptation takes place on two different time cycles. The research on TBI has been concerned with the rapid-cycle adaptation that occurs at the moment that bad outcomes occur. However, there is also a slow-cycle adaptation based on reviewing the personal track record of life experiences and arriving at decisions to alter priorities, commitments, or courses of action based on personal values (Erickson, 1963; Levinson, Darrow, Klein, Levinson, & McKee, 1978; Vaillant, 1977, 1993, 2002). The false all-clear signal of the broken executive system disengages the first kind of adaptation, and the obsolete self-concepts it protects discourage the second kind of adaptation (Damasio, 1994), without altogether preventing it from taking place.

Most survivors gradually develop a partial awareness of deficit (Prigatano & Johnson, 2003). Any physical disabilities or deformities become recognized in a matter of days (Boll, 1982). Memory deficit is usually recognized after several months (McKinlay & Watkiss, 1999). Some survivors recognize other deficits, including tendencies to respond slowly or to say things that are regretted later (Schutz et al., 1984). This research documents the recognition of certain universal mental abilities as being impaired (Prigatano, 2005).

People often have individualistic ideas about themselves that are not tapped by this research using universal categories (Bem, 1992; Kelly, 1955; Marceil, 1977). If they are allowed to explain their self-assessment in their own words, additional concepts can emerge (Nochi, 1997). For example, some survivors show indirect evidence of awareness through their sensitivity to being seen as inferior and their efforts to compensate by presenting themselves as favorably as possible (Nochi, 1998a). Others characterize themselves as impaired in vague or indefinite ways because they are unsure that they understand their condition or fear they may have forgotten key incidents (Nochi, 1997). Still others indicate that other people see them as impaired or doubt their capabilities (Nochi, 1998b). Some recognize deficits without realizing their seriousness and practical implications (Crosson, Barco, Velozo & Bolesta, 1989). Many see specific deficits without reaching the abstract conclusion that they are cognitively impaired (Schutz et al., 1984).

This half-measure of awareness (Prigatano, 1999b, 2005) appears to affect mood. As many as 60% of survivors are rated by relatives to suffer from a depressed mood (Draper et al., 2007; Lishman, 1987; Malec et al., 2007; Pollack, 2005; Prigatano, 1999b). At the same time, when asked if they are depressed, only about 20 to 25% acknowledge feeling depressed (McKinlay & Watkiss, 1999). Many of these individuals show symptoms of sadness, tension, reduced energy, inactivity, and other depressive symptoms, but without the general ideas of worthless self, world, and future seen in classic mental-health depression (Beck, 1967). They express similar dissatisfaction with specific aspects of their lives (Gordon et al., 1999), although rating overall life satisfaction as normal (Brown & Vandergoot, 1998; Burgess & Alderman, 1990; Mailhan, Azouvi, & Dazord, 2005; Oddy, Coughlan, Tyerman, & Jenkins, 1985).

If survivors can gain partial, delayed insight, there should also be partial, delayed adaptation. One study found family reports of insight and functional gains achieved 5 to 10 years post-onset (Sbordone, Liter, & Pettler-Jennings, 1995). Another found only "slightly dissatisfied" life satisfaction ratings at 10 to 32 years post-onset. With 29% working full time and 60% married or cohabiting, these findings suggest "a gradual adjustment to persisting difficulties imposed by brain injury" (Wood & Rutterford, 2006, p. 72).

Adaptation is not limited to practical and functional adjustments. People also adapt by making internal, emotional adjustments (Hartmann, 1939; Lazarus & Folkman, 1984), which can improve the quality of life after TBI (Eslinger, 2005; McGrath, 2004). Some survivors report gaining a broader perspective on life, greater empathy for others, enhanced spirituality, pride, and satisfaction in carrying on with life, and/or the inspiration to correct old bad habits (McGrath & Linley, 2006). These positive outcomes have been observed mainly in survivors who acknowledged some deficits and committed to work on personal recovery (Nochi, 2000).

Interim Summary

Most severe injury survivors experience permanent impairment of new learning and a dysexecutive syndrome that leaves them incapable of responding effectively to situations of high risk, high difficulty, and novelty. Unable to directly recognize these deficits, they usually try to resume their old lives. Because they mishandle too many high-difficulty situations (particularly in social life, family responsibilities, and school or job), most get gradually forced out of participation by dissatisfied partners and associates. Life gets narrower and simpler, until they are left with a simple and routine life that they can handle reasonably well. The therapy that is widely available at present does not prepare them to do more than this.

Over an extended period of time, some learn about aspects of the injury and the changes in their lives, and begin to look for ways to make the best of them. A few adapt relatively well. Their success indicates that the typical severe injury leaves enough cognitive capability to function successfully in a full life, but only if the new brain is programmed with self-awareness and readiness to adapt. The research on long-term recovery mentions very few successful adaptations, and when it does, it fails to delve deeply enough to explain how the survivors actually fix the deficits. These studies only suggest that fixing deficits must be difficult to figure out and/or to implement. The current understanding of how to fix real-world deficits has come almost entirely from the research on TBI rehabilitation.

Accelerated Recovery in the Unreal World of the Clinic

The best-developed programs use many psychological techniques to teach insight. While delivering the education in a supportive, trust-enhancing context, they train deficit recognition, self-monitoring, and the recognition of deficit-prone situations. Together, these steps prepare patients to notice real-life deficits, first as a part of homework, and then on their own initiative. At the same time, they learn generic coping strategies for each major type of deficit, so that they can become self-corrective. The most advanced patients learn the ideas behind the techniques, become able to design their own therapies, and go on to have great recoveries if they invest enough effort.

TBI rehabilitation programs are "unreal worlds" presenting coping lessons custom designed for rapid impact on an impaired, doubting learner. In the early 1980s, it was estimated that rehabilitation produced good recoveries (the capacity to interact socially, independence in the home and community, and readiness for some kind of job) for one third to one half of patients (Levin et al., 1982). However, this basic form of rehabilitation has been criticized because the physical abilities and well-learned habits on which most of the lessons concentrate are functions that recover naturally (Bond, 1975; Walsh, 1978).

What survivors most need to learn is how to get the new brain to adapt (Diller, 1987; Horn, 1992; Mayer, 1989). This section discusses the well-developed, advanced programs that directly treat adaptation.

Insight Training

"Acceptance of disability is a major variable being treated in a holistic outpatient treatment program" (Diller & Ben-Yishay, 1989, p. 170). Acceptance is hard-won: Insight comes as terrible news, and getting bad news accepted by a person who feels *sure* that it isn't true requires skillful psychological handling. "How does one make a patient concerned that they are unconcerned?" (Burgess & Simons, 2005, p. 224). The first stage of a holistic program is dedicated to this purpose (Ben-Yishay & Gold, 1990; Diller, 1994; Gordon & Hibbard, 2005), stimulating thinking about deficits long before the patients believe that they *have* the deficits.

Patients are taught to *spot* their deficits (Targeted Deficit Recognition) before they *believe* in them (Schutz, 2007a). The intake evaluation and every relevant therapy session spotlight the new learning deficit and a set of critical executive deficits, as well as deficits particular to an individual patient's injury. The Orlando program, which treated most of the great recoverers, labeled each major deficit with a single, catchy term (like *fishbrain* for the feeling of confusion that accompanies overload, or *impulsivity*) used by all members of the staff, so that the patient and family could begin to recognize and label the key "head-injured moments" (a phrase coined by Rachel—see Chapter Nine) within the first week (Giles, 1994). Patients kept a transcript of their tape-recorded intake evaluation report in their therapy notebook so that they and/or the staff could access the particulars about these deficits at any time during treatment. At this point, most (including the great recoverers, with the exception of Stephanie—see Chapter Seven) felt unimpaired and found the constant reference to the deficits annoying. The staff assured them that this annoyance was a normal reaction to the program. In psychotherapy sessions (a staple of holistic programs—see Gordon & Hibbard, 2005), deficit education was discussed at length. Often a "what if" (or conditional approach) was used. In essence, it was recommended to learn about the deficits "just in case" they turned to be a real problem in real life. Patients generally went along with this suggestion if a feeling of working partnership (also called a *therapeutic alliance*) had been developed (Mateer, 2005; Prigatano, 1994, 1999a).

The next objective of therapy was to teach patients to *watch* for the occurrence of their deficits (Alderman, 2003; Burke, Zencius, Wesolowski, & Doubleday, 1991; Cicerone & Giacino, 1992; Hart, Giovannetti, Montgomery, & Schwartz, 1998; Kennedy & Yorkston, 2000; Lawson & Rice, 1989; Levine et al., 2000; Malec, 1996; Webster & Scott, 1983). In the daily training exercises of group cognitive therapy, those who failed to recognize and identify their deficits got corrective feedback from up to 11 peers, one after another. They were also exposed to role models (Cicerone & Azulay, 2007)—senior members who diligently self-monitored and reported their deficits. Watching for deficits effectively and then admitting to them publicly was the only way to save face. Peer pressure of this kind has a powerful effect (Asch, 1952), and most learned to self-monitor effectively (Schutz & Trainor, 2007). Moreover, the more they followed these steps of their program, they more they began believing in them (Festinger, 1957).

At this point, they were surrounded by social influences that encouraged them to accept the program's principles and achieve true awareness of deficit (Ben-Yishay, 1996). Peers voiced these beliefs in program assemblies and often served as the primary teacher in the therapy groups. In many cases, family members also endorsed the program and pointed out deficits. Former members with successful outcomes gave presentations attributing their success to deficit awareness and urging current program members to reject their certainty about being unimpaired. In addition, the therapy sessions always taught a specific compensation technique to fix each major deficit. Those members who used the compensation generally earned better scores than those who did not. Psychotherapy provided assistance in using the compensations to address current personal concerns. The link between each deficit and its compensation was discussed so often that this, too, became familiar and well learned (Giles, 1994). Finally, members realized (or were advised by peers) that they would need to make progress in their therapies before being released back to work/school and driving. These external (extrinsic) influences and incentives usually got compliance and provoked self-questioning about how serious the deficits might be.

The last step in insight training is to learn where and when to look for the deficits (Targeted Situation Recognition) (Schutz, 2007a) so their real-life occurrence can be anticipated and prevented (Crosson et al., 1989). In this step, members completed a biweekly Error Analysis form describing where and how they had their head-injured moments. Seeing the deficits again and again in real life usually made it clear what was wrong and how serious it was, providing good reasons for them to adapt on their own (intrinsic motivation) (Schutz, 2007b).

Repair Strategies

How do you fix a broken brain? The experts in this field have not achieved complete agreement on a fully detailed game plan, although effective therapy cannot be done without one (Baddeley, 1993; Caramazza & Hillis, 1993; Robertson, Stuss, & Winocur, 1999; Shallice, 2000). Game plans are being field-tested (Rosenthal, 1999a), but they need to be more richly detailed to properly guide therapy design, and many important questions about them remain to be answered to the satisfaction of the community of specialists (Worthington & Walker, 2008).

The first step is to select therapy's basic purpose: to eliminate the impairment or to improve the use of the impaired brain. Many years of serious effort in exercising deficits have yielded discouragingly little evidence that severe impairments can be eliminated (Carney et al., 1999; Cicerone et al., 2000, 2005; Gordon, Zafonte, et al., 2006; Katz & Mills, 1999; Miller, 1984; Prigatano, Glisky, & Klonoff, 1996; Uomoto, 1992; Wilson, 2005). Hence, compensation (broadly defined as finding ways to work around the inevitable impairment) is widely regarded as the primary job of rehabilitation (Gordon & Hibbard, 2005; Katz & Mills, 1999; Malec, 1996; Trexler & Fordyce, 1996; Wade, 2005; Wilson, 2002). Unfortunately, much clinical time is still spent on drills administered for the purpose of cognitive restoration (Ylvisaker, Hanks, & Johnson-Greene, 2002).

Compensation is largely a matter of doing things the hard way (Dixon & Backmun, 1999; Evans & Preston, 1990). In fact, the most basic compensation amounts to simply trying harder at doing something in the familiar way—a strategy that is known to reduce impairment from brain disorders of all kinds including TBI (Dixon & Backmun, 1999; Prigatano, 1999b; Sohlberg & Mateer, 2001; Wood, 1987). In this usage, trying harder refers primarily to focusing attention and concentration to enhance executive control, which makes movements more precise and better timed (Fuster, 2002; Schmidt & Lee, 1999). In fact, the one form of cognitive exercise still widely practiced in well-developed programs, *attentional* drills (Cicerone et al., 2000, 2005; Gordon, Zafonte, et al., 2006; Malec, 1996), may be useful mainly because they enhance this executive component of recruiting attentional effort (Posner & Peterson, 1990), a skill known to improve through drills (Muraven, Baumeister, & Tice, 1999; Posner & Fan, 2007; Rothbart & Rueda, 2005). In a similar vein, students with TBI can be trained to learn large volumes of information when distributed practice and self-testing are augmented by the recruitment of concentration and mental effort (Elhardt et al., 2008; Schutz & Schutz, 2000).

Compensation is accomplished in several other ways (Diller, 1987; Diller & Gordon, 1981; Miller, 1984; Whyte, 1986): (a) an altered environment (simpler tasks, helpful devices, reminder signals, assistance —see Sbordone, 1990), (b) reprogrammed automatic behaviors (to stop problem behaviors or add missing ones) via behavior modification, (c) modified strategies that substitute intact skills and actions for defective ones, and (d) the full SMS cycle deliberately implemented one step at a time (Evans, 2005; Schutz, 2007a, 2007b). This diversity of methods may even be preferable to treat a disorder with such a wide variety of symptoms and consequences (Craine, 1982; Gross & Schutz, 1986; Wade, 2005; Wilson, 2005). The vast magnitude of dysexecutive syndrome effects justifies an emphasis on the executive steps (effort and SMS) whenever possible (Gordon, Cantor, et al., 2006; Schutz, 2007b).

The technological compensations that are almost universally recommended (Malec, 1996; Mateer, 2005) include entering large-volume information in a notebook or computer and using a written or computerized schedule or a schedule-programmable paging system for prospective recall and time organization. All of these have been shown to be effective even with very severe deficits (Donaghy & Williams, 1998; Schmitter-Edgecombe, Fahy, Whelan, & Long, 1995; Wilson, Emslie, Quirk, Evans, & Watson, 2005; Wilson, Scott, Evans, & Emslie, 2003; Wright et al., 2001).

Two contrasting procedures can be used to establish a compensation. A "painless" technique starts by giving the member enough cuing to guarantee the desired response, as in instructing a task step by step. Then, as training progresses, the cues or instructions are taken away so gradually that no mistake is ever made (Ben-Yishay & Diller, 1983b; Wilson, 2003). This method provides success experiences that encourage accepting both the training and the strategy (Elhardt et al., 2008; Goldstein, 1940/1963). Alternatively, failures can be deliberately planned to arouse natural motivations (worry, concern, or fear) that will later trigger the real-world use of the compensation (Schutz & Langenbahn, 1985) and stimulate brain activation to assist with the on-line problem solving (Gray & McNaughton, 2003; McGuinness & Pribram, 1980). These methods can be used in sequence: first, the errorless method can establish a behavior, and then the error-inducing method can structure reactions that will carry the behavior over into real life.

When improved self-monitoring has been established, most patients learn to readily recognize the effects of overload. Because overload is monitored and recognized internally, the transfer to real-world situations is accomplished with relatively little difficulty (Rath, Simon, Langenbahn, Sherr, & Diller, 2003). In fact, overload is the symptom that was reported most frequently as interfering with real-life activities in the Orlando program (Schutz, 2007b). Techniques for overload control (including anticipation, stimulus control, emotional modulation, and relaxation) are readily learned and applied (Schutz, 2005d; Sherr & Langenbahn, 1992; Simon, 2001).

Most well-developed programs include a module addressing dys-executive syndrome (Cicerone et al., 2000, 2005; Gordon, Cantor, et al., 2006; Kennedy & Coelho, 2006; Kennedy et al., 2008), most often by teaching a problem-solving formula as an executive compensation (Evans, 2001; Levine et al., 2000; Meichenbaum, 1993; Rath et al., 2003; von Cramon & Matthes-von Cramon, 1990). Others employ self-talk to organize the steps of problem solving (Cicerone & Giacino, 1992; Cicerone & Wood, 1987; Meichenbaum, 1993; von Cramon & Matthes-von Cramon, 1994). Still others address problem solving holistically, building component skills through content modules (Ben-Yishay & Diller, 1983b) or sustained mental effort (Schutz, 2007a, 2007b). This expression of effort refers to the extent and quality of thought invested in preplanning and in particular in the elaboration of anticipated outcome scenarios (Grafman, 2002; Picton et al., 2002; Pribram, 1991; Schutz, 2005a). These last programs provide no step-by-step instructions, assuming that preinjury methods of problem solving are retained (Goldstein & Levin, 1991; Schutz, 2007b) as procedural knowledge (Miller et al., 1960).

The Orlando program's approach evolved during the era of the exceptional recoveries, with the first five members trained on the use of a formula, whereas the last seven used their own, preexisting methods under supervision for effort and quality control. No ill effects were seen from relying on the members' own methods. In fact, the increased emphasis on effort and quality control was associated with slightly better long-term outcome (Schutz, 2007a). However, this approach must be considered only a working assumption until further research examines it.

In the second phase of training (Fitts & Posner, 1967), compensations are practiced to reach full proficiency. The length of this phase depends on the levels of impairment and motivation (Prigatano et al., 1986, 1990; Schutz, 2005b; Schutz & Schutz, 1999; Sohlberg & Mateer, 2001; Wood, 1987). As members become proficient at fixing their deficits, they also become more willing to admit to them and more adept at seeing them in others. In this phase, the psychotherapy shores up this new confidence in the adaptive behaviors and starts to apply them to meet personal needs under the therapist's guidance (Prigatano, 1999a).

The third phase focuses on the real-life situations into which the compensations are to be systematically transferred (Fitts & Posner, 1967). Neglect of this phase is a major barrier to program success (Diller & Ben-Yishay, 1987; Dixon & Backmun, 1999; Gordon & Hibbard, 2005; Wilson, 2000). Again, there is a lack of consensus on how this objective should be accomplished. Some programs plant compensations in the real-world situations by doing the therapy in those settings (Diller & Ben-Yishay, 1987; Guercio & Fralish, 1998; Hart & Hayden, 1986). Even more "situated" therapy is done in real-life situations from start to finish, with actual role partners serving as the trainers (Diller, 1994; Uomoto, 1992; Ylvisaker, 2005). This approach can be used for adults with limited insight and motivation as well as young children, but its effects last only until the survivor relocates, a profound flaw (Katz & Mills, 1999; Schutz & Trainor, 2007). The alternative approach trains the patient as a therapist so that compensations are self-generalized (Crosson et al., 1989; Meichenbaum, 1977; Rath et al., 2003; Schutz, 2007b; Wood, 1990; Worthington & Walker, 2008). Most patients learn to recognize their tendencies to have head-injured moments in certain states of mental or emotional strain, when doing awkward tasks, when working with difficult partners, or in unfavorable settings (Mateer & Raskin, 1999; Schutz, 2007b). The most ambitious approach teaches general concepts for the deficits, compensations, and situational vulnerabilities, so that trainees can *construct* self-treatments and resume self-managed adaptation (Goldstein, 1940/1963; Hart & Evans, 2006; Schutz & Trainor, 2007). The Orlando program employed a one-page Error Analysis form with menus for selecting the type of error, features of the situation in which it took place, the primary compensations needed, and a section for a narrative corrective plan. Completed forms were reviewed and critiqued by a family member, and then discussed in a group therapy session. Continued use after discharge was recommended (Schutz, 2006a).

The psychotherapy given in the third phase of training, in addition to reinforcing the lessons of the cognitive therapy, addresses key psychological recovery objectives. As survivors dismantle their preinjury self-image and discard the associated hopes and dreams, they have an urgent need to replace their old self with an acceptable new one (Prigatano & Ben-Yishay, 1999). Psychotherapy helps to develop a new way of thinking about their accomplishments and prospects. As they approached graduation, many program members began to accord themselves a new kind of respect for their participation in the program: "This was the hardest thing I have ever done." This bolstered their confidence about undertaking real-life challenges. Finally, the injury has impacted their life purpose, and they must begin to redefine that purpose (Pollack, 2005).

Outcomes

Follow-up research indicates that holistic programs improve all major functional abilities (Boake & Diller, 2005; Cicerone et al., 2000, 2005; Cicerone, Mott, Azulay, & Friel, 2004; Gordon, Zafonte, et al., 2006; Katz et al., 2006; Malec, 2001; NIH, 1998; Schutz, Rivers, & Ratusnik, 2009; Trexler & Fordyce, 1996), particularly for patients with the most insight (Ben-Yishay & Prigatano, 1990; Diller, 1994; Ezrachi et al., 1991; Prigatano, Klonoff, O'Brien, Altman, & Amin, 1994; Sherer et al., 1998; Trexler & Fordyce, 1996; Wehman, Targett, West, & Kregel, 2005). Brain imaging finds unusually large executive zones activated when successful patients rally mental effort to perform hard tasks (Glenn, 2006; Laatsch, Thulborn, Krisky, Shobat, & Sweeney, 2004; Levine et al., 2002; Maruishi, Miyatani, Nakao, & Muranaka, 2007; Scheibel et al., 2003; Strangman, 2006). This "compensatory hyperactivation" is a network-organized brain's adaptation to injury (Dixon & Backmun, 1999, p. 65). The symptoms of other executive brain disorders are also controlled by this executive hyperactivation (Peterson et al., 1998; Schulz et al., 2005; Schwartz & Begley, 2002).

This "effort effect" can be triggered externally even at the beginning of therapy, when a simple effort cue (Burke et al, 1999; Campbell, 2000; Levine et al., 2000; Rath et al., 2003; Sohlberg & Mateer, 2001) or a wager optimizes performance (Lashley, 1963; Parente, 1994; Thornton et al., 2007). Upgraded quality control can also be triggered by a prearranged sound (Manly et al., 2004; Robertson, Tegnér, Tham, Lo, & Nimmo-Smith, 1995), a phrase-length self-instruction (Burgess & Alderman, 1990; Webster & Scott, 1983), or a command to self-monitor (Schloss, Thompson, Gajar, & Schloss, 1985; Sohlberg, Sprunk, & Metzelaar, 1998), apparently eliciting greater activation (Posner & Fan, 2008) and effort via self-consciousness about performance quality (Carver & Scheier, 2001). Such simple, therapist-initiated effort-management compensations even elicit normal-range performance at times (Prigatano et al., 1986).

Self-triggered hyperactivation of the executive system would be a potent game plan for recovery (Prigatano, 1999b; Strangman, 2006; Schutz, 2005b, 2007a). It is theoretically reasonable: An active network can substitute for an inactive one as long as both connect to the same system (Grady & Kapur, 1999). The emotional and executive-attentional networks both interface at the central executive's on-off switch (see Feinstein, 1999; Fuster, 2002; Goldberg, 1985; Pribram, 1960), and both normally activate the recruitment of effort in situations of urgency (Gray & McNaughton, 2003; Miller & Cohen, 2001; Pribram & McGuinness, 1975; Stuss et al., 1994). Therefore, it seems possible to bring the dormant executive system on-line by creating a feeling of urgency. Patients occasionally display executive function spontaneously when coping with situations that naturally arouse the sense of urgency (Schutz, 1989).

Thus, training seeks to consciously, deliberately summon the urgency and effort that activate the executive in the critical, real-life tasks where it is needed (Ben-Yishay & Prigatano, 1990; Gross & Schutz, 1986; Schutz, 2007b). Successfully treated patients are expected to watch out for problem-prone workplace, scholastic, and interpersonal situations (Kennedy et al., 2008), and, when entering such situations, to fully activate the mind to work out an effective solution. They should also set aside time to reflect skeptically on the quality of their current life, and to decide on how to improve things whenever life is not working out as they intend (Schutz & Trainor, 2007). Holistic programs lack the major research resources needed to study how former patients actually do these things in the real world (Fordyce, 1994; Gordon & Hibbard, 2005).

The Orlando program invited graduates to come back later and update the program about their current lives, and almost 250 actually did so, but the data obtained from these conversations were limited. The project that led to this book began when the senior author proposed creating a free recovery group for untreated survivors, with successful, former patients serving as the trainers. He invited the 15 graduates with the most distinguished recoveries to join a task force developing this new model, and 12 agreed to help. While the task force was meeting, each member gave an extended interview discussing how he or she had recovered. Those interviews, edited only to organize the statements into logical sections, are presented in Chapter Four to Chapter Fifteen. In these chapters, they describe the adaptations they achieved and maintained.

One final note concerns the program changes that took place when the exceptional survivors were in attendance. Administrative policies forced radical cutbacks in the program after the first five exceptional graduations. The team decided to cut the program back farther than necessary, so that the aspects regarded as essential curative ingredients (therapeutic partnership, TBI education and psychotherapy, high-intensity feedback, effort management, error recognition and correction, and situation recognition—see Schutz, 2007a; Schutz & Trainor, 2007) could be increased by 50%, while eliminating what seemed to be the less-important therapy modalities and program activities. Much phase two and phase three training was replaced by homework and family involvement. In essence, therapists did less for members and required them to do more for themselves. The modifications reduced therapy intensity by two thirds at first and by four fifths at the time Jomo attended (see Chapter Fourteen). This much shorter program got essentially the same results, with a slight improvement in the competitive employment rate at follow-up (Schutz, 2007a). In addition, 7 of the 12 exceptional outcomes were obtained under the new, reduced program. These results suggest that the curative factors were probably well chosen.

The success of this therapy approach helps to explain why so many families and professionals who do not specialize in TBI have had so little success in trying to encourage recovery. The teaching and training methods of normal life—correcting errors, simplifying tasks, instructing and cuing correct responses, providing repeated practice in using skills, and rewarding successes—have no direct effect on the adaptive processes that need to be fixed, and bear little resemblance to the therapies that have improved recovery. Normal-life methods do not teach survivors to disbelieve and ignore the powerful "all clear" signal from the broken SMS, or to substitute the recognition that anything important now must be done more carefully, more thoughtfully, and with more effort than ever before (Dixon & Backmun, 1999; Luria, 1948/1963; Miller, 1984; Wilson, 2000; Wood, 1987). Although a therapy program that invests heavily in credibility and massed feedback would have a big edge in breaking through that signal, any survivor *could* decide to force insight, recruit effort, and resume adaptation on his or her own.

Why Recovery Can be Studied Properly Only in Real Life

> Only the study of recovery in real life accurately captures survivors' sense of purpose, which is what activates their full potential to adapt.

The most successful recoveries are the product of inspired effort (Diller, 1994). Traditional laboratory research methods are poorly suited to examine such highly personal and individual phenomena (Schutz et al., 2009).

A fundamental limitation of clinic treatment and outcome research studies is ecological invalidity (Brunswik, 1955; Long, 1998; Sbordone, 1997; Tupper & Cicerone, 1990), the failure of exercises, tests, and outcome questionnaires (Schutz et al., 2009) to inspire full effort because they are not true to life (Evans & Preston, 1990; Guercio & Fralish, 1998). Most patients do not care how well they arrange colored blocks to match a picture (Wechsler, 1955), build creative designs from Tinkertoys (Lezak, Howieson, & Loring, 2004), play games like twenty questions (Delis, Kaplan, & Kramer, 2001), participate in role plays (Ben-Yishay & Gold, 1990), or rate statements on a seven-point scale. They are asked to pretend that these activities are important (Retzlaff & Gibertini, 1994), but in dysexecutive syndrome the ability to bind thoughts and efforts to such imaginary purposes is lost or at least limited (Goldstein, 1940/1963), as behavior is excessively reactive to the environment (Goldstein, 1942; L'Hermitte, 1986; Wood, 1987).

Moreover, different functional abilities matter to different individuals (Burgess & Simons, 2005). Idiosyncratic interests and accomplishments are often among the most inspired activities in a person's life, but research cannot discover them unless it examines their real lives in their own terms (Nochi, 1997). This represents a specific instance of a more general point about research methodology: "In order to investigate the impact of intervention, clients with brain injury may need to be asked about specific activities with relevance to their lives (using narrative) techniques that produce authentic data in order to assess changes in disability" (Sohlberg, 2005, p. 95). The most important phenomena of recovery are simply too personal, too individual, and too subjective to understand through any method other than the survivor's own explanation.

Chapter 3

Fifteen Who Broke Down on the Road Back

High-intensity treatment fails to help a significant minority of patients. This chapter describes 15 of the Orlando program's treatment failures. Poor recovery occurs when patients continue to use drugs and alcohol, refuse treatments, or participate only halfheartedly. Damage to the right rear quadrant of the brain also tends to have a poor outcome.

As a baseline from which to examine successful long-term recoveries, these are stories of 15 former patients who are classified as treatment failures, chosen from the program's follow-up database on the basis of the length of time from injury to last contact. They are functioning much like many untreated, long-term survivors described in the follow-up research studies—unemployed, with limited or unrealistic career plans, experiencing behavior and adjustment problems, and poorly adapted to post-injury life.

Kenny was a college student from a rural Michigan single-parent family. Once an overweight, unpopular child, he worked hard on his physical conditioning after graduating from high school. He became buff and well developed, with a nut-brown tan from his summers as a Florida lifeguard. Having made himself attractive, he could enjoy the flirting, and his last girlfriend was an exotic dancer. He also became involved in long-distance road racing, and was training for a triathlon when a speeding car ran into him, throwing him high in the air to land on his head. At this time in his life, he was also struggling to make the transition from community college to the university. A bright young man, community college had been easy for him, but he had failed out of the local university because of his casual study habits. He had been readmitted and was in his first semester back at the time of the accident. The injury was quite severe, with a coma of 6 weeks and contusions in the left frontal and right parietal lobes. He was not especially interested in rehabilitation, and so uncooperative that he was discharged without meeting his treatment goals. As recommended by the treatment team, he moved back to Michigan to live with his mother, a school principal. When he left he was not driving, having failed his rehab driving evaluation by refusing to cooperate with the examiner. Within a year he passed the driving evaluation at his new hospital. After his second stint of rehab, he was given a volunteer assignment to supervise an elderly man who had suffered a stroke. He then got hired as a playground aide (through his mother's influence), but was fired because of odd behavior. At 10 years post-onset, he moved back to Florida, living alone in a mobile home owned by a family member. He agreed to reenter treatment and attend a brain injury group, but he was only marginally cooperative with this therapy and expressed open contempt of other group members. He stated the intention to get a job within 2 weeks. Two and a half years later, he arranged his first hiring interview, which he sabotaged. Although he was able to manage the household on his own, he barely did so, running out of food and going days without eating on occasion. He also had several minor auto accidents. He received several offers of friendship and some overtures from an eligible woman, but he spurned these and led an isolated existence. He quit doing his therapy exercises, gained weight, and developed problems with walking. Although he talked about correcting these problems, he did nothing about any of them. At 14 years post-onset his mother contracted a terminal illness. At this point, as he finished his therapy, he said he was disappointed but not dissatisfied with his new life.

Denzel was holding vigil in the waiting room as his wife was delivering their third child. Suddenly he slumped over and fell to the floor. An internal carotid artery had disintegrated, cutting off the main blood supply for the right half of his brain. He would have died had this happened anywhere but in a hospital. He was cooperative with his rehabilitation, but his effort was halfhearted at best in both his physical and his cognitive therapies. He stubbornly refused to set any long-term goals other than to resume his former life. After rehab, he was unable to resume his high-paying, white collar job. He shunned offers of vocational help, preferring to wait at home until he healed and resumed his old job. Four years later, still living in his mother's living room, he was still waiting. His wife had separated from him, and he saw nothing of her or his children. He spent all day watching television. He refused to do the home exercises his therapists gave him at discharge, or other any physical activity, and was developing complications from the lack of activity. He still had no interest in looking for work. His plan was still to "heal up," although he knew that his doctors had declared his healing over long ago.

Jericho was a budding star in the field of microbiology, developing the most promising program of research in the top Chicago laboratory that hired him after he got his PhD. His injury was complicated by brain surgery to remove a blood clot. The surgeon slipped and cut through both of the main arteries supplying the front of his brain. At hospital discharge, he was sent to live with the only relative who could care for him, his sister in Orlando. A contagiously friendly and exuberant patient, he charmed everyone in the program. However, he was easily distracted, got carried away by his silly (hebephrenic) sense of humor, and did not even make marginal progress in his therapies. He also did no homework, even after his sister had been called to meet with the staff. The sister was employed full-time, and did not become involved with his therapy. After the team exhausted all possible interventions to help him to participate, they discharged him from rehabilitation unimproved. Seven years later, he encountered his former neuropsychologist at a head injury conference. He was still living with his sister and had never worked. He was no longer excited and outgoing, and he admitted that he had been treated for depression in recent years. He was unhappy with his empty life, but he tolerated it and was determined to survive it.

Todd shot himself in the head in a suicide attempt over a relationship breakup at age 18. He was something of a "slacker" in rehab, with a low level of motivation, though he was cooperative and friendly. He was suspected of smoking marijuana while attending the program (a violation of program rules automatically leading to discharge), though the suspicion was never confirmed. His single-parent mother was invited to participate in his rehab, but she elected to remain at a distance. After graduating, he refused the entry-level job recommended by his vocational counselor. Instead, he enrolled in a training program in computers advertised on television. He was able to finish this program also, but could not find a job. He enrolled in another trade school program for training as a junior executive in the hotel industry, but again there was no job at the end of the training. He then took a training course to work as a salesman, but this also failed to land him a job. Eventually he took still another trade school course in electronics, but remained unemployed at 8 years post-onset. He continued to live with his mother, with a social life limited to his family. He was discouraged about remaining unemployed but denied depression.

Brady was a child tennis star who enrolled in a prestigious Florida tennis academy where a number of international champions had trained. He expected to rise to the top of his sport and become a millionaire one day, and his family hoped to share in his good fortune. While playing on a hot day without replacing enough fluid, he suffered a stroke. Although the brain damage made him slow and visually impaired with a blind spot, he was cocky about returning to tennis. His father echoed his optimistic expectations. They ignored the doctors' warnings, claiming that the doctors did not know tennis. In rehab, Brady was jovial but disruptive, making a limited effort and skipping many of his homework assignments. He believed his body was healing, and felt he had no problems with his mind. His final scores in all cognitive therapies were poor. After leaving rehab, he secured a tennis scholarship to a private college and played small-college tennis for several years, but never got back to the championship level. He invested the funds from his lawsuit in a series of businesses, each of which he attempted to run without success. Eventually he returned to his home town and moved back in with his parents.

Jeb was a charming, handsome university student living in a fraternity house at the time of his car accident. The right half of his brain was crushed by the impact, and he was nearly blind from the resulting visual impairment. Jeb refused to acknowledge any cognitive deficits no matter how badly he did in his therapies; he had an excuse to explain every failure, claiming to be tired, or distracted, or uninterested, or improperly instructed. Peer feedback about his deficits made no impression. At one point, a list of the excuses he made to explain away his errors reached over a hundred in less than one week. Presenting him with the list made no impression. His visual problem and limited efforts to overcome it prevented him from participating in many of his therapies. His lack of effort and refusal to use any compensations undercut his performance in the other treatments. His parents were brought in to discuss his lack of progress a number of times, but they felt unable to challenge or discipline him because of their extreme sympathy. They helped him to do everything that was difficult. His mother and sister even did his therapy homework for him. As his program wound down, he was advised to focus on developing an entry-level job, but he and his family rejected this advice. They wanted him to go back to school and complete his studies for his degree. When he was discharged from the hospital, he moved back into his old room in his parents' home. He attended classes at the university with his mother or sister walking him to the classroom and back to the car each day. With their help, he was able to finish his last year and a half in 5 years. After getting his degree, he took a job as a telephone solicitor, but was fired within the month because he was unproductive. Two more entry-level, minimal status white collar jobs also failed within a month. Finally, he got a "supported" job (that is, one designed for a person with disabilities) as a greeter at a local hospital, but again lost it in less than a month after several incidents. He blamed the loss of each job on his employers' failure to train him properly, and learned nothing that might help him to get another job. Demoralized at this point, his parents admitted that they had helped him so much that he really had not learned any independence skills in the 6 years since onset.

Thomas was a business student who had severely bruised both sides of his brain in his car accident. His father was a successful businessman, and Thomas had every intention of making himself equally successful. In therapy, he was earnest and sincere and got along well with both his peers and his therapists. He worked harder than any of his peers and met all of his therapy goals. He returned to school, but because he did not plan his daily schedule as recommended, he didn't get all the necessary studying done and almost flunked out. Initially, he blamed his noisy roommates for his problems in school. Counseling helped him to admit that he was allowing himself to function in a disorganized manner; he gave in, used his day planner, and graduated. He then went through eight jobs in 10 years, beginning as a trainee for a management job and ending up as a salesman in a lumber yard and then as a gofer in a business run by a friend. His father kept an open offer for Tom to join him in his business, but Tom felt that he would be admitting defeat if he took it. So he continued to seek the same kinds of jobs in which he had been failing, with no change in plans that might give him a better prospect for success.

Manny was in high school when he had his car accident. His brain injury was one of the least severe in his group, and he was friendly and got along well with everyone at the day program. However, he did not make enough effort to compensate even for his relatively minor symptoms in therapy. He gradually increased his level of effort with much urging from his therapists, although it was felt that he never exerted himself enough to reach his full potential. At the end of his program, he decided that he didn't want to go back to his high school, and instead got his GED in a community college adult school program. He moved to another state, lived alone, and took and got fired from six jobs over a span of 8 years. He wasn't always sure why he had been fired, but when it was clear, it was always about his impulsive behavior, his too-casual attitude, and his lowered productivity, never about his competence to do the work. At the 8-year point, he decided he needed a new plan, but the change had nothing to do with his deficits. He concluded that he had failed at work because he didn't make enough money on these jobs. So he moved back to Florida to live with his mother, and borrowed money from her to undertake a training program in massage therapy. At last report, he was about to start training.

Matt was a married realtor in his late 30s who was just beginning to earn the big money when he dumped his Harley, bouncing his bare head over the asphalt. He was very drunk, which made his bifrontal, left temporal, and right parietal lobe contusions bleed profusely, and he remained in a coma for 6 weeks. He awoke with serious language problems and bouts of uncontrolled emotion. He got so loud and hostile during therapy that his speech therapist discharged him on the spot. He also got angry in a therapy group, left in a huff, and walked several miles home. Although he blamed drinking and driving for "ruining my life" and swore he would never drink again, he resumed after getting permission from his father. Spurning advice and urging from his wife and fellow patients to quit before he lost control, he had his third DUI accident in 3 years. He eventually yielded to pressure to sell his Harley, and swore off alcohol a second time. Four months later he was back drinking and smoking marijuana. He worked as a part-time dishwasher in a fast-food restaurant. By 4 years post-onset, he and his wife had divorced. By 7 years post, he had been psychiatrically hospitalized for bipolar disease (manic-depressive psychosis), jailed for assaulting a police officer, and while awaiting trial, arrested for smoking a joint on a public street. He used the last funds in his savings account to buy another Harley. At 9 years post-onset, he was unemployed and selling his home to avoid foreclosure. At last report (11 years post), he remained unemployed and had recently attempted suicide.

Chuy had just graduated from high school and was working as a summer youth counselor at the time of his accident. He was driving his brother home from music lessons on a rainy day when he lost control of the car and it slammed into a light pole. Chuy spent a week in coma, while his brother was killed. When his parents finally told him about the death 2 months later, while he was in inpatient rehabilitation, he was stricken with grief and self-blame. He had not recovered from the emotional trauma 8 years later. He held a number of jobs over the years, and talked about going to college, but he did not attempt it until 7 years post-onset. He had failed at his first attempt, and was on probation on his second attempt at last contact. He was involved in an emotionally explosive, self-destructive, long-term relationship for several years. He continued to drink to intoxication, despite knowing that drinking got him into trouble on several occasions.

Toby was unconscious for only part of a day following his traffic accident, and his limited medical records did not indicate any focal injuries. However, he complained of many cognitive problems and performed inconsistently on cognitive exercises during his 6-month treatment stay. He was always friendly and maintained a positive attitude, even when he failed in his exercises from lack of effort. His vocational counselor got him a job as a commercial vehicle driver, which was scheduled to begin on the day after his graduation. On his first day at work, he crashed the bus and was fired. This was his last full-time, competitive job. After several months of unemployment, he joined a support group for head injury survivors and served as an officer for many years. At 18 years post-onset, he volunteered as a minister at a community church and worked occasional gigs as a musician. He described himself as happy with his new life, and seemed to be truly happy.

Louis was in his mid-20s, unemployed, and living with his mother when he had a severe injury from a car accident. He was in a coma for 4 weeks, with a large focal injury from a hemorrhage on the right side of his brain. His early recovery was unusual in that he made little effort in inpatient or outpatient rehabilitation to try to regain the ability to walk. Although his therapists believed that he should be capable of walking again, he never did so. He remained in a wheelchair 10 years after his accident. His outpatient rehabilitation was marked by a lack of effort on other therapies also, and he was discharged in a state of total dependence. His mother remained his devoted caregiver, doting on him in every way. He remained unemployed and dependent on her. When she became disabled by health problems of her own at 10 years post-onset, he refused to help her.

Delta was an accomplished weightlifter in high school before her car accident. She was a marginal student, and her severely alcoholic single mother had little success in getting her focused or structured. She responded well to the structure of the rehabilitation program, and got along well with her therapists, although it took a great deal of therapist attention to inspire her to full effort and homework remained a problem throughout her treatment. When she went back to school she abandoned her compensations. Her aggressive behavior came close to getting her expelled after she threatened a student and struck a teacher. She got her diploma via a nontraditional program located off campus. The next 4 years she remained sedentary, living alternately with her mother and one of her short-term boyfriends. She was able to get hired for various entry-level jobs, but none of them lasted more than 3 weeks. She admitted to losing her temper with her employers' demands and quitting impulsively. She was also smoking marijuana on a daily basis, but could not see the connection between her drug use and her unemployment. She came back for the aftercare group but attended only three sessions before dropping out.

Kristi finished high school and gave birth to a daughter out of wedlock before her car accident, which left her in a coma for 2 weeks. In rehab she was friendly but moody and unmotivated, with poor follow-through on homework assignments and an undisciplined approach to dealing with the practical problems in her life. After therapy, she and her child moved into a back room in her sister's home, and they were still living there 3 years later. She attempted to find work, mainly in jobs as a secretary/receptionist, though she had no experience in that field, as all of her previous part-time jobs had been blue collar. At follow-up, she was in extreme poverty, and had been unable to get a job after failing 22 interviews. She had not asked for any feedback from the potential employers about why she was rejected. She continued to look for work in the same kind of jobs, and had no new plan to improve her chances of success. She was despondent about her financial problems, feared losing custody of her daughter, and admitted to depression.

Nolan was 17 when the car he was riding in got wrapped around a tree. In many ways, his old life had been ideal: Socially popular, a star athlete with pro prospects, he was so stylish, tall, handsome, and well built that he had been accepted to train at a famous modeling agency. His parents participated in his therapy, but father was focused on his sports career and mother was very permissive. In therapy, Nolan was cocky. He expected to recover completely and saw no reason to learn to compensate for anything. On this basis, he did not take the feedback seriously, and did homework only when his mother helped him with it. He almost flunked out of the program, graduating only with the pressure of an emergency family meeting. At school, his family got a homebound teacher permanently assigned to teach him all of his academic subjects, against medical advice. Later he reported that this teacher had fallen victim to his charming ways, and had given him test answers and gifted him with high grades for little work. He intended to rejoin his school team, but after going to one practice, he found playing so painful that he gave up sports. He visited the modeling agency, but they didn't welcome him back with the enthusiasm he expected, so he gave up modeling. After high school, he lived with his parents and worked part-time in his father's store. Four years later, he tried community college. Undisciplined after his free ride in high school, he failed remedial courses in his first semester. After using his full rehab strategies at the urging of a new girlfriend, he got a high-B average. However, an ugly confrontation by a harsh professor convinced him to drop out. His father then arranged with a family friend to train Nolan as a building inspector. He completed a grueling week-long training course and exam, and started as apprenticeship. However, after criticism for mistakes and poor productivity, he got fed up and quit. He went back to his father's restaurant. Nolan remained in contact with a few of his old friends, continuing to smoke marijuana with them. He participated sporadically in a therapy group, but quit therapy after the group confronted him about giving up so easily. At 6 years post, he moved to Thailand to live with his new girlfriend and her wealthy parents, but he soon returned to the states and his dad's shop. He is still living at home at 11 years post-onset and working for his father.

What went wrong in these 15 recoveries? First, their effort was limited. Only Thomas and Delta worked hard in any therapy sessions, and only Tom followed up well with homework assignments. Brady dropped out of therapy against medical advice. In addition, they did not seem to bond with other trainees, nor did they take pride in their program accomplishments. Brady acted aloof, as if he were already a sports star. Kenny came across angry and alienated, rebuffing others' suggestions and help by announcing that he didn't care what they thought. Todd and Kristi all came from low-achieving backgrounds, and none of them expected to succeed in therapy. Nolan wanted attention for being cute and charming, but not for recovery. A therapeutic community program does not work for people who feel too good for it, or those who feel it is too good for them. For both types, even massive feedback rolls off their backs.

Eight of the 15 cases (Jeb, Brady, Matt, Todd, Denzel, Kenny, Louis, and Thomas) had right posterior contusions. They did not process feedback normally, and their self-image was locked onto a picture of the old self. Flooding them with feedback simply gave them a bad attitude toward treatment and their therapists, while they continued to believe in their own "big picture." Right posterior focal injury is associated with poor progress in all kinds of rehab (Schutz, 2005a). It destroys the effectiveness of education-based therapy, although the latest versions of the program found some success with several patients who had this injury.

Substance abuse was ongoing in seven of the recoveries. Matt resumed alcoholic drinking and multidrug abuse. Delta became a daily, heavy drug user. Kristi and Chuy continued to get drunk. Nolan and Manny also used drugs and drank to excess, though how often was not clear. Individuals with a history of addiction do not do well in rehabilitation programs in general (Gronwall, Wrightson, & Waddell, 1990), and the negative effect of substance use on recovery was discussed in the last chapter. A history of drug use creates a pattern of handling problems by escaping into intoxication rather than by coping (Carver & Scheier, 1994). That urge to escape can become even stronger after a head injury. The best illustration in the author's clinical series comes from an executive chef at a gourmet restaurant who had lost his sense of smell and taste in his accident. Desperate for any option to stay in his profession, he was delighted when a distinguished authority on Soviet rehab techniques offered to consult with the treatment team, and felt optimistic that it would be possible for him to return to his career. However, his 6-year habit of smoking high-grade marijuana on a daily basis had been interrupted by his injury. He planned a holiday visit with drug-using friends, and was warned that he faced testing when he came back and would be expelled if he tested positive. He never returned, passing up his only chance to get his career back. Getting high proved to be more important to him than recovery.

Here is another way to look at the problem. Recovery requires tolerating an immense amount of distress and pain, forcing the search for the damaged self and wrecked life and then keeping them always in plain sight without flinching or turning away. At the same time, the person cannot give in to pessimism, hopelessness, or frustration while learning how to beat back the deficits. Building a new career or relationship takes humility (to find a proper match), patience, and a feeling of urgency to repair the mistakes made along the way. Facing these threats and challenges squarely takes character. Workplace behavior can be retooled so that it does not break social rules only by a person of strong character. Other features of good character are also needed, such as holding back impulses, delaying gratification, and resisting the temptation of urges and easy ways out (McCall, 1975; Shapiro, 2000). Adolescents or young adults who were neglected, indulged, spoiled, allowed to get high, or asked to shoulder little responsibility as children often do not develop the character needed to meet these requirements. Good outcomes tend to be reserved for the families that require responsible conduct (Schutz & Lewis, 1985).

The 15 cases reported in the next 13 chapters represent the opposite end of the spectrum: Their progress exceeded expectations. In the most important respects, they returned to functioning at their preinjury levels.

PART II

Great Recoveries as Individual Efforts

Chapter 4

The Story of Riley

When Riley was in the hospital, a good recovery seemed unlikely. He was a middle-aged, blue collar man with a history of hard partying on multiple substances. He had essentially no family support. His injury left him with severe disabilities of physical, cognitive, and language function. Most people injured at his age are crippled and remain crippled for life, opting for disability benefits and a handicapped existence. The direction that Riley chose instead, and the things he has accomplished in the process, are not just unexpected but unprecedented.

1. The Old Riley

"I first entered the work force when I was 15 years old. I did this because my older brother moved on after my father passed away, leaving my younger brother and myself with my mother. I came from a very large, poverty-line family in Louisville; my parents never even owned an automobile. I hated being poor and going to school wearing the same clothes every day. Most of my family didn't make much of themselves, but I was determined to better myself. I worked after high school for two years, until I graduated, when I got a job in a factory. After one year of college, I became a construction laborer and stayed with that company for six years. Even then, I had an uncanny ability to recognize knowledgeable people and learn from them. My supervisor was willing to teach me about the business, and I made it a point to learn as much as I could from him. It paid off for me—three years later I was the assistant superintendent, and later I moved up to construction supervisor. Then I went into business for myself, mainly as a carpenter contractor, though I also built a few houses. I always had between 10 and 20 helpers working for me. I took good care of them, and I didn't put up with any backtalk from them. If I needed to, I could whip any of them.

"When I was a teenager, my mom lived in a shack—I helped her get a mobile home. When I was 23 years old, with the help of a couple of my brothers, I built my mom a new house free of charge. In the mid-1980s I married a lady who had a child. I raised her son as my own.

"I was an independent contractor for 12 years. As a small businessman, I ended up doing pretty well financially. After work, I was a hard-drinker who made the rounds of the local bars and got involved with recreational drugs. I was in shape, I looked good, I had money to spend, and I had plenty of women. I thought of myself as a self-made man and a success. That was important to me. Then I made a big mistake and lost my business, and it took me more than a year to get it back. And it was at that time that I developed my self-discipline, which helped me with my recovery. I restarted my business, and had it going well for about a year and a half when I got in the accident."

2. The Accident—13 Years Ago

"Coming home from a bar just before midnight on December 17th of 1994, my car was hit head-on by a drunk driver in a speeding Geo Metro. My friend was driving. He ran from the scene and disappeared. I guess he didn't want to get questioned about the accident. I remember nothing about the accident, of course."

3. The Injury

He had large contusions in the left temporal, parietal, and frontal lobes, each associated with hemorrhage and swelling. He came out of coma with right hemiparesis, extreme weakness of the right side of his body, including both his arm and leg. This symptom appeared to be the result of brainstem damage. While in the hospital, he was confined to a wheelchair, and his arm was limp and had to be kept in a sling across his chest. His diffuse injury was associated with 2 to 3 days of coma and 7 days of post-traumatic amnesia.

4. Early Recovery

"It's amazing the mind games we play with ourselves when we're in the hospital. After I woke up, I said to the nurses that I had to get out of there—I had to put through my payroll. The nurse said, 'You can't do that—your brain's broken!' At that point, I was determined to get out of the hospital as quickly as I could. After a while, I realized that my leg wasn't working, and I knew I couldn't go back to work like that. I wasn't ready to accept that my body was half-broken, that I would have to live my life as a physically disabled person. But I remember a couple of nurses coming into my room to talk with me, and asking what I did for a living. When I told them, they said, 'You'll have to find something else to do.' I guess I accepted my condition to an extent, because I said to them, 'I want to go back to school.' That was something I'd always thought it would have been good to finish, so I decided to do it now. In one side of my mind, I realized that there was a good chance I'd be paralyzed for the rest of my life, and I needed a new career. My right side is still partially paralyzed and remains weak. Still, I keep hoping that one day my body might start functioning again if I keep pushing. I know it's never supposed to happen, but I still haven't lost hope altogether.

"When I got out of the hospital, I had to move in with my brother and his wife. I stayed with them because I had been told that I needed somebody to keep an eye on me for awhile. They took advantage of me, taking my disability checks and keeping most of the money for themselves. I knew what they were up to. For awhile it was a choice between putting up with my brother stealing my checks or living at the Salvation Army, so I put up with it. Then I literally started planning my escape. I had kept my old apartment. I called Social Services and got them to pay my rent with the agreement that I would repay them when my Social Security officially kicked in. I arranged transportation to get down to the Social Services office. Finally I finished making all the arrangements, for the power to be turned on and everything, and I moved back to my own place. For the next 6 months I rode the city bus to everywhere I needed to go until I got approved to drive again.

"I have to live by self-conducted therapy. I had to teach myself to do even the basic things in life with my left hand. I must eat with silverware in my left hand, and bathe, dress myself, and even write and type with only my left hand. Going to the grocery store was hard —I could hardly use my right arm at the time. I had to buy small amounts of food—only what I could carry in my left hand. Going to the laundromat was hard for the same reason. Bathing required me to make some adjustments—I fell down in the shower a number of times. When I had to wash my leg, I had to find a new way to do it. I ended up sitting down to wash it. Since then, I've learned a way to do it standing up. As far as washing my back, I found a brush that would reach back there. I had some digestive trouble. I had to experiment with my diet and that's when I started exercising. I didn't bug people for help. I asked so many questions anyway.

"As far as cooking, I've always been a pretty good chef. But the dishes were a problem. I don't like dishwashers. I had to learn how to wash dishes in a different way—I don't believe my therapists gave me any help with that one. I had to do the dishes four or five times a day instead of once a day. It was physically difficult enough that I needed to stagger it out. Getting dressed—I had to learn how to do things in a totally different order. I put my socks on first, now, sitting down, and then I put my pants on. I have to lay down to button my pants up. I have to be careful to tie my shoes tight as a drum because I don't want them to come untied while I'm out doing something. When I tie the shoe on my bad leg, I have to either lean into a corner or sit down— that's why I don't like to have to do it out in public—it's embarrassing.

"I had to become more of an organized person. I had to make cleaning a part of my daily life. That's not a manly thing to do, according to how I was raised, and being a construction worker that's almost unacceptable. When I was younger, I kept my place clean, but I'd clean up everything on a particular day. Now when I leave for school I put the stopper in the tub, fill it with bleach, and let it sit through the day. I've learned a lot of tricks for cleaning like that. Making my bed—I make sure I set up my bed in the corner, which makes it easier to make the bed. Taking out the trash—I always make sure I have trash bags that tie shut. The last 5 years, I don't think I've ever made a trip just to go to the dumpster. I always take the trash out when I'm leaving to go somewhere. I kill two ducks with one stone. It just takes being more organized. When I make a trip to the grocery store, it's not uncommon for me to have a trash bag in one hand, and three empty water jugs. I'm always planning ahead, looking at what I need to do. I was never that organized before. My life has definitely changed in that respect."

Riley was wheelchair-bound and completely dependent when he started in the outpatient program. His right arm was completely nonfunctional. His speech was limited and almost unintelligible. He spoke in a soft voice, his pronunciation hampered by dysarthria and expressive aphasia. Even when his words came out unimpaired, many people did not understand him because of his thick Kentucky accent. Because the senior author had trained in Kentucky, he understood Riley's speech better than most. The program's junior neuropsychologist had a similar advantage, having grown up in Kentucky. Riley bonded with these two men after some conversations about the University of Kentucky's basketball team. The depth of fan loyalty to this team is legendary; hence, the bonding was not unexpected. "In the outpatient program I quickly took a liking to (them). I think it had to do with their Kentucky background. I also appreciated that both of them were hard-working. As a hard-working person myself, I respect that in other people. And they both put their heart and soul into helping other people. Anyway, I quickly came to trust them. And the fact they both encouraged me to go back to college, as old as I was and out of school as I was for almost 30 years, it meant a lot to me. [They] taught me to tape record the information I needed to learn. That got me into the habit of tape recording all of my classes, which I still do. When I told my asshole brother that I was going back to college, all he said was, 'You can't write.' I said, 'I'll learn to write with my left hand if I have to.'"

Riley's proposal to go to college seemed unrealistic for a man who worked in construction all of his adult life. The obstacles were formidable. First of all, the aphasia would make it difficult to process the language information on which college education is strongly based. Second, Riley talked like a construction worker, using a kind of grammar and phrasing that is unacceptable in college. Third, his study habits had never been particularly strong, and for many years he had been accustomed to doing things his own way. To develop the style and discipline required for college would be a Herculean task, one at which most blue collar young adults routinely failed. Yet Riley was determined, and he was clearly a hard worker. His potential to achieve this "nearly-impossible dream" would hinge on his insight.

"At first, I couldn't admit the fact that there was a problem with my mind. I thought all that was wrong with me was physical. I didn't realize I had memory problems, comprehension problems, that I was slow in thinking. I had always been willing to make plans, but after the injury I was bad at the planning itself—I didn't think things all the way through to the point where I could get successful outcomes. When [the two neuropsychologists] gave me the results of my testing, I realized that I had cognitive problems. I didn't totally accept it at first, but they kept telling me about them in my therapy sessions, and I listened. Then when I went to Valencia [community college], I could see my cognitive problems affecting me—I wasn't understanding things to their full limits. Of course, I still catch new problems all the time. Last week, I was supposed to do something and I totally forgot what it was. When I realized what I had done, I said to myself, 'Man, you need therapy!' Another rude awakening came when the business school didn't accept me. Actually, they told me that they were going to admit me, but they delayed the acceptance and then told me that I didn't get my paperwork in on time. To me, that was just another reminder that I still had problems."

Stress is a particularly difficult problem for him, not just mentally but physically. "The stutter in my speech increases whenever I am in a stressful situation. When I am under a lot of stress, I also have nervous reactions to loud noise. Those nervous reactions cause the muscles in my arm and leg to tense up, which causes me to lose control of my limbs. When this happens, I limp and my arm becomes clumsy."

Early in rehab, soon after we began discussing the issue of college, Riley asked if we felt he could succeed. We candidly sketched out the long odds, and detailed each of the obstacles he would need to surmount. In his characteristically cautious decision-making style, Riley announced that he would need to think about it.

"One day I reached a turning point. While talking to the social worker, she asked me about my past. So I just decided to tell her the truth. I told her about drinking too much, and about trouble I had gotten into, and every other thing that was screwed up about my life. Her eyes got real big and she swallowed hard—I think she was shocked at the problems in my past. Once I said it, I thought about it myself, and realized that I hadn't done such a good job of living my life after all. And I got determined to make a new start for myself, and to do things right this time. I decided that my best chance was to put my life in the hands of my therapists, so I did."

We agreed to decide about his prospects for college based on how well he did in the program. If he met all of our therapy challenges at a high level, he would receive our endorsement for higher education. Some of the program's most difficult therapy tasks were included in the preacademic protocol. "The compensation strategies include me needing to remember to write things down or tape record anything I need to remember." Riley gradually mastered the disciplines he needed, and graduated with our recommendation for college.

5. Accomplishments of Recovery

"Going back to school at community college 8 months after my injury was hard. I was a scared puppy—I didn't know if I'd be able to handle it or not. Being around all those young people, and being on a cane for a period of time—it was a big adjustment for me. The first semester it was hard to even get myself to go to class each time. I felt like I stood out like a sore thumb. I was ashamed of myself. At that time I could hardly talk—I didn't talk well at all. I was crippled. I felt like I didn't belong in college.

"As far as schoolwork, I had good preparation being taught proper study skills in therapy, though it was hard tying the things I had learned in therapy into the educational world. I tape recorded all the classes and made good notes. In that class I had to give one or two speeches. That was difficult. I think I did a pretty good job. I was ashamed that my speech was bad. I hated standing in front of the class where everybody could see the crippled guy. I gave a lot of presentations over my years in college, and I've gotten used to it gradually, to where I no longer feel intimidated. Last semester I gave an excellent presentation in my behavior management class—everyone commented on how excellent it was—and it was! People might say—what's the big friggin' deal about giving a speech. But I was a construction worker, and giving a speech at college is like going from one extreme to the other.

"Most of my life, my way of balancing my checkbook was to make sure I deposited more than I spent. That was it. I intended to keep my checkbook up to date afterward. At first, I forgot to write down a lot of checks. I worked at remembering to write them down and got very motivated. It took me a couple of years before I had made myself consistent at it—I'd get it straightened out, turn my attention to something else, and the checkbook would slip up again. Finally I got on top of it.

"When I first got home from my injury, I wanted to get back to jogging—I used to be a pretty good runner. I was still on the cane, so

I started out by walking. A quarter mile, up to a half mile. I got off the cane. Then I was able to do a little jogging. I would not be denied. I went into an exercise room in my apartment complex, I did about 400–500 sit-ups a day. I still do, but they're good sit-ups now. I'd work out on the machines, and that's helped my jogging a lot. It's stabilized and improved my control of my upper body.

"I'd say I fell down while jogging about 10 times over the years—the last time was 6 months ago. I'd just get up and keep jogging. One thing that helps me is my not wanting to admit I'm disabled—that's why I keep pushing myself. Jogging is difficult what with my being hemiparetic. It's painful, because I use my muscles and bones in a way they're not designed to be used. The muscles on the inside of my leg are weaker than the ones on the outside of my leg. I run with my foot turned out, which gives me better control of my leg. It's hard to swing my leg—I have to throw my leg forward each time by swiveling my hip. Then I lock my knee. The foot lands heel first, and the side of the foot, and it rolls forward to the ball of my foot. When I try to jog with my foot normally prone, I drag my toe. Because I run that way to compensate for my right side, it makes my left side hurt from overuse. It's frustrating to put myself through so much pain and still run so slow. I handle the frustration by keeping my mind on my accomplishments. That's how I've been able to run 14 miles. My long-term goal is to run a 26-mile marathon. My short-term goal is a half marathon in 2½ hours. To meet my goals, I've become very careful about what I eat so I can lose weight. I've learned to be a patient guy to deal with my problems —I've learned to appreciate small gains. How I motivate myself—if I can get myself through a 26-mile marathon, there's nothing I can't do.

"When I got my BA, I thought I would go on to get my MBA. And that didn't work out—the local university with a graduate school of business didn't accept me, though they said it was because I sent in my application too late. But I didn't do anything for a year and a half."

While going to university in another region, Riley telephoned regularly. Once or twice a year, he related a current problem and asked for advice. He always put the advice to use, and reported back on what he had done in the next phone call. When told about the start-up of a new post-program support group, he joined it, driving 70 miles each way 1 day per week. He soon presented his plan to go to graduate school and study for his MBA. The group questioned this plan, since he had not gotten a job with his bachelor's degree in business. "I realized that going into the business area, which was what

I had always done and always expected to do, maybe wasn't the right direction for me. I talked to a counselor at my school and she recommended speech therapy. I brought that up with the group, and they encouraged me to go ahead with it. So I enrolled at a nearby university in the speech department and after one semester transferred to a university with a program in speech therapy to get a second bachelor's degree.

"My neuropsychologist warned me that to be a speech therapist I'd have to finish fixing my own speech impairment. I knew that my speech had been pretty bad before, and that I'd made a lot of progress with it, but I really didn't realize that it was still a problem. He told me to listen to myself on a tape recorder, and I had to agree. Since then, I've been working on slowing down, because I pronounce words much more clearly when I go slower. I try to get myself well prepared to speak clearly before I start talking. That strategy has made a big difference.

"Here's how I've done grade-wise. At the community college, I was on the Dean's list, and got a 3.7 overall. At my first university, 3.2. At my second school I went for one semester and got a 3.5. After four semesters at my present university I have a 3.9. The former department chair told me that I'm a shoe-in for grad school—I can get into any school I want.

"I volunteered to help out in a program for autistic kids to earn credits to join a speech organization. After I had earned the credit, the doctor who ran the program asked me to keep doing it. After I had done it a few more times, I saw that the kids were getting some help from what I was doing. I kept them in line more than the other volunteers, but they also seemed to love me—like I was their daddy—after a while. I guess I look at people differently, now. I know what it means to be hurt. That makes me sensitive to people in a new way.

"After my injury I was a moderate drinker, and thought that was OK. Eventually, after a discussion of my support group on the negative impact of alcohol, I realized that it was affecting me—make me function at less than my best. I finally realized that this stuff has got to go—if I want a full recovery, it has to go. Once I saw how I functioned without it, I had no desire to ever have any more of it.

"In the group, my neuropsychologist explained to me that my injury has given me a tendency to get overly suspicious. It's a problem that people with left parietal injuries get—what people are saying doesn't make sense, it doesn't add up, so you come up with your own suspicions about why. I'm learning to recognize that I do this, and how to correct my thoughts. It could create problems for me if I didn't fix it, so I'm going to fix it.

"One thing I haven't succeeded in yet—(I'm) not in a relationship. I lead a lonely life. It's frustrating to know I can do something yet not as yet have succeeded in it. I know I have to succeed in it to better my recovery. It's a part of a successful recovery. What makes it more difficult to have relationships when you have an injury is trying too hard. I keep thinking, why would somebody want me? I know that I look different than other people do, which makes it hard to feel any confidence in my ability to establish a relationship. I'm learning to change my thinking on that—I'll have to do that if I'm going to find the right person."

6. Methods of Recovery

"The way to recover—hard work is at the top of the list. I've always been an extremely motivated person, and I'm very motivated now. After I had my problems, I became capable of a fine-tuned kind of dedication. Also, I try to compete with my peers whenever I can. I'm driven by my desire to overcome my impairments and limitations, by my desire to be a complete person again. It comes down to being tough-motivated, strong, disciplined, accept small steps in your recovery. When you fall, literally or figuratively, get your ass back up and go again. Learn from your mistakes. Accept advice of people who know what they're talking about, and use it.

"You have to learn to do things the best that you can do them, which involves doing them a different way. You have to be willing to try new methods of doing everything until you find a method that fits you. Every day, I realize there is room for improvement in my methods—a better way of doing things. Every time I take notes off of the tape player, I think there must be a better way to write an outline that summarizes the notes more effectively, better organized. I'm always looking for new ways to get enough rest and to eat properly to help my jogging. In dealing with other people, I always try to communicate better, for example, to make sure I don't talk without thinking about what I'm going to say first. I always try to copy others who communicate well. I've turned into a perfectionist—before my injury I was a perfectionist about my work, and I had a good reputation because of it. But I didn't worry about how I did anything else. Now I'm a perfectionist across the board. Every day in my drive home from school, and when I'm jogging, I review my life, and see what I've done well and what I need to do better. I come upon a lot of things I want to improve on. I even do it at home, when I'm walking around the house. I find this way works better than writing down my plans and self-evaluations. When I get negative feedback, I make myself realize that some people are trying to help me and I use it as motivation to work on myself.

"I'm extremely picky about how well I do in my schoolwork. Some of the other students have begun to copy me by taping their classes. I laugh at them—taping is just one tenth of it. It's what you do with the tape. You can't just play it back. I make an outline of the notes I take off of it. I perfected the process of taking notes. It amazes me how quickly I can do it now. It took me 4–5 hours a 1-hour tape. Now it takes me 2 hours. When the other students see my notes, they freak out. They don't expect an old guy like me to have such carefully prepared notes.

"I've learned to take more time to think about what I'm going to do before taking any action. I inspect and review my plans to make sure they're adequate."

Asked about dealing with his emotions, Riley reported, "I had a real hard time controlling them for a long time. I worked at improving it and I am getting better at it. There are several reasons why I'm working to improve my control. First of all, I have to do it to get a complete recovery. It makes me a better person to be able to talk to people without losing control of my emotions. It's not a manly thing to do to lose control of your emotions. It's a sign of weakness, and I'm not willing to be weak. When I get emotional, my thinking is not as good. A lot of times, I make decisions that aren't in my best interest in the long term—I pacify my desires. If I control my emotions, I make myself do what's in my best interest. It's a part of doing the right thing.

"I think God has a plan for me. Maybe that's why I had the accident. Look at the way I used to live my life—drinking and driving. I drove 225 miles to Miami in 2½ hours. I used to get plastered and drive. Isn't it ironic that I got injured as a passenger in a car, and it changed my life. Maybe God said, you're living wrong and I'll get you straightened out.

"If I finish grad school and run a marathon, those will be the ultimate accomplishments for a head-injured person. I want to show the world what I can do. In my mind, I want to show my brother—even though I'm disabled, I'm a lot better man than you. I can do things you could never do!

"Generally speaking, I'm pretty damn happy these days. Still things I'm not happy about, relationships being one. I realize what I've accomplished, and I see successes each and every day. I have a long-term goal I'm reaching. Now I'm getting myself to give myself credit for the things I've done. I think of myself as a lucky son of a bitch—lucky to be alive!"

The Neuropsychological Perspective

Riley was admitted to the trauma center at Glasgow Coma Scale level 3. His acute CT scan showed left frontal, temporal, and parietal contusions with edema, and some transtentorial herniation. He underwent intake testing for the cognitive rehabilitation program 7 to 8 weeks post-onset. He was a pleasant and cooperative subject, although difficult to understand due to his pronounced dysarthria.

Focal attention and working memory were within normal limits, indicating that he was admitted to the outpatient level at a time when he was capable of participating adequately in the program. Executive deficits were quite prominent in his test protocol, including difficulty in learning to break old habits, a very strong tendency to repeat incorrect responses, and a strong tendency to rush and consequently to overlook targets. His scores on measures sensitive to dysexecutive syndrome (mazes and word fluency) were severely to profoundly impaired. He showed surprisingly strong performance when asked to learn verbal passages, with normal performance in the immediate condition and mildly impaired performance in the delay condition. Word-list learning was mildly to moderately impaired in both the immediate and the delay conditions, with impaired accuracy of recall increasing the functional impact of his memory disorder. For nonverbal information, his immediate and delayed recall of simple material was borderline, while for complex information he performed at the severely impaired level. Most of the measures of processing speed were severely impaired. His poorest scores, on the most complex, problem-solving measures, were depressed deep into the profound range of impairment. In addition, his access to verbal information from his general fund of knowledge and for word meanings was moderately impaired. Reading comprehension was profoundly impaired for accuracy, essentially at the random guess level, as well as markedly impaired for processing speed. Hence his language and academic skill limitations presented direct obstacles to his intention to pursue a college education. Psychological testing indicated additional obstacles, including extreme acute stress and psychological overload, with evidence of affective lability and depression.

Riley made slow progress through a high-intensity program, receiving extended regimens of traditional speech, occupational, and physical therapies as well as a full cognitive rehabilitation program. No matter how much he might have been suffering internally, he remained affable, cooperative, and motivated for recovery. He was usually willing to accept suggestions of compensation strategies, although he was susceptible to withdrawal of cooperation when he felt that his therapists were condescending or manipulative. However, he was willing to discuss these concerns with his neuropsychologists, and consistently accepted their encouragement to make the best personal use possible of these therapies even when he disliked the therapist's interpersonal style. It was extremely important to allow Riley to save face, as his pride was easily wounded by excessively harsh criticism or sarcasm. Because his overall attitude toward the program remained positive, he was able to make steady progress.

Riley remained in contact with his two neuropsychologists for several years, and enthusiastically joined a post-rehabilitation group they started together as well as the task force for the development of GiveBack. He often sought advice to deal with problem situations, and always reported later on that he had either tried it out or adapted it to his purposes. Although such extended contact is not a normal part of the rehabilitation protocol, and can sometimes indicate unhealthy dependency, in this case his excellent outcome argues in favor of the support.

Chapter 5

The Story of Hillary

Hillary hated being told what to do. She always did things her own way, and managed to succeed in everything she did. Her self-determined style was obvious even when she was a hospital patient. She entered the program cracking jokes and voicing a cocky confidence that she was fully recovered. Because of her strong independent streak, she despised the directiveness of the cognitive program. She fought the insights and instructions every step of the way. And when she graduated, she wanted nothing more than to forget the program and move on with her life. But instead she used everything she was taught, and built a remarkable recovery.

1. The Old Hillary

"I grew up in a large, close-knit family—six girls and four boys and we're all still best friends. That background made me a strong person. In my family, if you want something, you have to do it yourself—no one is going to carry you along. I was eighth in line and whatever they did I wanted to do. I beat every one of them in sports. I liked to win. It's a power thing, I guess. I was the strong-willed one. I paid every penny for my own college education. My dad figured if I wanted an education, it should be up to me. I think that's a good child-rearing approach.

"I always believed in trying your hardest, and if you don't make it, you regroup and find another way. The first time I tried out for basketball I didn't make the team. And I was determined to figure out what to do to make the team the next year. And I did. If plan A doesn't work you just have to make plan B. And to make plan B, you have to figure out what went wrong with plan A.

"I got my bachelor's degree in health education. My competition sport was racquetball. I gave some lessons, and taught the sport at Valencia. I was a driven player, ranked in the top 10 in Florida. I worked for awhile in the wellness centers at two local hospitals as an exercise physiologist. When I had the accident, I was in college working on my MA in health education. At that time, my mother was succumbing to terminal cancer."

2. The Accident—16 Years Ago

"I was coming down a hill, and at the bottom, the road exited out to a four-lane road. I'm sure I was going real fast, faster than I probably should have. According to a witness, my front wheel hit a curb, which threw me straight forward over the handlebars and I hit the pavement head first. I tried to get back up on my bike, and that was when I had a seizure. Then the paramedics showed up and took me to the hospital."

3. The Injury

Hillary hit her head in the left frontotemporal area and suffered a contusion and a hematoma at the site of the impact. Her brain rebounded inside her skull, producing a hematoma on the opposite side in the right parietal area. She remained in coma for 11 days, and had post-traumatic amnesia of 3 weeks. "They told my parents that I was going to die. Then they said I would be a vegetable. They said I would never walk again."

4. Early Recovery

When she reached inpatient rehab, Hillary was very impaired in her communication skills. "I remember that I couldn't name a tennis racquet. I couldn't name a violin or a unicorn. And I knew what they were, and it killed me." She was impatient to work through her physical disabilities, and did so quickly. By the time she got to outpatient therapy, she was walking unassisted and demanding to go home.

Outpatient therapy was an even greater annoyance. "It bugged me that I couldn't drive. I had to ride in a van, which meant following a transportation schedule. I didn't want to be there in the first place, and they made me wait to get a ride." Hillary was a strong-willed, outspoken patient who wanted nothing to do with outpatient rehab. "Leave me alone—I'm fine." Her cognitive progress was also striking. She tried to use this fact to argue that she had no cognitive deficits at all. Then she protested, "I'm going to get better. Let me do it on my own." "I insisted that I absolutely would not go through rehab under any circumstances. I was perfectly fine. Finally I agreed to do the evaluation, but there was no way I would go into the program." After considerable discussion, she relented and agreed to start the program under protest.

Even though she ended up receiving almost 6 months of therapy, Hillary was always ready to argue that she should be released today. Slowly—and grudgingly—she admitted her cognitive deficits one by one. A fellow patient, an arrogant, boastful teenage athlete (Brady, see Chapter Three) "insisted he was fine and wasn't willing to listen to anyone. He was more stubborn than I was. I didn't want to be like him, so I guess that helped me to look at my problems. I came to accept that the injury had made me very impulsive. I didn't think ahead, didn't look at the whole picture, bit off more than I could chew. I didn't process everything I saw. So I'd say, 'All right, I'm impaired. Now hurry up and teach me what I need to learn—let's go!' A lot of times the therapy in the groups seemed too easy to me. I'd say, 'I'm so much better than anyone else, I don't need it.' But then they'd ask you to teach somebody else, and that was when you'd really learn it. When you can teach it, that's when you really know it. Towards the end I realized that it had been good for me to be there. People have to get to that point, where they value what they learned and plan to keep it in mind after they get home." She performed well in her outpatient program, and the team agreed that she was ready to go back to college.

5. Accomplishments of Recovery

After finishing her last semester with a 4.0, she received her BA degree from the university with a major in physical education. She had planned on to graduate school in PE, but she had a change of heart: "I wanted to help out other people with the head injuries. I tried to get into OT master's program—Holy cannoli—that was way more than I could chew. While I was waiting to hear if they accepted me, I took some classes that were prereqs. I was able to handle the classes, but they wouldn't let me in [to grad school]. Then I came back to Orlando and started working at the Wellness Center again. I knew the job, but it was a challenge to try to get along with some of my coworkers—I have a temper. It worked out well, though. I made Employee of the Year for the corporate division. I was there for 10 years before I finally left.

"I met my husband there. I've been married for almost 9 years. Marriages work—though it's taken hard work. My approach to being a wife—give 100%. I was ready for a relationship. And he loved my dog and loves his kids. We have a boy and a girl, ages 7 and 4.

"I got back into racquetball and won my first tournament. I practiced a lot first because I wanted to make sure I was really ready. I didn't want to be impulsive. I have a new attitude toward the game: I play the game because I like it. That's how I win—by enjoying myself. That's a change for me.

"After 10 years at the Wellness Center, I got fed up with the benefits. We had been doing personal training for teachers and principals, and a principal kept encouraging me to come and work for her. At that point, she had a position open for a health and fitness teacher. I asked my friends in the teaching business, and they all said, 'Don't take it!' There were a lot of problems at that school. But I was impulsive on that decision: I took the job, and I really struggled. There was no teacher training, and no one was willing to help me get my bearings. It was the other way around—teachers dropping my kids off early, picking them up late, loading me up with two or three classes at a time. The classes were huge. I said, 'I'm a tough person. I can tough it out.' I had headaches every day. I hated it. Hate is a strong word. I was determined not to quit on the principal, so I worked out the year. Through a friend, I found out about a job opening at my current middle school—a great job at a great school. I was hired as a health teacher—personal fitness and life skills. I was careful about everything I did, because I wanted the job to work out. I made up all my own curriculum. We've taken the initiative to start some new programs: Wellness Wednesdays—no junk food, a hydration program, a Make-Your-Own-Smoothie program—teaching them how to build a healthy drink that tastes great.

"Teaching these kids the right lessons about how to live their lives is important to me. I pass along to them the lessons I've learned in my recovery, without telling them where I learned them—be prepared for anything, do your best, learn from your mistakes to improve yourself, don't let anybody discourage you. Sometimes you can get it across to the whole class all at one time, sometimes it has to be one-to-one to a particular kid. I also have an unusually well-behaved class, at least that's what the substitute teachers all tell me. We have a system in my class. Mess up one time, I say, 'Don't do that again.' Everybody needs a second chance. The second time, they see the look on my face, and they don't want to do it a third time, because there are consequences the third time. You have to have a system like that for kids this age—they'll behave only if they know what to expect. Tough? Yeah, I guess I'm tough when I need to be, but only when I need to be. I think it's working out well for me. My goal is to get chosen as the Teacher of the Year. I've heard that the principal is telling some people I might get it this year.

"I did Toastmasters recently. I was a guest twice and won the impromptu speaking both times. I had to think and make a plan—open with something—anything—to catch their attention, then close it, and don't talk too fast. I still talk too fast sometimes, don't I?"

After graduating from rehab, Hillary never returned or called for any additional help or guidance. She did return at our request to give an inspirational presentation to other patients who were in the program. She also offered to help in the development of GiveBack. It has always seemed one of her top priorities to do as much for herself as possible, including in her recovery.

6. Methods of Recovery

Hillary is reluctant to make a big deal out of her recovery. Like the others with exceptional recoveries, it took encouragement to get her to detail her accomplishments. She also began with understatement when I asked her how hard it was for her to recover. "How hard was it? I was glad to be alive. It was a challenge. I have to try harder than ordinary people to get everything done correctly, to be aware of myself and my actions. I have to have higher standards than other people do."

Is there anything you've ever done that was harder? "No. It was the hardest thing to do. It's not like you finish a race and you're done. You're never done. You can't say, ' I've conquered this.' You conquer it as you go.

"The motivation came naturally—I like challenges. I think I learned to be compulsive about thinking ahead—I was always a person who planned ahead, and I just had to do it more carefully. My memory would be a problem for me now if I let it, but I use my methods of organization to handle it. For example, I have to memorize the names of 150 new kids twice a year. But I have ways to help myself do that. I have assigned seats—that helps me remember their names. And when they run the mile, I record every lap. I have their name and number on a sheet, and when I see them cross the line I look up the number, and doing that over and over again helps me to learn the name. Memory is only a problem for me when I have too much going on at one time. Then I get bombarded and forget things. If I have time, I write down the things I will need to remember—I write them ALL down— I'll always do that. When I get too many little sheets of paper I stick them on a big sheet of paper. Organization. Sometimes my husband helps out in organizing who does what for which kid, and who does what chores around the house. Teaching has tested my organizational skills and it comes naturally to me. now. I built my organizational skills because I was aware of (having deficits in) them. You have to be aware of the deficit. You have to admit the areas of your deficiency or you can't get better.

"There are some deficits I still don't like to admit to myself, like impulsivity. I keep that one in the back of my mind. If people say something to me about my having done something impulsive, I take a look at it and fix it. I've learned to be careful about what I say—to the kids, the parents, my coworkers. In my business you have to think about what you're going to say. In marriage, that's important, too. It's become a habit to keep my guard up all the time. And sometimes I don't show my feelings. I come across real serious, and don't look excited even when I feel that way. My coworkers will kid me, 'You DO laugh!'"

Hillary offers this advice to survivors: "Nobody can recover well unless they learn where the damage is. They don't need to know the big words (to diagnose the lesions), but they have to know what they need to control. You make a plan for how you're going to do that, and a backup plan, and a backup plan for that. How can you be sure to be aware of everything, how can you know how you're making the right moves? If you're married, you can get guidance from your spouse. You can keep working on it and you can get better and better, and it gets easier to do.

"When I was in therapy, I was religious, but not as much as I am now. I had left the Catholic church when I was younger, the only one in my family to do that, and joined the Methodist church. When I discovered that I had survived a near-fatal accident, I figured that it had been God's doing and a part of His plan, and I assumed he saved me because he had a purpose for my life. Was it to get married and be a good wife, to have children, to be a teacher and perhaps touch someone's life? I didn't know what it was, but I figured it was there, and that was an inspiration for me. But as far as asking for God's help, no, I didn't really do that. I expected myself to deal with things, and I did. Now, as I look back on it, I know I had His help, but I wasn't thinking that way at the time. Now I've become much more involved with the church—I teach Sunday school and work with the Fellowship of Christian Athletes."

Asked if she was still the same old Hillary or a new Hillary, she didn't hesitate. "I'm a new Hillary." Then I asked if she could choose to be the old Hillary again, would she. She stopped and thought about this. "I'll be the new Hillary. I'm much more easy going. I'm happy to be able to do whatever I can do, and I wasn't before. I really like the person I am now."

The Journalistic Perspective

Hillary comes across like a "jock" approaching middle age. Her short-cropped hair is starting to fleck with grey. She looks you in the eye and talks tough, with a gravely voice and a direct manner. As the topic got more personal, her speech got "punchy" like a coach giving last minute instructions to his team. When talking about her injury, she stayed with that "tough guy," matter-of-fact demeanor. She made it sound like her injury was an old racquetball foe, one she was determined to outlast. Then at the end of the discussion, her eyes dropped, and she looked up with a sly little smile. The message was, "I hate this injury, but I'll be damned if I'm going to deny my deficits." She gave no other hint that being injured got to her.

The Neuropsychological Perspective

Testing was performed four to five weeks post onset. The most prominent feature of her protocol were profound impairments on the word fluency test and delayed recall for narrative passages, consistent with the maximal left anterior focus of her injury. Her immediate recall for passages was moderately impaired, consistent with her difficulties with attention (discussed below). A severely impaired performance on Woodcock-Johnson Antonyms-Synonyms, as well as a moderately impaired performance on Woodcock-Johnson Analogies, revealed unusual difficulty in accessing her linguistic knowledge base, as performance on these tests is usually well-preserved in TBI (Schutz, Tucci, & Raymond, 1987a). She also evidenced severe impairment on the Visual Search and Attention Test, showing a slowed decision-and-response-execution process that remained at the same level when she was re-tested for driving readiness three months later. Her pattern of performance on Purdue Pegboard also had localizing significance, as she showed moderate impairment on the dominant (right) hand condition, normal-range performance on the nondominant hand condition, but a substantial loss of efficiency in the severe range of impairment for the bimanual condition, this last being a common finding in patients with frontal lobe involvement (Lezak et al., 2004).

Her performance on tests of focal attention and working memory was moderately impaired for even the simpler measure (Digit Span in the forward condition), and remained at this level three months later, with her test behavior indicating a susceptibility to emotional interference that is often seen in subjects who "overstrive" on this procedure. On the more demanding measure (Digit Span in the reversed condition), her score improved from the moderately impaired level on initial testing to the normal level three months later. These scores are interpreted as indicating that she was not fully ready for cognitive rehabilitation due to residual acute attentional impairment at the time of admission, although she was able to participate in the program through effortful concentration.

Even at this early point in her recovery, Hillary demonstrated surprising strength on the most challenging tests, the Category Test and Tactual Performance Test. On the former, her score was at the borderline level. On the latter, she was moderately impaired on the first, dominant hand trial, but improved to within normal limits on the second (nondominant hand) and third (both hands) trials. These tasks, which provide tangible ongoing feedback about the quality of performance, seemed to elicit a strong competitive response which facilitated her processing.

Measures of nonverbal perception and nonverbal learning and recall were areas of strength. These included a measure of perceptual accuracy, the NYU Shape Cancellation test. She also performed just below normal limits on mazes.

Psychological testing employing a measure of premorbid personality designed by the first author (Schutz & Schutz, 1989) found markedly elevated scores in achievement motivation, conscientiousness, interpersonal ascendancy, extraversion, optimistic attitudes, and well-socialized behavior. These scores, which were verified by protocols completed by the subject's father and sister, indicated a strongly favorable prognosis on the basis of her personality traits.

Hillary was an exceptionally difficult patient from whom to gain cooperation or the acknowledgement of insight, and ultimately the "battle" was ceded to her in public. It was assumed that Hillary was learning many things that she did not admit. The most useful format for the training of her higher level skills was to challenge her to design her own confrontation task, and then to self evaluate. Because she had been working as a wellness instructor before her injury, and planned to continue in that vocation as a career, it was agreed that she would simulate a wellness presentation to the high-level cognitive group in her second month of treatment. We had agreed that we and she would regard the quality of her performance as binding evidence of her readiness to complete the program. Here is her written narrative summary of the experience:

"Teaching stress management to the SEI (social-emotional-interpersonal) group helped me learn a lot about myself. I learned that I have to do a lot of planning and organizing in order to go back to teaching again. To prepare myself before the lecture, I designed a pretest to have filled out by the group, so I would be aware of their knowledge about stress before teaching them. That helped me be aware of what ideas needed the most attention. Then, I designed an outline covering all the main ideas of stress management, so my lesson would flow smoothly (the standard strategy for expressive language deficits in this program). I used good eye contact to determine if they didn't understand my concepts (the standard monitoring strategy for pragmatic communication deficit). I also tried to talk slow and make the idea as clear and concise as possible. Because we were very stressed from the beginning of SEI, we practiced some relaxation techniques for the last 5 minutes to let everyone know what it feels like to relieve stress. I gave everyone a post test to see if they understood what I said and for them to recommend what I should do different next time so it would be easier to understand. Everyone did good and gave good feedback. Next time I will use the blackboard so we could make lists of topics as a team and have everyone give examples so everyone gets involved." Hillary was given feedback on the run-on tendency, the slight grammatical errors, the concreteness of thought, and the failure to fully address the topic in this written summary. She also acknowledged that she had spoken too fast and needed better organization, and agreed to continue her treatment. Later, she produced a high-quality, graduate-level paper on executive deficits to earn her graduation.

Chapter 6

The Story of Deloris

Deloris faced a bigger uphill battle than any other patient in this book. Her focal injury was large and situated in a critical area. Her diffuse injury, from anoxia, was profound. Coma from lack of oxygen is more destructive than coma from head trauma. As the oldest patient in the group, she also had to cope with the most limited natural recovery. Her life roles, as an educational professional with a complex, multifaceted job and a parent of teenagers, demanded the high-level cognitive skills that were most impaired. Only an "impeccable" recovery could have met her needs.

1. The Old Deloris

"I grew up in a cohesive community where I knew what was expected of me. There was never a burning feeling that I had to prove myself in order to be accepted. It was a close-knit community in which you had no freedom to misbehave, because everyone knew your family. I was the oldest child of two excellent parents, and my mother was ill during much of my childhood, in and out of the hospital and in and out of bed while my father worked nights, so I had to care for my sister and brother. I grew up quickly, but it was not a burden for me—I just assumed that life worked that way. Learning was always important to me—I have a great respect for knowledge. When I went off to Patterson College, I was humbled by meeting people who were brighter than I was. I earned my BA in education, with a minor in library science.

"I had not planned to be a school librarian. I looked for teaching jobs near my husband's grad school, but the job I was offered involved taking charge of an old-fashioned school library. I brought it up to date, and 3 years later got a highly competitive job as a librarian in an exclusive community. Two years after that, we moved to Florida. After working briefly as a secretary in city government, I started as a school librarian in 1975. Not long after that, I got my MA in library science from USF. I balanced my career with my roles as a wife and mother, and felt good about the way I combined them. In 1990 I snapped up an abandoned computer and converted it into my record-keeping system. At a new job in an elementary school, the principal asked me to take charge of the school's computer program. I became the person who installed and repaired the computers, or if it was complicated, sent them out and tracked the repair jobs. I also installed the software and trained the teachers to use the equipment. Training teachers to use computers is a lot like training little children—you have to deal with them diplomatically."

2. The Accident—12 Years Ago

"November 8th, 1993, was my son's 13th birthday. My year-round school had been on vacation for 2 weeks while my son and husband were busy in their schools, which were on traditional schedules. It was a Monday morning. I walked across the room, suddenly felt a tremendous sense of dizziness, and was told I fell to the floor, though I don't remember falling. For the next month, I have only little snatches of memory. I remember hearing paramedics. I couldn't open my eyes or talk to them, even though I tried to as hard as I could. The next thing I remember is being in the hospital in the ER on a low, flat bed. The doctor insisted that they were going to transport me by helicopter to the trauma center. Then I have a memory of a moment in the helicopter. At this point, I had no idea what was wrong with me. I remember they said that they were going to operate, and I wasn't worried about it.

"My next memory is at the hospital, getting a swallowing test. I remember having a dream and waking up to find myself in a diaper, and I had been incontinent. Next, I recall them telling me that they were moving me to the rehab center. That evening I saw myself in a mirror for the first time. I realized that I had no hair, a series of gashes in my head, and staples. That was when it first occurred to me that something very, very serious had happened, something I needed to investigate."

3. The Injury

"Rod told me what had happened after I was transferred to the inpatient head injury rehab unit. I forgot what he said, but I asked him again a few days later, and he went through it again. The fainting was caused by a subarachnoid aneurysm of the left anterior communicating artery, affecting my left frontal lobe. When they gave me an angiogram they accidentally tore open an artery and I bled to death in the scanner. They were able to resuscitate me, but I remained in a coma for 21 days. I developed hydrocephalus (fluid on the brain) and they did another surgery to install a shunt. That helped me to wake up. It was on the day of this conversation that my continuous memory returned, which was 32 days after my illness began. The neurosurgeon told Rod that I was only alive because I wanted to be—he called me a fighter and said I had a strong will to live."

4. Early Recovery

Considering that Deloris had died in the acute hospital from the accident in radiology, and had a very extensive coma, it was remarkable that she regained the ability to walk and talk within a couple of months. All of the inpatient therapists were encouraged and excited about her recovery. "I was doing OT and PT at the hospital. I had double vision that made it hard to read—that was frightening for me. I am a compulsive reader—a large part of my life revolves around reading. I helped to train a young librarian who had a car accident and was unable to return to work because she had trouble with reading." This was the first time it occurred to her that she might be unable to return to her own job. Her physicians were not expecting her to be able to go back to work; they assumed that she would retire. They were impressed that she continued to talk about going back to work, and for that reason alone, they were willing to continue aggressive therapies beyond the inpatient level. Patients with cognitive deficit with potential to return to work were routinely referred to the outpatient cognitive program. Deloris had done well enough that she was recommended as a candidate. They made a referral to the senior author, who visited her on the inpatient unit and accepted the referral.

"One day they asked me to get on the exercise bicycle and I did maybe 10 minutes on it. I had a visitor, and they guided me to one of the therapy mats to visit with her. When I stood up, for the first time I felt sharp pains, so severe that I couldn't even walk properly. I went straight to bed, stretched out, and the pain went away. The next day I was fine for about an hour, then the pain came back. The more I noticed the pain, the stronger it got. I started mentioning it to the therapists. One of them tried a heat treatment, but that didn't fix it. The next day she brought in a diagram of the muscles of the backside where I was having the problem, but that just increased my agitation and anxiety. The Medical Director gave me muscle relaxers, pain killers, heat and ice treatments, and extra pillows, but the only thing that made me comfortable was stretching out in bed. I got released from inpatient on New Year's Eve." In view of her urgent desire to go back to work, and her readiness to be trained, it seemed appropriate to begin teaching her the basic compensations even before she started her outpatient treatment. In any event, if she was unable to remain seated, it would not be possible to test her or to administer the group treatments that formed the core of the outpatient program. The hospital sessions functioned as a kind of "home school" while she got ready for outpatient.

At this point, she had regained a normal ability to speak. In fact, her conversation sounded intelligent, with well-constructed sentences and the frequent use of big words from her sophisticated vocabulary. When patients regained fluent speech so quickly, the inpatient staff often figured that they were nearly intact cognitively, and this is what they assumed about Deloris. "At that point, I felt fine, except for the pain in my butt, so I had no interest in getting any more rehab. I thought other people obviously needed it more than I did. The therapists mentioned that it would be good for me to get therapy next door with the Cognitive Program when I became an outpatient, but they didn't make it sound particularly urgent. But after meeting with the team, Rod and I agreed that we should give it a try. Rod advised me to go through 2 weeks of testing, and give the treatment a week, and if I wanted to stop at that point he would support me. My backside was very painful during the meeting, but they were optimistic that the pain would subside. I wasn't so sure.

"After I finished the 2 weeks of testing, which I found interesting intellectually, and then we had that meeting with everyone. At that time, I believed that double vision was my only problem other than the pain—that once I could see better everything would coalesce. I remember a test where I was asked to copy a complicated drawing and later reproduce it from memory. It turned out to be much harder to do than I had thought. That gave me a sliver of awareness that there might be something wrong. After the testing was completed, they showed me a chart, and I saw that some of my scores were below average, which meant that I had some problems. The tests said I was having problems with organization, which had always been my bread and butter. But I also realized that I would come out of this OK. The speech therapist said I had gotten the highest reading score she had ever seen at this program. That came as a big relief to me."

When she started in outpatient therapy, her behind was still so painful that it curtailed most of her treatment sessions. She had been able to tolerate inpatient sessions of 20 to 30 minutes pretty well. But the outpatient sessions were a full hour long, and she needed to bail out after a mere 15 to 20 minutes of sitting. "I can remember laying on the couch with Letty [the clinic's office manager], tears streaming down my face. It was in the waiting room. People would come walking in and I would be there crying." She tried to grit her teeth and make it all the way though each therapy, but soon became "distracted, unfocused, and fretful." The treatment team began to wonder if we would be able to do therapy with her at all.

All of the traditional, medical pain control modalities had failed. This sometimes happens with patients who are too tough for their own good, as well as too intellectual, which seemed to be the case here. A much different protocol is needed for patients of this kind. The senior author received permission from the physicians to try this protocol, and then brought it up with Deloris. "He said 'I'm going to give you what you need to get better, but not now.' I had hope, but I felt impatient because I had to wait for my cure. The next time, he gave me some specifics and I put them into practice, and it really worked. I became able to sit through whole sessions, and my pain started to dissipate. Soon I wasn't having any problems with it." The procedure required her to pay attention to her symptoms and her weight bearing pattern, aided by signals from a kitchen timer. She was required to lower herself to a sitting position slowly, rather than to plunk down as was her habit. She remained on this protocol for approximately 6 months.

"My sister was coming for a visit, and he warned me, 'You're going to relapse.' I said I wasn't. He bet me 25 cents that I would." Deloris interrupted the storytelling interview to pull a 5-by-7 gold picture frame out of her purse. "And here is your 25 cents in a frame. Sometimes when I fear that I'm going to overdo, I remember that I can't —because I want to keep your 25 cents." What made Deloris's no-longer-aching butt important was that it reinforced her trust and confidence in her treatment. "His stock went way, way up after that! It also taught me that I had permission to be imperfect. For me, that was like recreating my life! I could leave a note for myself, or put a sign on the door, or put my papers on the floor so as not to forget them. I had permission to do all of this stuff, and make the accommodations I needed to make, and it was OK to do it. I never would have allowed myself such luxuries before."

The new rapport permitted insight training to move forward rapidly, as Deloris began to accept feedback at face value, which is highly unusual in postacute rehab. "In the next week or two it slowly dawned on me—I couldn't deny that my mind was impaired. It took my breath away sometimes, and made me extremely nervous from time to time. I had to acknowledge that there was work that had to be done. I found that I was having memory problems. I was required to play an old video game called Breakout, and I couldn't turn the dial fast enough—there was a disconnect between what I wanted to do and what I could make myself do. When I finally mastered it, that game taught me that there are things I don't do that I can do. To this day, when I come across something I'm wretched at, I say to myself, 'Here comes another Breakout moment—maybe I can master this, too!' A lot of what I was doing was frustrating—highly frustrating. It took awhile for me to realize that I just had to buckle down and get it done."

Once she started accepting insight without any question, Deloris became the model patient. With her compulsive traits and "nerdy" study habits, she made full efforts to learn her compensation strategies, develop, and apply them in doing her homework. She then used them in sessions following all approved methods to the letter, and giving maximum effort and quality control. She moved through the rehab curriculum, mastering every exercise, with astonishing speed. It was as if the aspects of the injury that hold all other patients back had been taken away. Unlike other patients, Deloris was giving rehabilitation "that old college try," with excellent results. She finished her program in 3 months, whereas most patients required 5 months.

5. Accomplishments of Recovery

"The school invited me to a party in my honor held a month before my rehab ended. They presented me with a reclining chair I could use to take my rest breaks. [I took] a rest break after every half-hour of work, at least when I first got back. They made me feel like a queen. They had refreshments, a little skit, every person on the faculty was there at least for a few minutes. My principal came up and said, 'Deloris, we've missed you so much.' He said four computers were not working, so I said, 'Let's look at them right now.' I had to walk almost a quarter of a mile—farther than I had walked since my injury. We got there, he told me what the problem was, I told him what to try, and we did it. Fixed the machine in under a minute. He smiled, I smiled, and in that moment we both knew I'd be OK when I got back. I knew I wouldn't have to worry about working with the computers. I could concentrate on finishing my therapy.

"I was released to go back to work half-time. I needed to make arrangements for transportation, because I was not driving. My principal was very flexible. I arranged for rides to and from work. I made up a kit of the special things I would need to take with me and put it in front of the door at night, so I wouldn't forget to bring it with me when I left in the morning. I took a clock with me that had a 5-minute timer on it to remind me of when to take my 5-minute breaks. I brought a pad to jot down how I was feeling, and how I was breathing—I had discovered that I actually forgot to breathe sometimes when I got into my mind too deeply—and to make notes to myself to remind me of my upcoming chores and my track record for the day—my successes as well as my glitches. During my break, I was also instructed to drink a full glass of water. It was an unusual routine, to say the least, but it worked.

"We had long ago scheduled an in-service for my teachers, and we could not get anyone to help out, so I checked about going back to full-time duty a week ahead of schedule. We set up a plan to make sure it wouldn't overstress me, and it worked out well. A week later, on my wedding anniversary, I transitioned to full time.

"About 18 months after I went back to work, I signed up for an in-service by a nationally recognized behavior modification expert. I took the class, took the exam—200 passed out of the 2000 who took the exam, and I was one of the 200. Two years after that I decided it was time for more mental stimulation, so I signed up for a state course to become a realtor. I had no plan to work as a realtor, but I wanted something I had never done before as a challenge. I took the class and passed the final exam with an 85. That proved to me that I could do it. Three years after that, both my kids were in college studying engineering, and they would come home and talk calculus to one another just to tease Mom. So I enrolled in community college to take a basic math class, and I am currently studying statistics. Next term I will be taking precalculus. I do these things not only to keep my mind sharp, but to prove that I can handle a new challenge.

"Through June of that year, every half hour my alarm went off, the kids left me alone, I went in my office and sat on my chair. I went back to full-time, and did everything I had done before I got sick. When I started the next school year, there were new people. I wondered if I should let them know that they were dealing with a brain-injured person. The first year I told a lot of people. The next year I told a couple of people. After that, the only one I told was my administrator, just so I could let him or her know about the strategies I needed to use to deal with my deficiencies. The second principal was so impressed that he suggested I write it up and send it to the author of *The Seven Habits of Highly Effective People*. My next principal was in awe of my coping strategies. I discovered that explaining my injury doesn't get in the way of my relationships with my supervisors. I don't get and I don't ask for preferential treatment. I told my current assistant principal recently, after working with her for several years, and she told me she had no idea I had any deficiencies. It turns out that they not only respect me for getting the job done, they also realize that for me to do an ordinary job takes more than an ordinary amount of planning and effort.

"A couple of years after my discharge, [I was invited] to come back and talk to the family group. That was extremely profitable for me. I had slipped away from using the technique of writing out my plans, but going back reminded me of how important that had been for me, and I resumed doing them. From day one, it has been my strategy to review my mistakes in my head, so that I can figure out a way to correct them. I think about them, I change what needs to be changed, and I move on. I have to be careful with this strategy, since I can be very self-critical and used to beat myself up mentally for the smallest mistake. Now I am very aware that beating myself up is a thing I should never do, since it only makes it harder for me to cope.

"Three years after I left the hospital I realized I was doing two full-time jobs every day, being a librarian and being a technical computer person, and I wasn't doing either of them as well as I wanted to. There just wasn't time to do them both well. So I approached my principal, and we made some adjustments to make my work flow better. Later I came back and requested that he hire a second person. I chose to stick with the librarian job, although I still try to keep up with computers and help people out with their computer problems when they ask.

"Toward the end, [I saw] an eye doctor out of concern for my field of vision. The doctor said that as long as my eyelids were held up, I was fine—I had a symptom of droopy eyelids called ptosis. That took care of the problem temporarily, but I went back several years later and the problem had gotten worse. The doctor performed eyelid surgery (blepharoplasty) and everything came out fine."

Her self-improvement program goes on as she studies calculus in adult school, math having formerly been her nemesis in school. Most amazing is the change in her personality through the treatment. She realized that she was living a narrow, bland life and simply decided to force herself to open up. Like the others, Deloris didn't stop at fixing her cognitive deficits—she decided that she needed to fix everything in there, in order to make her life all that it could be. She has become a much more multifaceted person, open to her feelings, and willing to share them with other people. Recently she told a dirty joke at a Give-Back meeting. Recovery has many different facets.

6. Methods of Recovery

"In addition to getting permission to be imperfect, my problem with my backside, and the treatment I got for it, taught me to get in touch with my feelings. Before I didn't even use words for feelings. Now I can tell when I get that pain in my backside—somebody has done something to make me angry, or done something I'm uncomfortable with. Now I have full access to it and can deal with it. It makes me much more successful as a human being. And I don't have to dust the furniture every week if I don't want to, and I can be angry with my husband if I want to.

"Before my head injury I was a Christian who did not attend church on a regular basis. During recovery you have to have an enormous faith in something. Mine was myself and God, not necessarily in that order. When I came back to consciousness I felt this warm, soft cocoon wrapped around me. When I think back on it, I think that feeling came from the prayers people had said for me. When I was still in rehab, I went shopping and a little girl recognized me, came up to me, hugged me, and said, "I'm so glad to see you back. We prayed for you." To this day I don't know which church it was. The kids had found out I was sick and I think I was prayed for in every church in Osceola County.

"I have experienced what I believed was the presence of God in my life, though it happened 20 years ago. I was sitting by myself on the bus, and suddenly experienced God telling me that my life was going to work out. Since my injury there have been times when I have been feeling sorry for myself, things not going the way I want to go, and I kind of get a slap in the head that says, 'Just keep at it.' It's in my head but it's not my voice.

"I ask God to help me make decisions, to help me understand my feelings, to help me understand what is going on around me, and more often than not I get clarity and calmness in return. I've never had to scream at God. He is an active part of my life. My relationship with God is there—I don't have to be in church to get the feeling that God is with me." Did you make Him a member of your treatment team? "I prayed every day, about what was happening to me. I was asking for guidance, asking for help. So I guess I did—I just realized it.

"There have been one or two moments when I said, 'Why me, God?' They didn't last long, but they were extremely powerful. To this day when I pray I say, 'God, let me do what you left me behind to do. I should have died several times, but I'm still here. There must be some reason for that. God, let me do Your purpose, let me do it to Your satisfaction, let me do it well.' I don't know why He left me here. I see so many kids at school that look so lost and forlorn, and all I have to do is smile at them, and it seems to fill them with a good feeling. It looks like they've never been praised, never been acknowledged before—when I do that, and they look at me with such gratitude, I wonder if that is my purpose for living."

Here is Deloris' advice for survivors: "Take the time to stop and think. Deal with each thing that comes up. Don't ignore it, don't pretend it's not a problem. Allow yourself the quiet time to think about it in depth. You need to accept that you have the problems, and then fight to improve. Allow yourself to feel good about the victories. Then move on to a new area of deficit, remembering that you conquered the last one. I guess it's a process. Keep at it. If it doesn't work, recognize that fact, and find another way. Keep going until you find something that does work. Like having a place to put things that need to go into the car. And list making—I was always a list maker, but now I am a list maker par excellence.

"Don't beat yourself up. I have always been able to accept the reality of my life. But being realistic doesn't mean settling for how things are. I'm brain injured, and I accept that, but it doesn't mean I can't improve myself and my life."

Here is her advice for family members: "Patience. I wonder if I could have found the patience to say what needs to be said without the anger, or the self-righteousness. You've got to guard against that. And the instant response—you family members need to stop and think, too."

The Journalistic Perspective

As befits her job at an elementary school, Deloris is an all-purpose matronly figure. Having worked with children for so many years, she is proficient, and knows how to handle them constructively. That her injury did not change, but it has obviously affected her at a deeper level. She doesn't allow the kids to see that, but it can be picked up by looking closely. She was kind enough to share with me an experience she had right after returning to work, when she became paralyzed with fear at seeing a student tip back in a chair. She had a vision of the child falling backwards and cracking his skull on the hard ground, "spilling blood and brains all over my nice, neat carpet." Since then, she has shared this vision with her students, but presents it as a dream she had, ending with a warning to them not to tip back in their chairs. To them, it's an entertaining story. It can also be seen as an allegory of her own experience. Her injury went, in her words, from painfully ordinary to life-threatening just like that. And even though she's done a fantastic job of putting herself back together to the point of seeming ordinary, she knows how quickly it can all change again.

On rare occasions, Deloris wanders outside of her well-established routine. For a personal challenge, she took a community college precalculus course, and she passed it on her first try with a C. When she received an e-mail invitation to the GiveBack Christmas party, she copied the directions down on paper instead of printing it out. The party was being held at a home she'd never visited in an area with which she was not familiar. She spent 3 hours driving around and looking for the address before she gave up and went home. She couldn't call the party, because she hadn't copied the phone number. It never occurred to her to call her husband and ask him to get it for her. This is the same ultra-competent woman who can still handle children and computers perfectly. Her life is filled with contradictions like this one.

The Neuropsychological Perspective

Although it is not possible to definitively reconstruct the medical facts of her accident, it is clear that she lost consciousness while at home, struck her head on a table as she fell to the floor, remained unconscious for 10 to 15 minutes, and then was found to have sustained a left anterior cerebral artery aneurysm. The resulting subarachnoid hemorrhage was surgically evacuated, with the surgeon noting that the tissue in the left temporal lobe proximal to the bleed was grossly hemorrhagic and moderately swollen. A small left recurrent artery infarct was also visualized. Recovery was complicated by vasospasm of the proximal carotid artery and frontal headache. An angiogram damaged her iliac artery and distal aorta, which resulted in prolonged anoxic coma. A gradual increase in ventricular size was treated by insertion of a shunt at 3 weeks post-onset, after which her condition improved.

She was discharged to outpatient cognitive rehabilitation in the 3rd month post-onset. Her intake evaluation demonstrated moderate-to-severe impairment of focal attention. Immediate recall for verbal and visual information was found in the range from normal to mildly impaired, with delayed recall ranging from mildly to moderately impaired. Measures of processing speed ranged from within normal limits to severely impaired, with tasks requiring sustained attention showing the greatest deficits. Dynamometer grip strength was moderately to severely impaired bilaterally. Her greatest deficits, in executive and problem-solving skills, ranged from the moderate down to the profound level. She also showed marked impairment on occupational therapy measures of visual search and rapid eye-hand coordination. In contrast, her naming and reading skills and access to her fund of information was excellent. This pattern of test scores suggests that her anoxic coma was probably extended by hydrocephalus, as a 3-week, purely anoxic coma would be expected to produce more impairment of immediate memory and access to remote knowledge. Nevertheless, given her age (48), and the multiple insults documented in her medical history, a poor prognosis would be expected.

Deloris suffered so much acute gluteal pain during the final week of her inpatient stay and her outpatient evaluation that some of her tests could not be completed, and she was not able to tolerate full therapy sessions. She tried to "tough out" her therapy sessions but was rarely able to do so. The rehabilitation and medical staff attempted to treat her for the typical complications of acute treatment with no success. It therefore seemed likely that her problem was due to an atypical pain disorder. After carefully observing her behavior, it was noted that she sat down in a chair from a full standing position making no attempt to brake her fall, and that she did not weight shift from that time until the pain began. These behaviors were familiar from the treatment of fibromyalgia syndrome complicated by alexithymia, and this became her provisional diagnosis. Her strong and rapid response to the behavioral management protocol for this disorder confirmed the diagnosis. She also achieved good results from the long-term maintenance protocol, providing further evidence in support of the diagnosis.

Her cognitive rehabilitation was relatively straightforward. The high level of effort she characteristically employed seemed to explain the rapid return of her basic skills, and supported a strong response to the cognitive therapies. The program's emphasis on executive skills was well suited to her impairment and intended post-discharge responsibilities. Although she still demonstrated occasional impulsive behavior at the end of her treatment, she was discharged to part-time return to work quite early, and made an effective transition as she describes here. It was anticipated that her scrupulous use of the error analysis protocol would support further improvement on her own after discharge.

Although it was not surprising, it was impressive to see her continue engaging in active and vigorous self-therapy at more than 15 years post-discharge. For Deloris, the idea that self-therapy is a lifetime activity is more than just a catch phrase. Her personal commitment to the recovery process is clearly associated with the successful results she continues to achieve.

Chapter 7

The Story of Stephanie

Stephanie had one of the mildest injuries in the group, though it was still deep in the severe range according to the research criteria. However, she had a critical focal frontal lobe injury. Like Deloris, she had always been a hard-working, rule-following person, and this made her an unusually cooperative and willing trainee, giving her best effort in every therapy. When she finished the program, it was obvious that she would have a good recovery. However, no patient with severe TBI has ever accomplished a more impressive vocational recovery.

1. The Old Stephanie

"I grew up as an Air Force brat who moved around every few years, but I had no trouble making new friends or adapting to new schools. I was very outgoing and always had a bunch of friends—I could make friends with all kinds of people.

"I was, and still am, very close with my family. I was an active child, and my parents were very involved in my activities as I grew up: They ran the concession stand and were timers at swim meets, attended my band concerts, helped me with my homework, chauffeured me around to dance, horseback riding, piano and clarinet lessons, and church youth group programs, and Mom was my Girl Scout leader. I enjoyed living life in overdrive. I was happiest when I was overprogrammed. I did not like idle time.

"At the university I was active in a highly respected sorority and held several leadership positions, including rush and membership chairman. I was one of the student-ambassadors for the school, a member of a team that mentors incoming freshman, worked at the college radio station. I graduated with a BA in marketing and a minor in French. In a marketing research class in my senior year, I had the opportunity to do a group project at an entertainment company where I hoped to land a job. I did extra work that got me the opportunity to meet with the VP of advertising, and he invited me to submit my resume, and approximately 4 months later I landed a coordinator level position in marketing.

"Work became the center of my life. It was my identity. I worked at that company for over 6 years prior to my accident—a total of 10½ years. I worked in a variety of disciplines including corporate sponsorship, advertising, promotions, and interactive marketing. At the time of the accident I was a senior promotions representative. I worked primarily on negotiating and developing sweepstakes and contests with major corporate sponsors. I played a key role in developing one of their most successful promotions. Successes in special projects like this one helped to build my reputation as a committed worker who fought hard to get things done."

2. The Accident—13 Years Ago

"My coworker Sandie and I were heading back to work after a department Christmas lunch at a local country club. The last thing I remember was pulling out of the restaurant parking lot in my teal-green Saturn." Stephanie was wearing her seatbelt. The car was struck broadside, so the airbag did not deploy. Her head struck so hard that it left a dent in the steering wheel.

3. The Injury

Both frontal lobes were contused, including multiple contusions of the left frontal lobe. The diffuse injury produced a coma of 2 days and a memory gap of 7 days' duration. She also sustained multiple cranial nerve injuries.

4. Early Recovery

"After I woke up out of my coma and began to remember things again, my first memory is of lying in my hospital bed, surrounded by gifts and people streaming in and out like schools of fish. It was amazing how many friends I had—in the hospital, five to seven people were in my room visiting me continuously. College friends, coworkers, business associates, members of my church, the list seemed endless. People I hadn't seen in years came to see me. Flowers and plants poured into my room as steadily as visitors. It got to the point that when the nurses saw a florist coming, they would just point to my room! I ended up receiving over 40 arrangements!

"Everything seemed so strange to me that for many days I thought I was in a dream—a bad one. My visitors told me that I had been in a very serious accident, and that my car had been totaled. When I was tested by my physical therapist, I found that I couldn't figure out how to do a simple task like putting batteries in a flashlight. I kept trying to put three batteries in it when it took only two. I had to be seat-belted into my wheelchair, and even into my bed, because my balance was so bad. They didn't want to risk my getting out of bed during the night and falling. They said they had to belt me in because I acted "impulsive," a word that would seem to haunt me throughout my hospital stay, and even through outpatient cognitive therapy.

"In occupational therapy at the hospital, I sponge-painted a tote bag, which I thought looked great. I look at it now and it looks like someone in the first grade made it! I had to relearn how to coordinate the movements of my legs and arms in walking. I had to learn to force inflection into my voice so I didn't talk in a flat monotone like a machine. I had severe double vision, and had become (and still am) deaf in my right ear. There was a slight numbness on the left side of my body, and I had a tremor of my right hand, which made fine coordination tasks very frustrating. I also have a video of myself in one of my physical therapy session—in PJs, hair a mess, no makeup, in a wheelchair—not a pretty picture! I remember consciously deciding not to get dressed that day because, after all, I was dreaming . . . why change my clothes for a dream? It's good for me to look back at the video now, because I can see how far I've come. It's easy to forget how bad off I was.

"Right after the new year, I began to realize that it wasn't a dream. After that, I paid more attention to my therapy sessions. I remember thinking to myself, "You don't like what has happened. Just deal with it, because you don't want to stay in this hospital forever." As the days turned into weeks, I prepared myself each day to work hard in all of my therapies. One of my therapists said it was like I suddenly came to life. I didn't want to stop or take any breaks. I just wanted to keep working and challenging myself.

"When I was released from the hospital, I had to move in with my parents. I still couldn't walk on my own—my balance was so bad that I had to have support from a person walking with me who hung onto a big brown [gait] belt. I still had to be assisted with everything. I couldn't walk anywhere on my own, not even to the bathroom. My mom had to help me take a shower and I had a baby monitor in my room. Here I was 30 years old and my mom had to help me take a shower—what a humiliating experience! I decided not to fight it. I kept thinking, 'Resist and it will just prolong your recovery.' That statement rang in my head through the time I was in treatment. No matter how useless I felt a task was, I kept my thoughts to myself. Deep down, I knew that the doctors, nurses, and therapists knew what they were doing and had my best interests at heart, so I went along with them all the way.

"Being with my parents at that point was very good for me. Not only were they there to help me out, they could also drive me places and provide mental stimulation for me. My parents made sure that I didn't just sit around and watch TV. We went to the farmers' market, museums, the mall, did puzzles, played games, and of course they would give me chores to do. Empty the dishwasher; make my bed, small things—but big chores for me at the time. Actually, I was anxious to help out. I wanted to prove to myself that I could do these things which I had taken for granted in my former life.

When Stephanie appeared at the outpatient program for her evaluation, she was truly a strange sight. Like many patients, she had to wear an eyepatch to speed her recovery from double vision. Occasionally, a patient with glasses would wear them under the eyepatch, which defeated its purpose, or over the eyepatch, which looked somewhat odd. But Stephanie had adopted a unique solution to this cosmetic problem. To cover the eyepatch, she had cut out a blue piece of construction paper which was taped to the lens of her glasses, and on the paper, she had drawn a large eye with eyelashes. So when you looked at Stephanie, you saw a young lady with glasses, one normal eye, and one hand-drawn, blue construction paper eye. Her very blue, self-made eye stopped traffic.

Stephanie's unique homemade eye told two things. First, as a cosmetic repair it was a total flop, making her by far the strangest looking patient in the building. Social judgment was a weak suit for her at this point. Second, as a coping response, it was extraordinary. She had initiative and a willingness to try unique solutions to her problems.

"Before discharge from the hospital, I was assigned to return for the outpatient cognitive program. It started with a full day of neuropsychological tests. I thought I breezed through them. The tests seemed *so* easy. I felt I was passing with flying colors, and would prove that I didn't need any cognitive therapy. All I wanted was to go back to my job and my normal life. When I got the test results, much to my surprise, they told me I failed sections I thought I had aced. That was reality slapping me in the face: I needed the therapy more than I thought. Physically I was recovering very quickly, so I didn't think anything was wrong—it would all be back to normal in just a matter of time. It wasn't until I started the outpatient program, and learned exactly what a frontal lobe injury is, that I really realized just how much I needed the cognitive therapy. I had to put my life on hold while I worked on myself.

"The tremor in my right hand made it virtually impossible to write. Since I couldn't write to take notes, I brought a small tape recorder to the therapy sessions. I listened to the tape each night to transcribe notes on my word processor for the next session. Before the accident, I'd always been compelled to do my best at everything, and this was no exception. I needed to make sure my notes were thorough. I continued to use a tape recorder when I first returned to work, mainly in one-on-one meetings with people. It gave me a way to double-check my understanding of projects and ideas that were discussed in meetings. Gradually over time the tremor reduced, I learned to hold a pen or pencil differently and could take effective notes rather than having to record everything.

"Outpatient therapy was a long, arduous process. Classes were 5 hours a day, 4 days a week. It was like being back in college. I spent my days going from one class to another and doing homework. There were definitely days when I thought I would be there forever, that I would never graduate. When I did my homework at night, I would long for the stress of my job. I was so thrilled when they cut me back to 2 days a week at cognitive therapy, and let me go back to work part-time. In hindsight, I'm glad they didn't let me jump back into the work scene full-time. I guess they really *do* know what they're talking about!" Stephanie mastered every therapy to which she was assigned. She always finished her homework, and it was always done carefully and thoughtfully. She was promoted to program leadership positions, facilitating the high-level groups and teaching strategies and program philosophy to new members.

Like Hillary, Stephanie was anxious to get back to work. She worried about how her office was managing without her, and it seems likely that she was also afraid of being replaced, although she had been assured that her job would be waiting for her. Unlike Hillary, she inquired about discharge meekly, and quickly accepted the reply that discharge would require her to meet a sequence of standards that was not yet complete. If anything, she gave up too easily. This episode hinted that she would probably struggle with self-assertiveness in long-term recovery.

"When I graduated from the outpatient program, I felt a great sense of accomplishment. I had just completed 3½ months of intense therapy—probably the most difficult thing I had ever done! Now it was time for me to transition back into work, and to try not to let it be as consuming as it had been prior to the accident. The sensible, conservative side of me decided to take my transition slowly. I decided I'd much rather have a lot of little successes than one big success and several failures. No matter how small, I didn't want to fail—that attitude is still with me. Most of all, I'm thankful to have a second chance and I don't want to put myself at risk physically or emotionally by getting depressed. I don't think there's a person who has been through a situation like this that would ever want to go through it again, or even wish it on their worst enemy!

"Other than the fact that I had to wear a patch over one eye, I had no physical scarring or deformities. I looked very normal from the outside, but on the inside I was struggling with getting to know and understand the new me. Where I was once very self-confident at work, I was suddenly afraid of doing the simplest things like answering the phone . . . or making a cold call to a company to pitch them on a promotion idea. Not long after returning to work I got a message from a pushy, egotistical, confrontational guy who worked for a promotional agency. I wasn't sure I would be able to respond to his questions or comments the way I could before—I was no longer a "shoot from the hip" type of person. I went to the department head and asked him if he would return the call for me. To my dismay, he wouldn't do it. I was petrified.

"In outpatient therapy, they emphasized getting into the habit of preparing for anything that was difficult or important, and that has been a key to my success in the workplace. Making this call was one of the first times I remember putting this strategy into practice on the job. I dreaded coming across as incapable. So I sat in my office by myself and anticipated what he might ask and what my answers should be. I visualized the conversation, not just my end of it but the guy on the other end of the phone. I wrote a little outline of the things I needed to say, and kept it on my desk as a cheat sheet just in case I blanked out and needed to prompt myself. Finally I made the call and it turned out fine. I still do that kind of preparation today. When I have a big conversation coming up, whether it is with my boss, a friend, my boyfriend, or an employee, I take the time to outline my thoughts and role play the conversation. I might practice having an important conversation when I'm at home or driving in the car. The point of all this preparation is that when I make the actual call, I'm ready—I know what I need to say, how I need to say it, and what road blocks the person might throw up. I come across as someone who knows what she is talking about because when I've prepared properly, my brain is ready to show what I know.

"About that same time, I learned a big lesson about getting overloaded. A lot was going on that day, and I was trying to juggle multiple projects at one time like I used to before the accident. A vendor came into my office and I gave her some directions in warp speed mode. I talked really fast about a few different things and then asked her, '(Does that) make sense?' She just looked at me with her eyes wide, like I was some sort of monster. I realized that I needed to slow down and be more thoughtful about my conversations, and that maybe my body language or tone needed adjusting, too. One of my outpatient therapies called Contextual Processing taught us to predict what was about to happen after watching sections of a TV show. It taught me a new way to read situations. After this embarrassing interaction, I realized that I needed to do a better job of reading my surroundings, and taking stock of myself. I told myself not to try to do so much at one time, but I'd be lying if I said I never overloaded myself again.

"This deficit creates a constant struggle for me. The old me could spin multiple plates in the air without any of them falling. Gradually, I've redeveloped the ability to spin more than one plate, but sometimes the price I've paid is overloading myself so badly that I almost melted down on a couple of occasions. I get overwhelmed easier. I need more sleep, and I seem to get hungry more often. I try to listen to my body. When I don't get enough sleep, or when I get too hungry, or when I've allowed myself to have too much caffeine, I get moody, I don't think as clearly. I become quiet, and I can't carry my end of a conversation. As if that isn't enough, at those times, my double vision starts to kick in. I'm not much fun to be around. I can avoid these problems when I'm careful, and my goal is to make myself careful more consistently.

"On top of my problems in reading people and situations, I knew how prone I was to do or say something that seemed normal to me, but which in reality would come off as abnormal to everyone else. Knowing that planted a deep-seated fear in my soul. I had worked hard to build a good reputation, and I had so many people trusting my abilities that I couldn't stand to let them down. I took myself to task in terms of mental quality control. I triple-checked everything I did. If I wrote a memo, I asked one of my coworkers to read it over just to make sure that it made sense. When I was assigned a project, I talked through what I thought I needed to do with a coworker or my boss just to get some feedback. It took me longer to get things done, and for that reason it seemed imperative to get them done right the first time. Even today, more than 10 years later, I still question my perceptions of people and situations. I still wonder if I have it right when someone disagrees with me. I think this is why I feel compelled to make every-thing perfect—because if it's perfect, it can't be defective or impaired.

"I also had a problem with reversing numbers (a bad thing when you work with budgets!). The first few times I listened to messages on my voicemail at work, I wrote the number down without verifying it and then deleted the message. As it turns out, I wrote the number down wrong and had no idea how to get in touch with the person! I made the same mistake when I took phone calls—I'd take down their number and not read it back for verification. Well, after a few of these mistakes, I started listening to my messages twice and/or saving the message on my voicemail until I was sure I had the right number. When somebody gave me their number over the phone, I always repeated it back to ensure that I had written it down correctly.

"I feel incredibly fortunate to have received cognitive therapy. I learned about the aspects of my injury that I needed to fix, and about the challenges I could expect to encounter in my new life. They taught me the compensation strategies that I have fine-tuned over the years and incorporated into my life. Everything I do today depends on those strategies. It's become so natural that I am not even aware of 'using strategies' anymore, but there is not a day, and probably not an hour, that goes by without my employing a compensation strategy."

5. Accomplishments of Recovery

"After returning to work full-time for several months I was promoted to manager of promotions. I was the 'catch-all' for promotions that didn't fit into the categories like regional, local, or media promotions. This meant that much of my job was dealing with unusual projects. One of these was developing my company's first Web site. The Internet is something we take for granted today, but it was in its infancy then, and unfamiliar to almost everyone. I was blazing a new trail, something that doesn't come easily to the new Stephanie. But I persisted—I would not 'throw up the white flag.' I was bound and determined to prove to myself that I could do it.

"Internet-related projects boomed and before I knew it I wasn't doing anything else. My regular job of developing promotions morphed into a job as the director of a new department, interactive marketing, which included managing a staff of four. Suddenly I had jumped from being a little fish in a little pond into a bigger pond filled with bigger fish.

"In 1998 I accepted a job with a major competitor as marketing manager for the introduction of a new high-technology service. Once again, I was involved in blazing new trails, but this time it was in an industry that was brand new to me (something very difficult for a person with my injury). Of course, that fit me perfectly since I usually don't take the easy road on anything. I not only had to get to know a whole new group of people, I also had to learn a new industry language, develop new operational processes, and find cross-promotional synergies throughout the company. It was a high-pressure atmosphere, but again, I was not going to be defeated. I worked long hours, something I swore I would never do again. But to me it was a necessary evil because I had so much to learn, and it took me longer to learn and absorb it. The work eventually paid off. I was promoted to a department director-level position, which involved working with major corporate partners.

"After 5 years, I decided to do something more meaningful with my life. A friend of mine consulted for a major nonprofit organization for troubled teenagers in Virginia and knew they were looking for a director of sales and marketing. I was hired to help reestablish the marketing infrastructure and develop a proactive sales team. The job required me to move to Richmond, which I did without hesitation. The move was exciting but incredibly stressful at the same time. I had always lived in the same city as my parents. Moving meant leaving my family, friends, and a familiar city. In essence, I wiped out my entire support system.

"I am very proud of the work I accomplished in the year I worked for this organization. My team delivered a new Web site, created a brochure, course catalog, tabletop displays, a DVD, and miniposters, shot and produced four videos, and more. Additionally, I created the framework for a sales team. While the marketing aspects were familiar to me, I was new to this company, and again, it was difficult to learn about the product and their new industry language. Many of the people had been working there for years, and had been doing things a certain way. Understandably, they were resistant to change. Imagine being in my shoes: a perfectionist (and a head-injured one at that), who is under pressure and high expectations from a board of directors, is placed in an environment resistant to change and in an area where you have no support system. This is a recipe for overload. Although I often thought about 'throwing in the towel,' I never allowed myself to exercise that option—giving up meant defeat. I knew I would not leave until I had delivered on the major projects. I experienced tremendous personal growth in Richmond. Not only did I develop self-reliance by moving away, but I also rappelled off a cliff, hiked up a narrow, vertical trail in the dark and went whitewater canoeing, things I never thought I could do. I reminded myself that just 10 years earlier I had a hard time walking! I discovered that I am capable of so much more than I ever allowed myself to believe."

Stephanie created the storybook ending in her last contact at 13 years post-onset. She announced her engagement. This filled in the last blank in her remarkable recovery.

6. Methods of Recovery

"During my recovery I spent every waking moment doing something constructive toward my rehabilitation. I was bound and determined not to stay in this condition forever. I did homework during my lunch break at therapy. I worked on puzzles and played games with my parents in the evenings. I practiced my exercises for physical therapy and my vocal exercises for speech therapy. I think being a perfectionist and remembering the way life was prior to the accident were very positive forces in my recovery. Although I improved physically and cognitively, I was never satisfied. I always pushed myself harder, always working to do more than was expected of me. As I improved to the point that would have been considered acceptable to others, the memory of how well I did before made me push myself to do better.

"Work was my main motivator during the hospital phase of my recovery. I was frothing at the mouth to get back. Focusing on my homework, therapy, chores, whatever—I always pushed myself to do better than what was acceptable. I was also extremely cautious in everything I did. I don't like failure, no matter how small. I felt that my reputation, both at work and as a person, was on the line, and there was no way I was going to risk rushing into something without thinking it through or testing the waters first.

"I like to plan things out. I like surprises every now and then, but I prefer to plan so that I know what is going to happen and can anticipate challenges. In cognitive therapy we learned how to do GPAs [goal-plan-anticipate, the planning algorithm]. I've definitely ingrained this process into my everyday life—in fact, I have to be careful not to anticipate more problems than I could possibly have!

"Communicating on the job via e-mail was one of the best coping strategies I found. It allows me to think through my response or direction I give to someone. It also provides a written paper trail or archive for me to refer to when I can't remember specifics. I also find voice-mail to be helpful. If I wake up in the middle of the night remembering something or have a sudden inspiration to solve a problem, I call my voicemail at work and leave myself a message.

"The new Stephanie is not as quick-witted and outgoing as the old one. I'm still very positive, friendly, and funny, but I'm more intro-verted now. Where I used to do everything in large groups, I now pre-fer being with two or three people. I do a lot of things by myself, such as running errands, going to the movies, hanging out at home, or spending time with my dog. I miss the old me that was very social, but I don't dwell on things I can't change. I just have to make the best of the situation.

"I am very open about my accident. I have to be: When people find out that I am deaf in my right ear they almost always ask what happened. I tell them that I had a head injury, and needed to learn to walk and talk again, but I don't detail what is cognitively difficult for me now. Most people don't understand what a head injury is and I don't offer an explanation unless they ask. To them it is just a bump on the head. A few close friends know the details of my injury, but I usually don't share the specifics with someone new until I have earned their respect.

"Overall, I have become a much more compassionate person at work. Sometimes this new, more compassionate side works against me. I have a difficult time managing or working with negative, unmotivated, and/or confrontational people. I know that I am too passive in dealing with conflict: Instead of addressing it when it first bubbles up, I avoid it, which only causes it to fester and get worse, and I wind up feeling angry and resentful. I work continually to improve this. Before each meeting with an employee, I make an outline of what will be discussed. This process helps me to organize my thoughts, avoid getting pulled off track, and be sure to get all the issues and corrective actions talked through. I also learn from each confrontational situation something that I can use to prevent things from going that far the next time.

"When people look at me, I want them to see a person who gets her job done well. I am a stickler for follow-through, and I know that makes me come across as somewhat inflexible and too focused on the details. I will not commit to something unless I know I can follow through and deliver on it. Once I make a commitment, I get it done regardless of how many extra hours it takes me to complete the task. I have earned the respect of coworkers and superiors this way.

"My work is a reflection on me, and the quality equals or exceeds that of people who have not incurred a brain injury. I know that sounds cocky, but that's the bar I continually force myself to reach. I'm very proud of what I've been able to accomplish. Just because you are brain injured does *not* make you incapable of doing great work!

"As important as my career has been, I don't live to be the career woman from Hell anymore. I have more of an appreciation for life and people. I do things because I don't want to have regrets when I get older. For example, I'm planning to go horseback riding through Costa Rica." She recognizes that her social recovery has not been as complete as her vocational recovery. Although this result reflected a conscious choice to prioritize reestablishing her career in the first decade, she has recently devoted more time, effort, and strategy to enrich her social life.

"I've never gotten angry or depressed over my recovery. I remember thinking to myself: 'OK, you have two choices. You can feel sorry for yourself, slow down your recovery, and make life miserable for your parents and friends, or you can accept it and make the best of the situation.' I chose the second. It was weird—I always had a feeling that everything was going to be OK. It might take awhile, but eventually it would be OK. It was a kind of calming feeling. I guess it was God's way of saying, "Don't worry, I have a plan for you, and everything will be all right.' I always believed that everything happens for a reason, and now I really believe it. Maybe the accident occurred to open everyone's eyes as to how short life is, and how we need to appreciate the time we have with the people we love right now, because there might not be a tomorrow or later. Other times I think it was to get me to slow down and to make me enjoy life more. Maybe it was to make me a more compassionate person or to share my story with others. I may never know why, but I'm positive there was a reason for such a full, complete recovery."

Here is Stephanie's advice for survivors: "Stay positive. Attitude is everything. If I had let myself get depressed and distracted, my recovery would have been much slower—and maybe not as complete. You may not like what has happened to you, but you can't change the situation. No amount of anger or tears will wipe away your tragedy, but they will make your situation worse if you let them consume you. Accept what has happened and try to figure out what you can do to make the best of the situation—to make your life better."

Here is Stephanie's advice for family and friends: "Stay positive. Make the injured person feel positive about themselves. Recognize that the small improvements are actually huge accomplishments to the person going through it. Be proud of them, and make them feel proud of the accomplishments, too. Don't try to do everything for the injured person. Provide suggestions on where to go and what to do, but encourage them to make the decisions. Help them to feel like they are contributing. Feeling that others believed that I could do these difficult things gave me strength and confidence. I couldn't let them down, and I couldn't let myself down."

The Journalistic Perspective

When Stephanie enters the room, your eyes are immediately drawn to the varied hues of her richly red hair. Then you notice her business attire, put together "just so," and the stern cast of her eyebrows. She is the figure of a powerful, young executive. As she walks in, and only if you watch closely, you can see that her gait is just a bit unsteady and her head meets her body at a slightly awkward angle, telltale signs of an accident that once badly broke the person, who was put back together only more or less properly. When she starts to talk, you see the same contrasts. Her tones are precisely modulated and her words carefully chosen. She sounds like a person who measures every idea in all three dimensions before expressing it. But then, partway through her monologue, she trips over a word and by the end of the sentence she is still collecting herself. And by the end of the paragraph, there are still bits and pieces out of place. As with most of the role-model survivors I have met through this organization, the signs of disrepair are so subtle that I would not recognize them if I were not aware that they are there.

Several attempts to get a one-on-one with Stephanie got no more than a "Well, I don't know . . . " Finally, I ran into her at a GiveBack meeting, made sure to sit right next to her, and she threw up a psychic wall between us. Her eyes stayed fixed straight ahead or went off to the side I wasn't sitting on. I'd seen this behavior in survivors with less-than-Olympic-gold recoveries: hunkered down and avoiding confrontation with their deficiencies. Clearly she did not want to talk with me about what it was like to be head injured. Then she made some striking comments to the group, and I started thinking maybe she might be a medalist after all. She took command of the meeting like a top executive. She voiced a keen awareness of her problems, while giving the impression that she'd taken command of them, too. There was the veteran's sure handling of recovery issues that Deloris also showed, and the urgency for accomplishment I'd seen in Faith. But a deep unease also loomed over her, like Matt's fears. Burdened but brilliant and capable, she knew she'd come down a long road of recovery, while a far longer road vanished over the horizon. Does she feel as if she controls her injury, or does it control her? Will she ever end up reaching a destination that satisfies her? I don't know.

The Neuropsychological Perspective

The accident left Stephanie at Glasgow Coma Scale level 3 at admission, with multiple focal injuries including a left frontal contusion and a right frontal intracerebral hematoma. There was also a left parietal superficial hematoma. On physical examination, she showed bilateral gaze deviation to the right, with bilateral pupillary dilation and sluggish response to light. She experienced a respiratory failure in the field and required resuscitation and intubation. During transport, her blood pressure was low. The admitting note raised the question of cerebral anoxia and documented right temporal fracture. Although these features are all potential signs of poorer prognosis, the parameters of coma duration and post-traumatic amnesia, although well into the severe range, are still among the lowest in this group.

During her acute hospitalization, she demonstrated a number of signs suggestive of cerebellar/brainstem injury, including ataxic gait, left lateral nystagmus, diplopia, and dysarthric speech. Cranial nerve exam was positive for third nerve palsy. Auditory acuity was reduced on the right side, and remains so at present. She showed a left hemiparesis. Her third-day CT scan showed diffuse edema as well as continued evidence of the bifrontal focal injuries.

Her evaluation for admission to the cognitive rehabilitation program was performed at 1 month post-onset. Focal attention skills showed good recovery to her superior baseline level, indicating her readiness for full evaluation and treatment. Performance IQ subtest scores were only mildly impaired, whereas verbal IQ subtest scores were moderately impaired. Immediate recall for verbal information was moderately impaired, although for visual information it ranged from the moderate to the profound level. Delayed recall was mildly impaired for word list information and severely impaired for narrative passages and for visually presented information. Measures of processing speed, executive function, and complex reasoning were all found in the profound range. She also demonstrated mild deficits in access to her storehouse of knowledge.

During this period of time, Stephanie attempted to interact normally but became dysfluent and confused easily. The sentences that she could finish effectively were mostly simple, declarative statements, with the occasional compound sentence. Her organizational difficulties were manifested in a tendency toward empty speech. These symptoms cleared well during her 3½-month rehabilitation stay.

Stephanie was easy to treat: She was cooperative, followed through well on instructions, learned quickly, and gave her best effort on every exercise. Because her injury directly affected the expressive and problem-solving skills that were essential to her job in public relations (and more generally in service industry management), her therapy needed to concentrate on those areas. Her progress was so rapid that new curriculum had to be designed in some areas to reach the high functional levels at which she needed to work after discharge. She did not quite reach the criterion levels for problem-solving skills or perception of contextual information at the time of her return to work. In follow-up interviews, she reported a successful return to work with limited duties, a rapid progression to full duties, and promotion within 1 year of her return.

Chapter 8

The Story of Faith

1. The Old Faith

Faith's pictures were all over her high school yearbook—prom courts, lead roles in plays and musicals, class offices, and she was selected as the senior most likely to succeed. She came from a family of bright, energetic, successful people. Her father, a charming surgeon, is an office-holder in the American Medical Association. Her mother is a gifted musician and favorite performer at local shows. Even as a middle child among siblings with strong personalities, Faith was the "go-getter." She was the one who captured the attention of her busy father by giving public performances as a singer, actress, beauty contestant, and two-time All-American gymnast. When Faith went off to college, she continued to stand out in extracurricular activities. Grades did not come easily; she needed to be the hardest-working student in the family. She earned dual BA degrees. Her first job was as a community liaison for a major corporation. In her spare time, she coached grade school and high school level gymnasts.

2. The Accident—8 Years Ago

Faith and a fellow coach were demonstrating gymnastic maneuvers to their pupils in an auditorium with a concrete floor. While being tossed in the air to execute a complicated spin, she lost control and came down on her side, striking the concrete head-first with a terrible bang.

3. The Injury

The force of impact exploded one of the main branches of her right middle cerebral artery, a massive tributary of the carotid artery (supplier of most blood to the brain). The bleeding would have killed her quickly if surgery had not closed and trimmed the wound. The front and sides of her right temporal lobe were removed. Her right parietal lobe was bruised and swollen. Her diffuse injury produced an 8-day coma.

4. Early Recovery

In the hospital, Faith looked like a wet rat, curled up and shivering from the head pains produced by the ordinary sights and sounds of the ward. As physically depleted as she was and as miserable as she felt, she still asked for the maximum level of treatment available, and made an impressive effort to learn as much as she could. "I didn't want to do anything. I was so lethargic. But I wanted to get better, so I pushed myself. I had ice packs on my head, because it hurt so badly." When she wasn't in therapy, she introduced herself to her fellow patients, their family members, and the staff. Even in her bedraggled, confused state, she tried making friends with the staff, patients, and their family members.

While Faith was still an inpatient, she asked what to expect from recovery. Given the choice to hear the truth or comforting lies, she insisted on the truth. She was told that part of her brain was permanently broken, and a good recovery from this kind of injury is virtually unknown. If she were to have a good recovery, it would take an all-out effort. She promised the best recovery on record.

Patients with her injury feel certain that they have not changed, and that was how Faith felt at first. She was advised that the only way she could understand her condition would be to listen and learn, and ignore the feelings that the facts didn't fit her—she would have to totally deny her own intuitions. At first, she refused. "I fought against the idea that there was a 'new' Faith tooth-and-nail. I used to tell the physical therapist, 'I'm going to be doing back handsprings when I leave this place.' Now, I remember their faces going, 'You're not going to be doing any back handsprings.' It took me months to learn that I was living in a different world." She persisted in planning to resume the gymnastics even after asking her neurosurgeon for permission, and finding out that if she were to fall onto the mesh area it would kill her. As an outpatient, she convinced her personal trainer to help her do workouts toward that end. Finally, she gave up when she discovered that her "gyroscope" could not track her position when she spun, as she had been warned by her neuropsychologist.

"In therapy group, [I was accused] of having left neglect (a condition of ignoring everything on the left side of the world), which I adamantly denied. Then one morning, gesturing as I talked, I accidentally ran my arm under a felt-tipped pen—my left arm!" When the pen marks were pointed out, she said, "Anyone could have done that! But I didn't forget it. A few weeks later, I knocked a cup of water all over the conference table—it was on my left, of course. This time, I said, 'I guess you're going to accuse me of left neglect again. So I beat you to it.' I was being a smart ass, of course, but after that I stopped believing that I didn't have left neglect, and even started watching out for it. That doesn't mean I'm always on top of it. Sometimes even now I put things on my left side, promise myself that I can be careful, and then have to swallow my pride again when I knock it over. So the learning experience, the accepting of the deficits, that's a never-ending process for me.

Faith had a whole list of deficits, and at first she didn't accept that she had any of them. When she was confronted with being impulsive, she didn't think it meant anything because the same accusation had been leveled at almost everyone in her therapy group. "I just figured it was something said out of habit to all patients, like 'good morning' or 'good evening.' Not long after I knocked the cup of water over, I earned my release to drive. That was a huge thing for me— I hated being on a medical driving restriction, and couldn't wait to get my freedom back. On the day I got my clearance, I called the car dealership and got them to pick me up, along with my old car, and purchased a huge SUV with airbags. Insufferably pleased with myself, I went marching into group the next day to announce that I had a new car." Why did she buy a new car with airbags? "[S]o I wouldn't hit my head again." She didn't realize front air bags wouldn't protect the place where she got hit before; for that, she needed side-curtain airbags. But that wasn't the end of it. It turned out that "I had just bought the most dangerous vehicle on the road—the model where the tires explode and make the car roll over." It wasn't a lesson easily learned, "but that was my turning point. I began to see myself as impulsive from that day forward—and I could see myself doing plenty of impulsive things once I was looking for it. And of course, once I could see it, I became able to stop it. By the way, I got another car. It took me a few months, but the new one did have side-curtain airbags. And when I got into an accident in it, it kept me from getting badly hurt.

"My impulsivity makes me say things before I've thought about them. Sometimes I realize that I've blurted something out I shouldn't have said, but not always. How to stop myself? I can, but only when I'm not stressed out, but when I feel strong emotions it's hard to stop. My boss tells me that I get too passionate about my pet projects on the job—I think, 'How can you be too passionate about something important?' but that's the feedback I'm getting, so I accept it—I need to always assume that there must be something to the feedback I get from everyone. In all my relationships, with my bosses, my coworkers, my boyfriend, and when I'm tired or anxious, that's when I get impulsive and say things I regret. When it's been an easy day, and I'm well rested and not stressed out, then I can be the person I want to be, which means I say things the way I want them to come across. I also make sure I don't do any impulse buying. Before I make a purchase, I get the opinions of so many people. I'm not willing to make another big mistake like buying that SUV—no more impulsive decisions!

After the SUV incident, Faith made a maximum effort to learn about her injury. When told that the senior author had submitted a paper on her syndrome (Schutz, 2005a), she asked for a copy, and methodically went through it with a medical dictionary and a highlighter to identify every symptom. She kept this copy, and the symptom list she created from it, in her notebook and referenced it as therapy experiences brought the symptoms to awareness. Soon she was quoting from it to apply it to herself: "I have problems reading people. I have problems reading myself. My brain doesn't handle more than one emotion at a time, whether it be stress, excitement, sadness, whatever emotion. I have to tell myself, 'You're reading the situation wrong. You're reading people wrong. You're not interpreting their tones, their real meaning, because you're seeing the situation in a different context than they are.' The part of me that knows how to act, how to react, how to give and take is dead—completely. I try to borrow other people's brains: 'Does it seem like so-and-so is mad at me?'"

At first, like most patients, she complained about the clinic's requirement to make complete, detailed daily schedules a day in advance. But she also had an urgent desire to go back to work, and she quickly found that the schedules made her organized and productive again. Soon, Faith had become a daily schedule wonk. She was scheduled 24/7, just as the program recommended. But she took it a step further. Sometimes her boyfriend or her family didn't go along with her schedule. For example, when she went home on vacation her family argued that she shouldn't *be* on a schedule—after all, it was a holiday. She didn't accept that. She insisted on continuing her program during Christmas and Easter vacations. Her family telephoned begging for someone to call her off. Eventually we worked out a compromise. Faith scheduled multihour blocks of "chaos" into her daily schedule, and during those chaos periods the family could be spontaneous. But any other opposition to her schedule brought a stern lecture on recovery.

While she was in the outpatient program, she had "the freedom to be the old Faith—I said yes to every request and every opportunity, and I sang, spoke, coached, didn't get enough sleep, working in the gym till midnight all by myself. I let myself go without eating and drinking, and I ran around like a wild woman rushing everywhere I went. Then I had a seizure. In the hospital they told me that my body chemistry was all screwed up from lack of food and water. And when I got out, [I was told] that depriving yourself of sleep is a way to trigger seizures."

Her seizures were particularly frightening—she remained awake and aware as she fell, lost her speech, and felt body parts go numb and spasm. The experiences were intense and dramatic, and afterward she was exhausted and confused. However, she also panicked and got herself hospitalized time and time again. The second time, she told anyone who would listen that she wished she had died in the accident, and only a last-minute intervention by her neurologist kept her out of a psychiatric ward. In therapy, it was pointed out that chronic seizure patients rarely become this emotional and don't need to be hospitalized for an uncomplicated seizure. A new expectation was established: "When you can have a seizure, pick yourself up off the floor, and go on with your day, that will mean you are adjusting to your disability." In less than 6 months, she was able to do this, and since then she has taken all of her seizures in stride.

Patients with temporal lobe injuries often experience their emotions with great intensity. Severe focal injuries such as this one produce emotional firestorms in the head. Faith reported "breaking into sobs" and "bawling" several times a week at work, as well as in social situations.

A new expectation was needed. She was asked to imagine how others experienced her emotional outbursts. She recognized that these episodes "got old pretty quick" and contributed to her status as a "high maintenance" colleague and friend. She then set a goal to stop the outbursts in the workplace, and was successful. Later, she also gained control in public places. She still has outbursts in private and occasionally around acquaintances, but she has prevented them from affecting her important relationships and her reputation at work.

When she went back to work, she started on a part-time basis. Her employer, who had been a friend before the injury, realized that she got tired and overloaded easily, and tried to keep from overloading her. After she developed the seizures, she cut back her time on the job for a while. It was difficult for her boss and coworkers to cover the extra work she had always done, but they did so for more than a year. Finally, the time came for her to go back to full-time. Now, to do a full job, Faith could not complete her work in 40 hours or even 50. She had to work many extra hours, and came home exhausted at the end of a day. However, she didn't ask for a lighter load—she was determined to pull her own weight.

"I was really strict on the scheduling. The night before I sat with my day timer for at least 30 minutes planning out when I was going to eat, drive time to and from all my meetings, because I don't work in one building or place, and getting a driver, because at that time I was driving restricted because of my seizures. I used my alarm watch to keep myself on schedule. I was able to set timers to get me to my next meeting, to keep my commitments, to keep from spending too much time chatting, because I was the social butterfly of the world. It kept me on task and meeting my priorities. Whenever someone pushed something extra onto me or tried to change my schedule, I got angry and felt I was being exploited. Changes in my agenda would never have bothered me before. Mostly I just shut up and accommodated the requests, although I also griped about it. Without my schedule I was a total mess—I couldn't get anything done.

"I need to do things the same way all the time, or things will go to hell. I find myself getting distracted, or spending too much time on one project before moving to the next project. So even as much as you try, your brain doesn't have sense of time. You can't count on your brain to remember jack." As she was instructed, Faith always takes detailed notes, saves them, and uses her notebooks as reference books to look up the information when she needs it later. "Everyone always laughed at me because I wrote everything down, but I didn't want to miss anything or forget anything. I didn't end up forgetting important things but once in a blue moon. It always goes back to planning. If I did forget anything I wasn't organized enough or didn't write notes that were detailed enough. I will always leave some little thing out, even now. Like I showed up 2 hours late at the bridal shower on Saturday, but I must have confused the ending time with the starting time. So I'm still working on it.

"If there was anything coming up where I thought there was potential for emotional overload—something that was going to upset me or put me on the defensive, I would discuss what could go wrong, and try to come up with all the obstacles and find a good strategy for how to respond. I didn't ever want to get caught off guard, because that was always when I was at my worst. When I let myself get rushed or overbooked, my whole organization went right out the window. A stupid example—I wanted to buy a smoothie today after I finished working out, but because I rushed I left the money in the car, so I had to skip the smoothie. I jam-packed my day with too much stuff today, so it's still happening."

Eventually, her coworkers began to distance themselves from her. "My former best friends Nancy and Rita [her boss] were acting more and more annoyed with me, and my relationships with them had started to deteriorate also. I couldn't make sense of those relationships—they continued to say they loved me, but they treated me like crap. It was very puzzling that Nancy was so upset with me. She wouldn't explain, wouldn't give me any feedback more than once or twice. She said, 'Every time I try, it gets OK for a couple of days, then it goes back to the way it was.' I would say or do something that upset her. I didn't have any idea what that meant. She said, 'Faith, I can't begin to tell you all the things you do. It's easier to shove you in a corner and not deal with you.' Nancy ended up not speaking to her for a year, and their relationship is still strained. Others whom she thought of as friends shunned her. Her relationship with her boss grew tense and difficult. She had frequent arguments with everyone.

One part of the problem seemed to be that Faith was not aware of the extent of others' frustration with being imposed on by her symptoms and special needs. Another part was her tendency to ask for more favors than she gave (without realizing it), not just at work but in all of her relationships. Gradually, Faith's role on the job changed, from someone beloved and welcomed back into someone who was excluded from parties and lunchtime and after-work get-togethers. She had never been rejected in this way before, and it was both painful and infuriating. She became sarcastic about it, and this only made the problem worse. "I blamed them for screwing things up, because I was working so hard. [I didn't] realize how demanding I was—one of the hardest discussions I ever had, because I didn't want to believe that, and I fought the idea." Finally, after much discussion, she realized that her coworkers had real grievances about the way her limitations and behaviors made their jobs more difficult. When she got a new coworker, she made a special attempt to give as much as she asked, and this relationship has gone much better.

"I found that my relationships with my family had become difficult, too. They had always been argumentative and intense, but I remember one time when my brother wanted my sister next to him in the car—because that never would have happened before. So I realized that I was an outcast with my family too—it wasn't just a work thing. I needed to get better feedback from them. Because the thing is that you don't see what you're doing wrong to piss them off.

"With Rita, it's ended up awesome. She and I are good friends again, now that she no longer works with us. I learned I could be very impulsive and inappropriate even to my leader, even though she deserved it—and she did deserve it—but I would never have done that before. I should have taken it like a champ and shut my trap. But I couldn't shut my trap. I just let out my true feelings, but it was inappropriate behavior. I added a lot of friction to the relationship. She made me very paranoid—I used to think she was taking sides with the girls who always criticized me behind my back. I got stuck looking over my shoulder—Rita hadn't been that way before, and I took it as conspiracy, like they were trying to make me leave. In our one-on-one meetings, she listened to me and wanted to know what was going on. She never gave me any good feedback. She would quote things the other girls said to give me feedback, instead of speaking for herself. So that got me thinking it was a conspiracy (while in reality), deep down, she wanted me to succeed. All I could see in her was Satan." Faith believes that God resides in everyone. When asked why she was treating Rita as if He was not in her, the question caused her to stop and think hard. "I realized I was misjudging her. And things improved after that. I realized that this had been as hard on her as it was on me, and that she really wanted me to succeed. It was hard to see how hard dealing with me was on other people."

The relationship problem also affected her romantic partnership. Her boyfriend had been a great support and devoted caregiver. When she went home, "He did everything, I just laid around all day. He was at my beck and call. I couldn't have been blessed with a better caregiver. He came home from work, cleaned up after the cat, did everything." Unfortunately, he popped the question not long after Faith was released from the hospital, in front of her family at an Easter celebration. He ignored her mother's warning that it was too early. She put on the ring, but when she couldn't decide whether to accept his proposal or not, the ring was back in his hands the next day. Soon after, "We started fighting because I insisted on going back to coaching gymnastics, and he thought I shouldn't be doing it—it was too late at night, I had to stay there all alone, and I got worn out doing both jobs. The arguments became more frequent, he slammed doors, I pushed him, he pushed me. [We were both] called down for physical abuse. At that point, we were still working together. But he wasn't really a part of my life outside of work. I spent so much time coaching gymnastics that I didn't have time to spend with him, let alone fight with him. I kept myself so busy there was no time for a relationship. I also began to realize that we were moving apart. I didn't try to restore the relationship—I began dating other guys, and he had an affair. It seemed to take forever for us to break up. I felt pretty crappy about myself. I felt like I had failed, blamed myself for things not working out. I must have apologized to him 1500 times for not saying 'yes' to his proposal. There went the hope of ever being with anybody." Since the breakup, there have been two other serious boyfriends, but each relationship has gone through a period of intense conflict and ended unhappily.

Faith understands how her cognitive deficits are still creating problems in her relationships: "I need guidance and strategies to deal with the cognitive side of my injury. Other people in my life won't accept me as I am. Certain things push my buttons—criticizing me, threatening rejection. People misinterpret me and paint me into a corner. I go on the offensive. When that happens, my communication sucks. My temper gets up, ignited easily. I lose my patience. If I step out of the situation, I can see how frustrating I am to deal with."

At the end of her 3rd year post-onset, she was driving to work when she rear-ended another car, going fast enough to give herself a new, mild head injury. She was putting on makeup when she hit the other car. "I learned that I can't multitask while driving. Actually,

I should have known better, but I had to prove it to myself. Like everything else, I had to learn it the hard way. They can warn us, but we have to learn by actually making the mistake. I was just putting on powder—I don't even need a mirror to put on powder. I was clear headed, well rested, wasn't even emotional at the time. I wasn't even speeding. I just let myself get distracted. It was my second car accident since getting out of rehab. The first one was a fender bender—I was hurrying to get to Dunkin' Donuts, so when the light turned green I didn't look at the car in front of me, focusing on only one thing, and getting too excited. I realize now that I have to be so much more careful because I think about those wrecks. Both of them were real, brain-injured mistakes and could have been a whole lot worse."

Another ongoing area of difficulty is dealing with new situations and developing new skills. "I avoid doing it at all costs. Partly because I know it's a problem area for me. I see how steep the learning curve is—something as small as a little computer program—takes me double the time to learn, though once I learn it, it's OK. I get too overwhelmed with the new information. Moving to a new home—it was the scariest thing I had ever done. I didn't know the roads. The emotion—it's like panic—I have to take myself in hand, tell myself, 'You're going to be OK.' I would write the directions out to compensate, so I wouldn't get lost. When I moved in, not meeting people was a problem. I had already preplanned how to get around from my house. The real estate lady gave me a binder that has sections for all the important papers—like it tells me where to go in a hurricane. It amazes me how many things I got done—get a garage door opener, get it installed—I had it all preplanned, made a checklist. I'm amazed at how much I got done. The old Faith never could have done any of that—I would have had somebody else do it for me. I've gotten a lot tougher. I know how to arrange it all, now. The next time it'll be easy."

5. Accomplishments of Recovery

Faith made good on her promise to work hard in therapy. "I read the paper [describing my condition], took notes on it, in every group wrote down what everybody's injury was and what it meant, and asked questions when I didn't know what it meant. I would jump into the future and demand to know how this was going to affect me as a mother and wife. I wanted to know everything bad the injury was going to do to me so I could beat it before it beat me. I've been able to find examples of every symptom in my behavior, so I guess I understand my condition pretty well. I think I did a great job as a patient!

"While in outpatient rehab, for about 6 months, I was a volunteer at my rehab hospital. I did a lot of little jobs, but what I loved was I got to take the menus to each patient's room, get their meal orders, and take them down to the kitchen. The nurses would put me to work as a kind of peer counselor—they'd say room number so and so could use you, and they'd tell me about the patient and I'd go and talk with them, or buy them gifts. The best memory was the little girl who never said a word, and when I bought her an Eeyore doll, she said, 'Eeyore!' I cried. A woman who had a stroke said she loved jewels and I got her a tiara. They said she took her tiara and wand with her everywhere she went. So you really felt like you made a difference. I told caregivers to get involved, go to the family group, to learn about their loved one's injury, and to give them hope. Look where I am, I was where your loved one was before. Your loved one will get here." She didn't realize she was giving some of them false hope, because all of them wouldn't get as far as she had. "Then I was more careful about that part."

Faith remains an employee in good standing 4 years after her return, despite the total reorganization of her department and her job, and two changes of supervisor. She is a prominent figure in the company who maintains excellent relationships with the customers. She deals with senior executives frequently, and they routinely compliment her and praise her value to the organization. Recently she made a presentation to her director asking for a promotion and got it.

"I became a member of the diversity resource group for my company. They asked me to be president after I'd been a member for half a year. My supervisor suggested that I decline, so I did and took the finance officer position. I do a lot of brain injury advocacy. A vice president contacted me and asked me to mentor a brain-injured college student working on a summer internship. He wanted me to determine her capabilities and needs, make recommendations to her supervisors to help her to be more effective. I sat down with the general manager over her position and explained what the young lady was going through and how the managers could help. I made them get into her world and understand what a struggle she was having. It didn't work out well for her, but she still calls me. She says I was the only thing that made her feel like somebody in an otherwise miserable summer. 'You brought God back into my life.'

"A month after my surgery, I appeared at the church where I had coached to pay people back because the whole congregation had prayed for my recovery. That's when I started witnessing my story and singing spiritual songs at schools and churches. I'm still doing it. In my presentations, I try to create brain injury awareness, I share my struggles, who I was, who I am now. My message is: 'With God, all things are possible.' All ages—there's not one person there who hasn't at some point felt ugly, unloved, like an outcast, even like their life is not worth living, but when I share my story they can see that miracles can happen. I treat my recovery as I treat my walk with God—sometimes I do great, sometimes I don't, but they're both religion to me. Through inspirational songs and videos I get my message across. It's a great message—the story always moves the audiences to tears, and some of them stand up and tell personal stories of their own. I've received quite a few letters of support and friendship from people in the audience. They give me a lot of empathy, inspiration, and strength. 'When I have a bad day I think of you,' or 'I have no right to feel griped with my life.' I tell them, 'I don't accept that—your problems are everything.'

"In October of 2001 I was scheduled to sing with a Christian rock band at a NASCAR event. I drove all night, but I didn't get to sing. Instead, I had a grand mal seizure on the stage." That debacle brought her out-of-state bookings to an end, as she became aware of the risks.

"In the building where I used to live, there was a little girl who had been abused by her mother and was in her father's custody. I took her to gymnastics practice every week, spent as much time with her as I could. I guess I was kind of like a surrogate mom for her—that's what her father said to me. They made a place for me in their family. And of course, I would entertain and watch over all the little kids in the neighborhood—it was like a group." She seemed to enjoy being the children's "guardian angel," but was surprised and frightened when the father came on to her one day, and only gradually recognized that this situation could place her in some personal danger should the children's estranged mother appear. When she recognized the risks inherent in the situation, she gracefully distanced herself from the family without abandoning them.

Does she see herself as a role model? "Yes. It means pressure to me. I've taken on that role, speaking, and being on TV and in newspapers and being in the public eye. I realize that I can't fail. The head-injured community is counting on me and God's counting on me. I *can't* fail.

"In 2003 I began working with [a local program for troubled teens]. I created a program for pro athletes to visit, teach the kids to play the athlete's sport. They asked me to share my testimony, and the girls really appreciated the singing. We just really bonded. It's neat for them to see an older girl who's a survivor. I'd love to work there. They made me their public relations chairperson for their 20th anniversary gala.

"Last Friday I volunteered to visit a classroom full of autistic kids. It was wonderful—so rewarding, so scary. I got to spend one-on-one time with each one. It was exhausting, trying to keep up my energy to connect with them. But it was easy to make the connection. This little girl, Autumn, came and curled up in my lap. I thought it was the cutest thing in the world. She was on her way home, and she came running back in to the classroom to give me a hug. And I looked at the teacher, and said, 'You've got me Friday.' I got them tickets, and I'm chaperoning them for a day at the theme parks."

"I hope to complete psychotherapy as the last step of my self-repair work. Thanks to the brain injury I decided to deal with some of the scary aspects of my past to achieve the life I really believe God wants for me. I also read inspirational or psychological self-help books. I have to face some difficult truths about myself, and I will."

6. Methods of Recovery

"There is an upside and there is a downside to my injury and you have to look at both. Being brain injured rules my life. Life is harder. It's harder to cope with things like relationships, vocations, and family. It's harder to be accepted for who I am. It's harder to master relationships, at least to the point where I'm bearable.

"The single most important strategy for my recovery is the Error Analysis (EA) (see p. 55). That's what protects me from doing head-injured things. I've memorized the form. I write it on a napkin, on a placemat, or do it verbally in conversation with a friend. There is no other way to handle this injury—nothing else works. Then, when I know what I should do, the next time I'm in that situation, I sound a warning to myself. 'Watch out!' I mentally sound warnings a lot. Those will keep you from repeating stupid mistakes—the result of doing an EA. Like when I buy something I think of buying that SUV. Sometimes I don't do an EA when I should—it's not always convenient—that doesn't mean that it's right. When I've made the same screw-up three times in a single day, I tell myself I could have done an EA and that would have taken care of it. I'll keep making mistakes and I'll keep catching them. Keep your radar on, be humble and say, 'That was a brain-injured mistake' and don't let yourself make any excuses. The day you become prideful is the day you let things slide by and don't learn from them.

"When I need to do something complicated or important, I use the planning algorithm. 'Goal-plan-anticipate.' It's easy to remember. I ask for a lot of advice, and a lot of feedback. My therapy group has had my back. You need someone vocally to tell you, you're screwing up. There will always be more things for me to learn about my injury. I haven't stopped making mistakes yet, and I don't think that's going to happen any time soon.

"Sometimes I want to be the old me so bad, and I've got to accept that I'm not. I don't have the big social life I used to have, but then, when I think about it, how plastic and unreal that life was, how shallow it was, so do I really miss it? I miss being able to do gymnastic routines down the hallway at work. A prideful thing—something to show off. When I think through everything, there's not that much of the old Faith I truly miss.

"But I have had the chance to let go of old dreams, a chance to make new dreams and strengthen personal relationships with God and family and friends. I share what I have when I go to schools or meetings to tell my story. We all have our own silent epidemic; mine is a brain disorder, while someone else's may be an eating disorder or something else.

"The injury has made me a stronger and deeper person. Stronger because you don't know what you can really handle until you find out that you can cope with being in over your head. You have to accept compensation strategies, you have to acknowledge the professionals, and when you think you can't handle any more, then you get seizures or lose your best friend, and then you realize that God hasn't given you more than you can handle. You realize you're not this weak little girl anymore. My character's stronger, my faith is stronger. Even though I feel weak at times, I know my strength is there.

"I feel that the new me is so much better than the old me. I love people more than I ever did before. I totally feel people's pain. There's a man in our church that's going through depression. And we were just praying, and I put my hand on his back. I was like, 'I'll take his pain. I don't want him to go through this.' And I just started bawling. It was as if I could feel what it was like to be completely depressed, where medication wasn't helping him. And that broke my heart.

"What I want people to learn would be that you can get through it. That you need to participate in a group to receive that support. Just like alcoholics have that support so they don't continue to drink, brain-injured people need that support so they continue to work on their recovery, continue to try to make their recovery be almost like a religion in their life. And the second thing that I want people to learn is that when others don't help you or let you down, one hand has reached out to me every single time and has picked me up every time I've fallen. And that is God, that's my relationship with God. That's important to me because that's who I am, that gives me the strength to keep going. Sometimes I just need to go to church. It doesn't matter what church it is. It's like a safe haven for me. At home I have a special place of worship on my patio. I go out there to sit and talk with Him, sometimes for hours. Whenever I need Him, He's always there—to love, comfort, reassure, get me through a situation. I just have to remember to reach out for His hand. And I don't always remember to do that, especially when I need it the most. That's one way I'm still working on my relationship with Him—to remember to turn to him when I'm hurting.

"My injury was in His plan for me. Because who I am now is definitely better and will become still better than the person I was before. He has helped me to get closer to Him, and to live the life He really wanted me to live, which in a broader way is helping others, for His glory. The story continues to evolve, and it was all because I had that injury. I just have to be patient."

The Journalistic Perspective

Faith is thin but athletic. Her wounds are subtle, her symptoms hard to identify. The even features of a former beauty queen are still there, but years of doubt and frustration have left their marks. Her blue eyes are framed by a few premature wrinkles. Her shoulder-length blond hair, usually parted down the middle, now obscures the surgery scar on the side of her head. Perhaps her greatest stigma is that she doesn't look like the survivor of a traumatic accident. People she meets think she's normal. She's not. She explains that her short-term memory is virtually gone. Trying to recall appointments made in the past half-hour is like shaking hands with a ghost. She writes notes on her hands. Her purse has several alarms in it. She lays out her clothes the same way every day. At home, she can't turn a corner without seeing a Post-It note she has no memory of writing, reminding her of something she doesn't recall being asked to do. She carries a large portfolio with her everywhere, from home to church to her job as community liaison. She calls the portfolio her "brain," as if to make up for the one that no longer works right. There, she records everything: appointments, meals, prayers, even her quiet time.

The old Faith was everyone's friend, everyone's sweetheart, everyone's helper or confidante. She always knew the right thing to say. The new Faith can lose her "feel" for people, and with it, control of her social interactions. One morning she suddenly blurted out, "(expletive) off!" in the middle of an innocent conversation with a coworker. Later, she had no idea why that woman turned cold toward her. Her every remark may cost her another friend, leaving her puzzled about what went wrong. These outbursts have strained friendships and killed romances. Worse still, people find her behavior rude and insensitive, as if she didn't mind hurting their feelings. She does—she minds it a great deal. What they don't realize is that her damaged brain can't translate her good intentions into good words any more. The inevitable rejection makes her feel "like a leper, looking good on the outside, yet degraded, less than human." She has been sentenced to a life of struggle, able to look and act normal at times, but not able to keep it up.

The Neuropsychological Perspective

Although Faith's injury was from an indoor fall, it involved unusually high impact forces. She had been standing on her partner's upraised hand when he propelled her upward, and she executed a combination of spinning and twisting maneuvers. Her partner reported that he did not recall the precise events of the fall, but thought that she spun out of his grasp, and believed that both his attempt to grab her and her attempt to right herself might have accelerated the fall. When she struck the concrete surface with the right convexity, her body was still rotating. The skull's impact was so loud that she may have swung her head around toward the floor when she struck it. The force of impact produced a burst temporal lobe, rupturing part of the middle cerebral artery. It also produced bruising and edema on her lateral scalp and face. In most cases, this is a fatal injury. A paramedical team was on site to serve the competitors, and she was taken directly to the nearby level one trauma center. En route, the neurosurgeon was contacted and he took her to surgery immediately upon arrival. She was rated at Glasgow Coma Scale level 3 at admission.

This injury produced a subdural hematoma. This was evacuated, and the shredded temporal lobe tissue was surgically removed down to the lacerated artery, including the right hippocampus, in two surgical procedures. The underlying cortex may have sustained some pressure necrosis from recurrence of the hematoma on day 2. There was also intraventricular hemorrhage into the right lateral ventricle. The neurosurgeon also reported a large area of contusion and edema in the right temporo-parieto-occipital junction. As noted above, there was significant diffuse trauma, with 8 days of coma in the context of a rotational injury.

Neuropsychological testing indicated rapid recovery from the acute effects of injury, with normal focal attention, and near-normal performance on WAIS-R subtests and the Gates-McGinitie Reading Comprehension Test. She had some relatively serious difficulties with verbal learning and recall, both for narrative and for word-list information, as well as the expected problems with deliberate and incidental recall of nonverbal information. Her most obvious quantitative deficits were elicited by the most complex and difficult tests, where she showed periods of confusion, perseveration, disorganization, and inefficiency. Qualitatively, she showed substantial difficulties from emotional interference with concentration and off-task behavior, as well as many careless errors. In addition, she had transient difficulty with oversensitivity to auditory stimuli until she began to wear industrial earplugs, and a similar problem with oversensitivity to bright lights and distracting visual stimuli. When she became emotional, she often lost her task set altogether in acute rehabilitation, although this problem resolved well in post-acute therapy after being made the focus of self-therapy goals.

The neuropsychological treatment strategy was founded on a strong therapeutic alliance providing dependable assistance to solve many ongoing psychosocial problems with her family, friends, and love interests. Therapy was structured so that she received more powerful accolades and accomplishments from accepting insights than from rejecting them. This approach channeled her competitive fervor into rehabilitation achievements: She embraced the challenge to become the most outstanding program member, and consequently attained unprecedented gains for this kind of focal injury (see cases of this focal injury in Chapter Three). The most difficult treatment issue was prevention of social conflicts and gaffes. No amount of preparation proved sufficient to protect against problem behaviors and the deterioration of relationships. She did succeed in recognizing the neurologic nature of these problems more quickly, and in learning to use repair strategies to correct many instances of miscommunication and misunderstanding. However, the compensation process was incomplete and remained a functional problem on a long-term basis.

The onset of seizure disorder produced symptoms of posttraumatic stress. Education and supportive therapy were used to normalize her expectations. Relaxation therapy was employed to restore her sense of control over her post-ictal condition. She made rapid improvement and became able to tolerate her occasional seizures. After much adjustment of her anticonvulsant regimen, nearly complete seizure control was achieved in the 3rd year of the disorder.

Her record keeping after returning to work was outstanding. In addition to an unusually precise, cross-indexed daily scheduling system, she also kept narrative notes of key issues in her work activities, including a list of preprepared questions she posed at the outset of each follow-up rehabilitation psychotherapy session. She used the feedback from her cognitive therapy and psychotherapy sessions to more precisely target her deficit areas over time, such that by the time she had been back to work for 6 months she was consistently targeting and correctly interpreting the primary symptoms of neuropsychological interest.

Of 52 patients with right parietal focal damage, Faith was only one of two with fair or good recovery in all functional areas. She developed new assets to compensate her employer for her difficulties in coworker and supervisor relationships. She developed new friends, avocational involvements, and romantic interests at a pace approximating that at which she lost them. Because her eventual acceptance of insight and her implementation of compensations exceed that of any other patient treated for this condition, her outcome suggests that nonverbal, perceptually based behavior problems can be actively managed, if not eliminated, through diligent self-therapy.

Chapter 9

The Story of Rachel

Rachel was subjected to a vicious assault in her workplace which could well have killed her. Throughout the uphill battle of rehab, she remained determined to get back to her job as a psychotherapist and to return to that very workplace. Massive bifrontal contusions, severe diffuse injury, many cognitive deficits, the fact that her employer had hired someone else into her job—she would not allow any of it to stop her from getting back the job she loved.

1. The Old Rachel

"My dad is kind of my shining star. I've always been daddy's little girl. He taught me about toughness: I had to watch him go through hell with a triple bypass surgery, knowing he died on the table, that strong, vital, powerful man lying helpless in a hospital bed. I watched him struggle and come back tenfold. I always had the determination and drive he had, and that's how I made it through school. He egged me on more and more: 'You're doing something nobody else in the family has been able to do!'

"I'm a person who always wanted to succeed, wanted to be better than the rest. I always had clearly established life goals. I knew what I wanted, knew how to get it, and went after it full force. I was always interested in improving myself, both personally and professionally. I was extremely independent. I had my own way to go about things, and was usually successful with it. I was always adventurous and a thrill-seeker. Rafting and skydiving were two big passions. I was training in kickboxing, a form of karate. I'd probably do anything that was proposed to me—I make an effort to try anything at least once. I'm always a take-charge person, an in-charge person. It's helped me to take charge of my brain injury.

"I decided on a career in mental health when I was a sophomore in high school. Graduate school in social work was tedious and grueling for me—extremely hard work. I got straight As, except for a B in a course in research—that was a struggle! I was supporting myself, so I had to attend classes part-time, while everybody else went full-time. Because I was in school for 4 years, I got to take twice the number of internships that the others got, which provided me with excellent training. I knew I was destined to work with children, adolescents, and families—that's where my heart and spirit were—and I had been working in that field for 2 years when I was injured. My job at the time was with Teen Xpress, counseling underprivileged middle- and high-school students at their schools. I had to deal with more issues than I can list, and had to be quick on my feet. I tried to give them the stability that many of them did not get elsewhere."

2. The Accident—4 Years Ago

"My only memories of that day had to do with getting ready for work. I was the first to arrive at work. While I was unloading my car, I was approached by a panhandler. Somehow, he got into the office and assaulted me. The police tell me that they found a number of wounds on him, so I must have tried to defend myself."

3. The Injury

Her coworkers found Rachel barely conscious, her clothes torn and her face so badly bruised, bloodied and swollen that they could recognize her only by her curly hair. There was blood everywhere. She had been beaten savagely, struck so hard in the forehead that her frontal bone was fractured. The frontal bone is so thick and hard that it is virtually unbreakable. Her nose was broken, the bones around her eyes were crushed, and her optic nerves were affected. Her frontal lobes were both damaged, as well as her right temporal lobe. The right frontal lobe had a large contused area. Much of the cortex was surrounded by blood (a subarachnoid hemorrhage). She remained in coma for 16 days, and reported PTA of 41 days.

4. Early Recovery

When Rachel was transferred to inpatient rehab, it became obvious that she had experienced a terrible injury, and would have a long road of recovery. Like most frontal lobe patients, she was out of control. She spent many hours yelling for help, and cursing, at the top of her lungs. It took several days for her to settle down enough to be able to carry on a conversation. There was little reason to hold a conversation with her, because she remained in post-traumatic amnesia for quite awhile.

At this writing, she has few memories of her inpatient stay, and cannot remember much from outpatient therapy. "It feels like there's 6 months of my life gone. I was going in and out of coma, it was Father's Day, and my dad was singing the Eagles' song, 'Take it Easy.' He got stuck on a lyric and I sat up and sang the rest of it with him— it was a bonding moment for us. When I came to and helped him finish the song, he knew I was going to come out of the coma. He said it was the best Father's Day present ever. After the song, I said, 'I love you, daddy.'"

Like many post-coma patients, she constructed false memories to replace the information missing from the gap in her life story. "My best friend and her husband visited when I was in the hospital. They had been living in Chicago. I fully believed that I had lived in Chicago for a year, to the point of constructing memories of my life and my job there as a therapist who accompanied ambulances to accident sites. I told this story again and again, and they said I was so convincing that even my parents were tempted to believe me.

"I was forgetting to pick out my meals for the day, and putting on my shoes but not tying them—the nurses getting on me—and I realized that there must be something wrong with me. It came to a head in occupational therapy. The therapist gave me feedback that I was kind of slow functioning. I keep remembering, 'This is bulls____ —I can do this.' There's denial for you. On my bulletin board a card said, 'Aunt Rachel, get well!'—if my 3-year-old nephew knew something was wrong with me, I figured there must be.

"I questioned and asked my parents a million times about when I was getting out. Every time they left the hospital and said they would be back, I interpreted it that they would come back to take me home. Five or six times, I had it in my head that I was about to go home and had completely packed my belongings. My friends had to help me unpack again and again.

"I don't think I fully realized why I was there until I was being discharged. Then they confronted me with all my restraints: I couldn't go home, had to live in an apartment with my parents, with home nurse care, not allowed to drive, can't go to work—that said to me that I had lost my independence and my ability to do anything, and somebody else had to care for me. I hated that—having to live with my parents. I was ashamed of it, and it robbed my confidence and self-esteem. It bothered me to no end to have to be a 10-year-old again. It got to the point where I was questioning how old I was."

Operating on bad advice from the family attorney, Rachel's parents had her declared incompetent by a court. Although this is a routine procedure for demented patients, it is never done this early in head injury and is rarely necessary. Someone in Rachel's condition becomes competent again long before you can get the court to restore her rights. Unfortunately, they ignored our advice, and the results were traumatic for her. "I hated when my parents had me declared incompetent. I wanted to tell everybody where to go. It was like everything all at once—my driver's license, my home, and my life taken away from me, and then being declared incompetent. I couldn't even write my own checks or take money out of my bank account. That was what proved to me that I had lost my independence. I knew all the stupid red tape it would take to get my rights back, but it dragged on and on. 'Why is this s___ taking so long?' Somebody telling me I'm not capable to drive, or take care of myself—it boiled over to make me feel so incompetent. I ran off the mouth with my resentment and had huge attitude. Words cannot express how much I loathed sitting around the apartment my parents rented for us, waiting for dumb soap operas to come on. I was stuck—I couldn't go anywhere or do anything! I stayed with my parents for a month and a half, and then went back to my place. I wasn't restored to competency until the end of January of 2002, about 4 months after I got out of therapy.

Just before the meeting to discuss her intake evaluation results, it was explained to Rachel that her injury was very serious. She asked how it would affect her career, and she was told that her injury was so severe that there was no precedent for recovering to hold such a high-responsibility job as psychotherapist. She acknowledged that there were other kinds of social work that demanded less thinking on your feet, but she was not interested in being a case worker. She would not be satisfied with anything short of a return to her old career doing psychotherapy. This attitude is commonplace in early recovery and usually it's a formula for disaster, because most patients can never again perform at their old level. But given how hard she had worked to get her MSW, it seemed that she might have enough motivation for an exceptional recovery. She was told that only an exceptional recovery would accomplish her goal, and that as long as she progressed toward one, her goals would be supported by the staff.

"After that meeting, I was very pissed off. I went home and I cried. '[They don't] know anything about me and how hard I've tried and what I've studied and there's no way anyone is going to tell me that I can't do what I've sacrificed everything for.' I planned to come back and show [them] how wrong [they were]." This event marked the beginning of her fight to achieve her goal. Nevertheless, this insight into her damaged prospects for the future was painful: "During this thing I went home every night and cried myself to sleep, thinking what the hell else can I do with myself. I was feeling like everything and everyone was defeating me in my purpose." Yet she put on a calm face in therapy and refused to show any upset in public. "I was not a truly emotional person. I only let my feelings come out when it was safe. I was guarded about emotions. I wish I could keep everything inside now but I can't.

"Outpatient was stupid to me. The meeting in the beginning where my parents and I got the evaluation results and I had to tape it and type up the transcript forced more realization of what was wrong with me. I tried not to accept it. It seemed almost like I was watching a movie about somebody else, not about me. I was in complete denial that the test results were really true for me: 'If I have so much wrong with me, why aren't I feeling it?' I remember a fellow patient— a guy—and I thought, 'Why am I in with this guy? He's really screwed up.' But then I would screw up on little daily things around my parents and think to myself, 'Maybe that was part of it.' Those brain error moments that we had to write out (Error Analysis), I felt like I had a lot of those sometimes. With my determined personality to get things done and a perfectionist attitude, I got aggravated when people did better than me on assignments. It made me try harder—try my [expletive] off—because I wasn't going to let anybody one-up me."

"At the end of outpatient, I was able to move home. I felt I was gaining myself back. I felt more confident. My roommate took me out driving when she wasn't supposed to have. My vision was still pretty impaired. [It was] like looking at the world with a pair of pantyhose over my head. That's pretty close. Actually, I was scared s___less to start driving. But it helped immensely to go for a drive and not run into anything. My confidence also grew from getting good at the therapies. Even in Contextual Processing, I really started to get it at the end. I knew it was the hardest therapy they had. It wasn't so bad. I would play Taboo [a game used in therapy] with my roommate or a friend and now I'm damn good at that game.

"The whole thing was a totally hateful experience. A year and a half of my life completely sucked."

5. Accomplishments of Recovery

"The first one is being able to be in my house by myself and fix my own damn food the way I wanted to. I could get on my bike and go to the store, because I still couldn't use my car. I despised the driving service. I thought, 'I can drive.' Of course, my vision still isn't perfect. I feel after I started driving legally it was my way of practicing my vision more. Also I did a lot of reading to practice my vision. Remember that stupid little eyepatch? I still have it."

The recovery period was afflicted by added burdens from her personal life. Her grandmother committed suicide. Her best friend and her best friend's husband from Chicago both died—he shot her and then killed himself. And when these things happened, she didn't have her work in which to immerse her mind. "I thought about them day in and day out." With the help of her friends, Rachel worked on grieving each of her losses.

Another ordeal involved confronting the man who assaulted her and participating in his trial. It took the police many weeks to find him, during which time she and her parents had some concern that he might come after her. Finally, they found him through a DNA sample. He was a homeless, rootless career criminal with a history of violent assaults. "It was an extremely grueling part of my life—waiting through seven postponements and subpoenas, and having to relive the fear and concern each time it was supposed to go to trial. They allowed me to make a statement to the court at his sentencing hearing. It was a very emotional experience for me."

She kept her end of our bargain about achieving an exceptional recovery. She conquered every challenge we threw her in the program. When she was ready to graduate, the team endorsed her return to work, with the proviso that she receive supervision by a clinician who knew about her head injury for at least 3 months or until she was cleared. At this point, the administrators of her department became the obstacle. They attempted to discharge her, and backed off only after we sent strongly worded letters documenting that she would be able to return to her job. They had reorganized her program, and the new boss hired someone to fill her position. When she reported for work, he tried to convince her to switch to a program for AIDS patients, but of course Rachel would have none of that. "Finally after some threats from my dad, they decided to let me go back to my old job by creating an extra position." She received and passed her supervision.

Rachel had to adapt to a number of cognitive deficits to work as a therapist. When she did so, she didn't actually tell herself that she was doing self-therapy. She still doesn't always anticipate the deficits that affect her therapy. However, she is so committed to the quality of her work that when she bumps into cognitive problems she sets about fixing them, using the approaches trained in her rehab: "Sometimes I get to feeling overwhelmed during sessions and my mind blanks out. I use a technique called reflection, which allows me the time I need to pick up the thread of my thoughts where my mind got off track. To keep myself from blurting out things I wouldn't want to say, I guess I say less now and think about it more. My biggest problem is forgetting what's been talked about in the session. I now take much more detailed notes during the session than I did before. After the session, my progress notes are also more thorough, which I use to review what we talked about before the next session. If I think of an intervention I want to use later in the session, I'll jot that down on my note pad to make sure I remember to do it. I used to have back-to-back-to-back sessions, but now I usually give myself time to absorb what happened in the last session. Sometimes it's crunch time and I still have to go back-to-back-to-back. A couple weeks ago, I confused what one girl said with what the next girl said. I said to myself, 'That was a big brain fart!' and decided that I can't push myself that far. So I'm still wrestling with my limitations. Overall I feel a little less effective than I was before. That's why I'm always striving to learn new techniques to expand upon what I do."

After getting an MSW, a social worker needs 2 years of full-time, supervised experience to become eligible to take the LCSW (licensing) test, and Rachel had completed only about 1 year of supervision when she had her injury. So during her return to work, "I also had to have supervisory sessions for my license." When she had enough hours, she took the computerized licensure exam. "I studied for it like I would have done pre-brain-injury—by reviewing, reviewing, reviewing—just reading the same stuff over and over again without making any notes. When I took the test, I recognized a lot of stuff, but I couldn't pull back the information I needed. I failed it by four or five points. I wanted to pick up the computer and throw it. I was cussing out the computer in my head—it was the computer's fault. I got upset. I cried in the car. Then I started second-guessing myself, I'm not ready to be licensed yet. It only took a couple of days for me to pick myself up and say, 'I'm doin' it again, and I'm passing it this time!' I realized that I hadn't studied right. I had never gotten the study manuals for the test. The second time I made sure I got those. There was a class I took on test-taking strategies for the LCSW. This time, I took written notes, anticipated the questions they might ask, and tested myself on them over and over, as they trained me in rehab to do. I wrote out lots of note cards (flash cards) for every question. I memorized the stuff. When I took it the second time, I took off extra time from work to spend full days studying. My emotions came into it more, because I severely stressed out and I broke out in hives, and I thought I was going to drive myself mad studying. But I passed it the second time. When I got my score, I threw my hands in the air in victory—I think the other people in the room thought I'd gone nuts!

"The therapists said that after brain injuries, relationships tend to break up, and most patients can't form a new one—so those needs go unmet. I didn't accept that limitation. Although I didn't throw myself into dating at first, the idea that I supposedly couldn't succeed at it stuck in my craw. Then I had a few lousy dates. At that point, about 2 years after I was back home and with my life back on track, I came to the realization that my options for meeting a mate sucked. So I tried on-line dating, the kind where you take a personality test. That's how my fiancé and I met. After some e-mails and phone conversations, we got to the point of meeting face-to-face. I checked him out up and down. A friend who works for the police ran a background check for me. I had my guard way up, determined not to let him in until I fully knew he was the one for me. I found out he had a teenage daughter. A former relationship with a guy who had a teenage daughter—he hurt me bad. That made me even more careful this time. But he proved himself to me, in many ways. It turned out that he had been a single father raising his little girl by himself since she was 3 months old. He has a romantic streak: He proposed to me on Valentine's Day. First he went to my parents' house the night before, asked my dad for my hand, then he had this whole evening set up for us. We went to this restaurant, and as we left, in this beautiful setting, he got down on his knees, asked for my hand, and handed me a rose. I asked him what the rose was for because I didn't see the little box attached to it—there was a ring inside. I wouldn't agree to marry him until he told me whether his daughter had given him an OK. But she was thrilled at the idea— she and I have a good connection. So I said yes.

"My short-term memory deficit has created some problems in my relationships with him and with her. He has diarrhea of the mouth and he'll load me up with all kinds of information and expect me to remember—we used to have arguments about that. And my 13-year-old keeps saying, 'I told you about that,' or 'I asked you about that and you said . . . ' She talks constantly, and I'm supposed to remember all this s___. She takes it badly if I don't remember. But I can't remember s___. Since getting back together to participate in GiveBack, I've been thinking about my injury a lot more. I realized that although I mentioned the injury, I never really explained to my fiancé in detail what's wrong with me. So we had a long talk about it. Now he seems to understand better, and is more respectful to me. With the 13-year-old, I tell her that she'll have to tell me at the time what she needs me to know, and not expect me to remember."

Asked whether she and her guy had run into any problems with give-and-take, she commented, "My fiancé and I have had a million arguments about it. I don't remember all the things he does and I do remember everything I do. It's smoothing out lately. I'm seeing a therapist, someone I had worked with before, to help out with relationship issues. She suggested that we schedule a regular family meeting to air issues. I think that's good idea." He has given her free rein to discipline his daughter as she sees fit. "With a teenager, it's difficult with my coming in so late in her life, she has adjusted and accepted it. I'm tougher than he is, and notice a hell of a lot more than he does. I think it helps her that I've befriended her, but never to the point of giving up the authoritative position."

6. Methods of Recovery

"I continue to learn more about my injury since getting out of outpatient. I see little quirks, little brain-injury moments that I keep having and that I'm sure will continue. The challenge is there for me to fix each one and fix it right because I'm a perfectionist. Sometimes the first fix I try doesn't work, but I don't quit tinkering with it until I get it right. If it's something I can't fix until the situation comes up again, I write down what I did wrong to remind me when I revisit it to figure out a different way to handle it. I write down the failed actions so I won't repeat them. When I do therapy, I concentrate so hard to keep total control of my thoughts that I'm extremely tired at the end of a session. I notice that after I've been with kids all day I'm terribly drained and exhausted, and then I have to go home to deal with another one. I've arranged for a time-out time right after I get home— I need it.

"Things have happened at the job that make me want to cry. I have to remove myself from the situation, take a time out, to get back in control before the emotions spill out. Sometimes I'm sarcastic and it comes out whether I intended to or not. I either go to the bathroom or go into the counseling room and shut the door.

"I've proved that I can accomplish what I set my mind to. I put my heart and soul into everything I do. I know I have to figure out ways to do things differently if I'm going to do them better. I can do self-rehab. The biggest thing I see myself faulting on is short-term memory, especially when there's too much information coming in at once."

Until recently, Rachel has not thought of herself as a person with a head injury, nor has she admitted that she dwells in a different world from the one in which she grew up. But that is changing right now. "I'm beginning to come to live in the Head Injury World, but I'm not fully ready yet." For many survivors, 4 years is not long enough to make peace with the injury.

"I've always been a religious person—as a child and teenager I was involved with the church. In my late teens and early adulthood, I had no involvement. I'm not sure if it had anything to do with being head injured, but now I go to church with my fiancé and his daughter. I'm more spiritual than religious. I've always believed that there is some sort of higher being that is directing our lives and throws at us only what they know we can take. God didn't throw anything at me that I couldn't handle."

Has she become tougher since she had the injury? "Oh, yeah. I'm much more aware of my surroundings, the people in my life, the events in other peoples' lives. The cautious side of me is now more hyper-cautious. I think I'm stronger now than I was back then. I think I earned a PhD, master's degree, and bachelor's in character. Going through this has also taught me a great deal about how traumatic my clients' experiences might have been for them. I've discovered an amazing strength inside of myself. I wouldn't have imagined that the old Rachel could have handled this."

Asked if she would like to be the old Rachel again, her immediate answer was, "No. I'm happy with who I am. For a long time I wasn't. I'm extremely glad about who I've become, and what I've gained in the meantime. I'm always looking to better myself, to promote myself, and I see this as just a part of the process: To learn from my deficiencies and strive for something bigger and better. I'm proud of myself."

The Journalistic Perspective

Rachel hated the fuss we were making over her. She hated the prospect of helping in the development of GiveBack, although for reasons of conscience she could not turn it down. Getting her to think about being brain injured was like pulling teeth.

Rachel is a bright-eyed, assertive woman with black curls cascading over each shoulder. She dresses in aggressively casual garb. There is no mistaking her for anything but a professional woman, but at the same time, she takes her nontraditional role as a mental health psychotherapist seriously and avoids any appearance that might suggest a business career. Rachel tries so hard to be certain, outspoken, and ready to respond to anything that she occasionally gets caught with her transmission in neutral and her mouth halfway open. When this happens, she shakes herself bodily, as if trying to snap herself out of it. She is always trying her hardest to put distance between her injury and herself and never gaining an inch. This could go on for many years.

The Neuropsychological Perspective

Rachel was admitted to the hospital at Glasgow Coma Scale level 3. She presented with a severe, focal frontal injury, with extremely poor impulse control, marked inflexibility, unrestrained emotionality, and a tendency to rush through every task. In addition, she was adamant that she had no cognitive deficits as an inpatient, insisting that she was going back to work as soon as she left the hospital. She continued in this aggressive stance when she was interviewed for her outpatient intake evaluation. The only arrangement under which she agreed to the evaluation was a challenge. Warned that her injury was too severe to permit her to work on an ethical basis, she backed off one step. Although she made it clear that she disagreed with the evaluation, she was willing to submit to the objective test results as the deciding factor in the decision about entering the program. It was also noted that she became silent for extended periods of time during this interview, a behavior she later explained as due to her angry unwillingness to continue. Her speech showed notably poor emotional expression (expressive dysprosodia).

Testing was administered relatively late because of early medical complications. The tests were given at 11 to 12 weeks post-onset. A number of dysexecutive behaviors reduced her scores on a variety of non-executive tests. For example, she frequently delayed starting timed tasks. She became engaged in making erasures during timed tasks. She frequently became frustrated and ventilated her emotions while performing the testing tasks. She also demonstrated a discouraged attitude, frequently criticizing her own performance excessively or voicing an expectation to fail before undertaking a task. She tended to get stuck on a thought or a theme (ideational perseveration), to violate instructions telling her to avoid doing something, and to become disorganized as tasks grew more complex. For example, her performance dropped sharply when she moved from using one hand to using two hands for the same task. She also made frequent errors on building tasks by virtue of turning the pieces in the wrong direction, and occasionally built things that had the wrong overall shape, both of these behaviors serving as evidence of a nonverbal perceptual integration problem (Schutz, 2005a).

Basic focal attention and working memory scores were within expected limits, indicating a good early recovery and readiness for cognitive rehabilitation. Scores directly indicative of executive dysfunction (mazes, word fluency) were found in the profound range of impairment. Speed of processing was generally in the severely or profoundly impaired range, insufficient for driving safety. Quantitative measures of high-level perception were moderately to profoundly impaired, confirming the compromise of nonverbal perceptual processing. Her recall for verbal passages was moderately impaired in the immediate condition and moderately to severely impaired in the delayed condition. Although her test performance in recalling nonverbal information was variable, it was felt that her basic impairment was no worse than mild in this area. A complex problem solving task (the Category Test) elicited heroic effort and a score that was only in the borderline range, but this remained an area of concern for a crisis psychotherapist. Her psychological testing was marked by defensiveness and a tendency to passive-aggressive personality of the negativistic subtype.

These test scores were extremely discouraging to her vocational aspirations. It was truly difficult to imagine an individual with such serious, enduring executive deficits, as well as acquired impairment of interpersonal perception, would be able to resume a career as a psychotherapist. In cognitive rehabilitation, she was closely and stringently tutored to develop effective self-monitoring, and with her high level of motivation, she performed exceptionally well in learning to recognize her mistakes. This progress confronted her with ongoing evidence of her deficits, which was both upsetting and frustrating for her. Her only recourse was to master the use compensation strategies, to make the confrontation with her deficits less uncomfortable.

High-achieving, dominant personalities have the courage and commitment required for excellent recoveries, but they often find it hard to accept guidance and direction and to admit their new weaknesses. Their capacity to benefit from rehab often rides on that issue. Rachel probably would have gone on ignoring her cognitive deficits and would have skipped rehab altogether if she could have done so without endangering her career. But in the end it was more important to her to get back to being effective in her work than it was to protect her peace of mind. The process of forcing herself to see the whole picture of her damaged self was painful and protracted, and she continues to think about being impaired only when her mistakes force her to do so. But she could not be the person she needs to be without being completely honest with herself, so she did not stop short of that point. As a self-determining individual, it has also been difficult for her to acknowledge how much she learned from rehabilitation—she is just beginning to voice the realization at this writing.

Collaborating on GiveBack afforded an opportunity to observe her work as a cotherapist. It was clear that she successfully reprogrammed her terribly damaged brain to do effective counseling. Whether listening or speaking, she actively processes events and considers her options with maximum effort and mindfulness. During the counseling process, her mind is continuously occupied with the cognitive tasks of her profession.

Chapter 10

The Story of Abdullah

Abdullah lives in a small California town with a slow, semirural, unsophisticated lifestyle. It is difficult to picture him living there. Abdullah has the most remarkable, eloquent speech, like a Shakespearian actor or an Oxford professor. If this country is a difficult place for Muslims to live at this time, then surely the place he lives is more difficult than most. His life there is a kind of exile, because he cannot practice his profession in his adopted home of Florida. He is unhappy with this life. In fact, he has never stuck this long to anything he disliked so much. However, his commitment to developing his new career requires him to remain where he is.

1. The Old Abdullah

The eldest son of a devout shopkeeper from India, Abdullah grew up in Zimbabwe (the former Rhodesia). He found his family's kind of strict Islam to be difficult and demanding, but he tried to practice it in the best way he could. Abdullah had a keen intelligence and a tendency to question and doubt. Rather than to simply go to mosque and read the Koran as his mother and father did, he developed close relationships with religious scholars and teachers and studied the meaning of his religion in depth. He was a brilliant student, perhaps too much for his own good. He grew up virtually without self-discipline; he never studied and breezed through law school while earning an unfavorable reputation as a sloppy scholar with an attitude. When he got his law degree, no professor would write him a letter of recommendation, so he wound up with the lowest status job as a prosecuting attorney in a small, out-of-the-way province. This work seemed important to him and for the first time he began to give his best efforts to something. Once he learned how the system works, he became successful and rose to a position in a metropolitan office, even arguing before the Supreme Court. Rhodesia had deteriorated politically into a despotic dictatorship, and the unfair way in which the laws were applied bothered him deeply. He decided to emigrate to America, along with members of his family, to become an American lawyer. He applied and was accepted at a California law school program for foreign attorneys. He was living in Orlando with his sister's family and working as a clerical supervisor to earn money for his law school tuition when he had his accident.

2. The Accident—9 Years Ago

While driving, Abdullah was T-boned by a car that ran a stop light and struck the driver's side of his car. No witnesses were available to provide any other details of the accident.

3. The Injury

Though in coma for only 2 days, he suffered hemorrhagic contusions to both frontal lobes, right greater than left, and contusions to both posterior temporal lobes, as well as a left parietal subdural hematoma. The duration of PTA was 7 days. Testing showed severe organizational and learning deficits. Fortunately, his basic language skills were spared.

4. Early Recovery

"My first memory was the day I woke up and realized I had a brain injury. I was devastated at first. Then I got used to the circumstances, and felt I would be okay in time. And then I went to the inpatient rehab unit and took those tests. And then I realized, 'You're screwed.' I think initially that was my biggest disadvantage. From that point, I felt I was never going to be okay."

The senior author met Abdullah just before he was to be transferred from the inpatient unit to the outpatient program. The staff were gathered around the desk at the nurse's station, tightly packed together. When they cleared away, it became apparent that they had been reading a letter that Abdullah had written to the staff. It was a letter of thanks, gracious and beautifully written, almost poetic, composed at a time when he was still having trouble with simple conversations. The staff was deeply touched by this gesture and talked about it for months afterward.

Abdullah presented himself with great humility, a custom in Islamic cultures, but one that he took to extremes. He referred to himself as "the guy with a dented brain" and "the village idiot." His humility seemed to create a problem at times, because he became passive and self-belittling when he ran into difficulties on his therapy exercises rather than redoubling his efforts to succeed on them. Eventually he agreed that his humility sometimes was a cover-up, and that inside he allowed his pride to get the best of him. Although this was a problem all his life, he began to realize that it might be a bigger problem for him now.

In his written work, he was as sloppy and undisciplined as he had been at university. He did not write down all of his homework assignments, did not complete all of the ones he did write down, and did not put a great deal of thought into the ones he completed. It was clear that he was not attempting to do his best work. He also protested politely against being instructed to use compensations, claiming that he was able to figure out how to complete the activities in his own way. He seemed quietly rebellious in dealing with the key therapist, who tended to give instructions in a no-nonsense, military manner. Nothing that anyone said had a noticeable impact on his underperforming style.

This problem was particularly surprising and concerning in regard to his training in verbal information processing. Abdullah would be relying on these skills to learn American law and take the bar exam, and they were his biggest area of deficit. Yet he did not devote enough time and effort to taking careful notes and studying them in the recommended manner, and the scores he earned were very poor. He was still scoring in the 60% range on passages of only moderate difficulty when he stopped making progress altogether. After many warnings about expecting problems with the bar exam if he did not learn proper study techniques, he continued to underperform and was discharged.

Before he left, we took pains to make sure that he had the recommended procedures clearly written into his notes, and understood that he should keep the notes and refer to them later when he needed them. "I didn't use my strategies particularly well in therapy, but I got the framework, and I tried to use them on my own."

In his discharge meeting, he was told that his neuropsychologist expected him to pass the bar exam, but warned that he would have to improve his self-discipline first. It was predicted that he would flunk the exam until he did so. He was advised to keep taking it even if he flunked it 10 times, because he would eventually give in and prepare properly.

5. Accomplishments of Recovery

He was able to return to his former, clerical job, and after a transition period of part-time employment, shifted to full-time work and full duties. His supervisor's evaluation after 3 months was a glowing report, with no complaints or suggestions. He corresponded with the law school in California and arranged to start his course of study about 6 months after his discharge. He worked throughout the 6 months to save money, and then left for California. He did not have enough money to pay for his courses, but his sister's son regularly sent him money to help pay for them.

"To some extent my going to SF was not calculated—it was a desperation move. I told myself, 'The sooner I prove that I can't do this at all, the sooner I can move on.'"

The bar exam requires memorizing thousands of pages of complicated principles, rules, and important cases. There may be no more difficult test for which to prepare. But his challenge was even tougher: He would be sitting for the California bar, the mother of all bar exams. In addition to the 6 hours of multiple-choice testing that aspiring lawyers have to pass in all states, California requires 2 extra days of essay exams and live skill demonstrations.

At the law school, his intelligence impressed a professor, and she sent him out to take the bar after only a few months of introductory classes. During his preparations he made a careful daily schedule, but he did not use his study techniques. He tried to study by rote learning (reading and rereading the same material), a strategy that doesn't work after a head injury. There was also a problem in his approach to the essay tests—he plunged right in and started writing answers to exam questions impulsively, without stopping to carefully think through each question, consider his options, and organize his answers. He failed his bar exam by a considerable margin.

"I flunked and I was ready to quit. Then two things happened. The biggest booster was when the professor gave me a scholarship. She told me, 'I don't know what was there before your brain injury, but what you've got left is pretty good.' So I decided to make the most of it. She was my biggest cheerleader—gave me a lot of support. She kept telling me, 'You can do this,' even when I didn't believe it. So a lot of my recovery has been to satisfy myself that I'm okay. I'm still a little skeptical about it."

The professor convinced him to go back for a second try at the bar exam 1 year later, still in the midst of his course of study. This time, he made an intense study schedule: start studying at 8:00 a.m., two brief meals, three breaks to say prayers, and finish studying at 10:00 p.m. After analyzing his failure of the first exam with a modified form of the Error Analysis technique, Abdullah decided to purchase study materials to improve his multiple-choice test taking. "This essentially required me to devote my evenings to doing practice questions and answers. I would do 33 to 50 questions, all of them questions I had answered before, whether correctly or incorrectly. I thought by doing this I would learn the law." He passed this section on the bar exam "with an uncommonly high grade. [To prepare for the essay portion], during the daytime, I would go through each subject from start to finish, writing out the relevant rules and principles, hoping thereby to engrave them in my memory. When I tried to recall or recount the rules by themselves, I was unable to do so." Again he tried to use rote learning, and again it did not work. When he took the exam, "some of my essay answers were outstanding, although the remaining ones and the work samples were abysmally poor." He failed again.

While finishing up his course of study, he decided to volunteer to help people with head injuries. He found a support group and arranged for an interview. When he arrived, he was surprised and disappointed in the group. "They weren't even trying to get better. They were wallowing in self-pity. I never expected to see that!" The staff person who interviewed him seemed skeptical about everything. She did not believe that he had a head injury. She could not understand why a law student would want to volunteer for this organization. Abdullah got a little angry with her attitude. After the interview, he was not asked to join the organization.

Five months later, he took the bar exam a third time. Because the total score on his second try was pretty close to the passing level, "I did exactly what I had done before. The grades I received in this [third] attempt were the worst of the lot. I wanted to quit. I was drained, emotionally and mentally." After his spiritual mentor advised him to take the test again, he gave it one last try, more than 4 years after his accident. He did another Error Analysis, deciding to upgrade the strategy for his practice answers by focusing just on what the examiners wanted to read. He also reinforced his studying of the difficult-to-remember principles by writing up notes.

On his fourth try, "I made more effort to be careful, thoughtful, strategic, and less interested in showing off how clever I am or how hard I studied. I was a bit more methodical. I carried that approach through the whole exam. I believed at that point that with God's help I could give them the right answer." When he took the essay exams this time, he changed his strategy considerably. Instead of doing the questions one at a time, he read over all three questions, thought about them, then made very detailed outlines for each, and then set to writing out his answers. Midway through the first answer, double-checking his wording, he caught himself on the wrong track and fixed it. So he planned out his answers five times—reading, outlining, writing, double-checking, and rewriting. When he finished with time to spare, he made little upgrades until the time expired. Looking back on it, he realizes how much more careful he had become: "It was like I was watching myself write this time." And this time he passed. To our knowledge, no one with a severe TBI has ever prepared for and passed a bar exam, let alone the California exam.

It was difficult for Abdullah to find a job. His age worked against him. It is safe to assume that his religion was also a problem. His job search took place about 2 years after 9/11, when Americans with Middle Eastern features were still having difficulty with being allowed to fly on airplanes. After almost 6 months, he was able to secure a job as a public defender in a rural Central California town. His adjustment to his new life was difficult, and continues to challenge him. The town has few people of his faith and limited opportunities for social interaction. Some of his fellow attorneys have invited him to social events, but he declines because the events are scheduled against his evening prayers at the local mosque. For a couple of months, he saw a counselor to receive treatment for depression.

The job started out as a real problem. He had no secretarial help. He had to learn how to organize his preparations for cases. He became disorganized during trials. When he noticed his disorganization, he became upset, which reduced his organization further. He sometimes overlooked obvious strategies or questions that needed to be asked. He wondered if he had lost some of his cases because of these errors. He was not sure that his quality level was below that of the other lawyers in his office, but he was painfully aware that it was less than he had been able to do before. He wondered if he could ever be a decent attorney again. Secretly, he hoped he would get fired, and he even encouraged his supervisor to fire him on one occasion when a case went bad. Gradually, everything improved. He learned how to draw up strategies for his cases on the top sheet of his legal pad, which helped him to stay organized during the trials. He kept his emotions better in check. The quality of his work got better, and his track record of wins and losses improved. He became friendly with one of his coworkers, learned some of the other man's trial strategies, and found them to be useful. In his second year on the job, he seemed more relaxed and more optimistic. He planned to look for a new job in another kind of law and another part of California. The job he is currently doing (litigation—arguing cases at trial) is perhaps the most challenging kind of law for a person with a head injury, because it requires so much thinking on your feet. After he adjusts to his next job, he hopes he will be well enough established to be able to bring the family out to live with him, which was their original plan.

6. Methods of Recovery

Abdullah was reluctant to make any comments about his methods, protesting that he had really not accomplished that much. He felt sure that there must be others more accomplished than he. However, with some prodding, he made the following recommendations about how best to recover: "First of all, you must realize that you are completely out of your depth, that you are broken, that you don't work anymore. As Proust said, the only thing we really pay full attention to in life is illness. You must approach your illness with a single-minded belief that working toward recovery is your only option, realizing that you cannot be one who figures out the cure. You must depend on others to show you the way. Acceptance is the key. Unless you accept what has changed about you, you are stuck on square one." Abdullah admitted that it was difficult for him to let go of being the one in control of his own life when he was in rehabilitation. He struggled to make his own decisions, and only gradually and reluctantly came to the realization that he would have to listen to others and try out what they suggested. "I thank God that I had my accident where I had it, because I needed the help and guidance I received from the doctors and therapists at the hospital I was lucky enough to be taken to. Getting the right medical help is essential. I still don't have all the answers."

"One thing I believe is essential—you cannot do it without family. A song I remember from my youth—you are the wind beneath my wings. My sister and my nephew said whatever you want to do, do it, and we will be there for you. If you want to go to California and study, go. If you want to take the bar exam, go.

"On the job, I try not to rely so much on inspiration. I just try to put things down in advance, so that my plan is written down and I can follow it when I need to, and I don't try to wing it. It's important to sketch out my strategy in advance. To deal with the unexpected, I try to imagine what could go wrong beforehand. I can extrapolate most of the things that could go wrong, and the consequences if it does. That way, I can be prepared.

"I try to learn from my mistakes. The last case I lost, I had assumed certain things. Some of the jurors thought I was a bit too stiff. I thought, okay, I have to be more attuned to how it looks to them. Being the kind of person I am, I always want to be fresh and novel, but sometimes, that is not the best way to get things done. Sometimes you have to get out the old recipe and do it the way you did it before. It's a willingness to say I don't have to be original every time. In other words, worry about the results more than about the means. Remember what you are here for.

"I haven't figured out how to manage my emotions yet. I know there's a problem there, but I can't put my finger on it. I feel like I'm a permanently roiling sea. People think I'm hard and cold, and I say to myself, you should live in my brain for a few minutes. It helps me to try to look beyond the task I am working on and see things in the broader perspective. It's emotionally less expensive when you realize you're not the center of the universe."

Asked if it seems to him as if his brain has fixed itself, rewiring itself so that it functions more normally, he said no. "I have to struggle. You have to make effort. You have to be persistent. You have to try. Even if God puts food in your mouth, you have to chew it. Some effort is required." He was asked how much effort life requires from him now. He looked up, and his eyes misted and he smiled sadly. "Oh, man . . . " He composed himself. "In normal life, few of us really have to go into overdrive. I was always a very lazy chap. I now believe that I can work hard enough to make my life work. Potentially, it doesn't depend solely on me. I'm not the hero of the story. The hero is God."

Abdullah is certain that his religion was at the heart of his recovery. The experience of his injury has taught him to accept the will of Allah in the way that a devout Muslim is obligated to feel. At first, he had difficulty in understanding why it pleased Allah that his life was so trying. He knew that it was his spiritual duty to trust Allah's will, but he struggled to do so. That has changed. "One of our scholars said, whoever imagines that God's kindness is separate from the blows of fate is short-sighted. If you could see God's wisdom, you would not choose to live life any other way than the way He has chosen for you. One of the things my injury taught me is that I am absolutely unable to do anything without God's permission. As humans, all we are is imagination. To actually translate any of that into reality, we are incapable without the help of God. The prophet taught us that there is no power, save God. That phrase is one of the treasures from Paradise. Very often God makes us taste our failures repeatedly until we see this reality. That is what happened to me. We are taught that our inability to comprehend Allah is our comprehension of him. I knew this before my injury in an intellectual sense, but I did not experience it. My injury made me know it in my heart, so that I can now worship God as if I see him right in front of me, with a sense not of belief but of conviction."

He was asked if he would prefer to have lived his life without a head injury. If he could do it all over again, would he have the injury? "Oh, yes. If I could have gotten this understanding in any other way, I would have taken that, certainly. But the way I was living my life, I could not have learned what I needed to learn in any other way. My spiritual advisor told me, 'You worry about your work and let Allah worry about your head injury. Never mind curing your brain injury— Allah can re-create your brain.'"

Abdullah believes that Allah could have fixed his brain good as new in the twinkling of an eye, but He did not do that. He gave Abdullah the power to learn to run his new brain properly. He feels that this task is ongoing—he is still learning how to use it, and he is still not entirely satisfied with how he is making it work. Finally, he continues to feel that he should be doing something to help others who have had head injuries. He plans to find a way to help organize recovery aid for those in his area during the coming year.

The Journalistic Perspective

Abdullah was so gifted at formalized, complex, and artful diction in the Queen's English that he should probably be writing this section in my place. He would undoubtedly describe himself with more eloquence that I can. Abdullah was a study in contradictions—short of stature, humble in dress, and soft spoken, with huge, dark eyes that seemed to take in everything. He often spoke about himself as "the village idiot," but he possessed a gifted mind that effortlessly gave out one apt parable after another. It was not easy to get beyond his formal façade, and his experiences with American prejudice after 9/11 left him cautious. After a while, it became clear that he was deeply embarrassed by his injury and its effects on his competence. He seemed to feel obligated to be as brilliant as he could manage, yet he never seemed brilliant enough to satisfy himself. He had to settle for doing the best he could, and it did not sit very well with him to do that.

The Neuropsychological Perspective

Abdullah was admitted to the trauma center at Glasgow Coma Scale level 3. His intake evaluation for the cognitive program was performed at 5 weeks post-onset. Although he was a cooperative subject, he tended to intrude off-task comments, some of which were tangential. He also made frequent self-disparaging remarks and sighed frequently.

Recovery of focal attention and working memory to within normal limits indicated his readiness for the cognitive program. His reading comprehension and access to his general storehouse of knowledge and word meanings was within normal limits. Key indicators of executive dysfunction (word fluency and mazes) were found in the moderately impaired range. His learning and recall of verbal information was moderately impaired on immediate presentation but severely impaired for delayed recall. Learning and recall for simple, visually presented information was mildly impaired, as was incidental spatial memory. Most measures of processing speed were moderately impaired. On a measure of complex nonverbal problem solving his performance ranged from severely impaired (on the first, dominant hand trial) to moderately impaired (on the second, nondominant hand trial and the third trial, on which both hands are used together). On the relatively demanding Halstead Category Test, his performance was borderline. His normal-range clinical profile on the MMPI-2 and his highly defensive configuration of response bias indices predicted a relatively poor response to rehabilitation.

Had Abdullah been a clerk or a janitor, his prognosis would have been at least fair, although he was old enough to make age a significant negative influence. What made this recovery difficult was the extremely high level of aspiration. His deficits in essential memory and executive functions were daunting obstacles for the study of law.

Treating Abdullah was something of an ordeal for the staff, as no amount of encouragement or criticism could motivate him to make adequate preparations for any of his homework-intensive courses. He did not learn to master the use of the Error Analysis technique because he was unable to recognize sufficient errors, and his extremely respectful family did not feel comfortable in pointing out errors to him. Despite many discussions of the importance of the study skills training procedures for his intended course of study, he never employed the techniques with sufficient effort to meet even the high-school level criteria for learning effectiveness. Ultimately, it became necessary to inform him that the staff expected him to fail his bar exam because of his casual attitude toward preparation. We took pains to make sure that he left with a complete description of the study strategies, and predicted that he would eventually use them in the intended manner when he realized that he could not succeed without them. In this case, the strategy worked.

Chapter 11

The Story of Samantha

Samantha is a person who stands out in a crowd. When she has an opinion, she speaks her mind. If she feels something needs to be done, she does it. If something gets in her way, she deals with it. This is hardly the stereotype of a person disabled by TBI. The challenge for her has been to keep her life organized so that she can do the many things she wants to do successfully.

1. The Old Samantha

At 19, Samantha was a 2nd-year community college student on a full academic/athletic scholarship. She was a leader on her softball team. She lived at home with her parents and younger sister. A willful teenager, she saw a counselor with her mother when she was in high school to work out problems in their relationship. Although she was always a better-than-average student, she was diagnosed with dyslexia (i.e., verbal learning disability) at age 13. She coped with her deficits by tape recording her class lectures and reviewing the tapes at home, taking notes, and by reading textbooks out loud. She was enthusiastic about the value of these strategies. Bright enough to get good grades without needing to do much studying, her main interests were her sports activities, her social life, partying, and country line dancing. Her life was simple and easy, and she lived it one day at a time, with no worries about her future.

2. The Accident—10 Years Ago

A weekend of fun in South Florida ended when she was struck in the head. She had been a passenger seated in a chair on the deck of a speeding cigarette boat when her head was rammed frontally into an overhanging tree limb. The limb was stout enough to shatter her frontal bone, one of the strongest bones in the body, and to fracture several other bones in her face. She was not knocked unconscious, but she was dazed and confused. She was taken to the emergency room of a local hospital, and immediately choppered on to the nearest level one trauma center.

3. The Injury

There was relatively little diffuse injury. When she had arrived at the trauma center, she lapsed into coma and remained comatose for a day and a half. She suffered 2 days of post-traumatic amnesia. However, there was considerable frontal damage. There were contusions on both sides, with a wide, deep contusion and a large blood clot inside of the brain on the right side. There was also a blood clot sitting atop the right frontal area and pressing down (a subdural hematoma). The fractured frontal bone was associated with a cerebrospinal fluid leak.

4. Early Recovery

In the acute hospital, she showed all of the classic behavioral symptoms of a bilateral frontal injury: poor frustration tolerance, irritability, diminished motivation, wandering attention, inflexibility, forgetfulness, and reduced communication. She also lost the sense of smell (anosmia) and had difficulties with balance. "For the first 2 weeks, I went in and out of awareness. My mom would come in and I would know who she was, and then the next time I wouldn't know."

Her memory of inpatient rehabilitation is spotty. "They would tell me to remember 'house, turtle, and brush,' and I would tell them to screw off." She recalls the ride to Orlando with her mother, which took place 1 month after the accident. "I was unhappy about the arrangement—they told me that I couldn't drive, and that I would be stuck in one place 40 hours a week."

Her first memory of the outpatient program is of the intake interview with the senior neuropsychologist. She took an immediate dislike to him as soon as he began to talk about how serious her injury was: "This guy is making a mountain out of a molehill." At the trauma center, she had been told only about how well she was doing (or at least that is all she can recall being told). The idea that she had deficits and limitations came as an unwelcome surprise, and one she did not accept. However, she resolved to do whatever this strange doctor required as quickly as possible until he released her back to her real life.

During this interview, she became visibly irritated whenever her mother corrected or amended her answers. It was obvious that she wanted to represent herself, and that she felt entitled to do so. She also became uncomfortable when her mother described her deficits.

She had taken a full neuropsychological test battery during her hospitalization in South Florida, and she reported many detailed memories from that testing. She remembered doing badly on a decision-making test, and when it was administered to her again, she thought long and hard before giving answers so she could do better on it. This was seen as encouraging evidence of a willingness to use strategies and make extra effort, important ingredients in a good recovery.

She has no recollection of the feedback meeting from her evaluation. "I think I had tuned them out at that point." She recalls arguing with her mother after the meeting. Mom insisted that she enter the program and follow their medical advice completely. "At that point, I needed her to call me out, and she did."

In therapy, Samantha was a self-starter and a hard worker who usually kept her negative thoughts to herself. "They were going to make me earn scores on some 40-year-old Atari game in order to get permission to drive. I thought that was crazy. Then I got my ass handed to me the first two times, and I realized that it was needed. So then I just worked on it until I got it right. I knew I could do it—it was just a matter of when. I told my mother to pick me up an hour late every day so I could put in extra practice on it. As soon as I passed it, I ran out and scheduled my eye-hand coordination test so I could get my license back. I didn't make any effort to remember what they were trying to teach me at that point, I just wanted to get it over with and move on."

She sometimes argued that she did not have the symptoms the testing indicated, particularly impulsivity. During the therapy exercises, she used compensation strategies as instructed, but in a somewhat half-hearted way. On the other hand, she used them vigorously and effectively when she was challenged by the prediction that she would be unsuccessful. With this in mind, the senior neuropsychologist took on the role of the "bad cop" to push and goad her while his junior colleague played the role of the "good cop," offering support and listening to her frustrations.

"I had decided that I was going back to school. I didn't care what the 'big' neuropsychologist said. He said that he wasn't sure I was ready. He told me, 'Brain-injured people set themselves up for failure.' I didn't care what he said. I was still determined to do it. In fact, he just made me more determined. Only later did I realize that he was saying that to light a fire under my ass. I took my last class at community college while I was still in rehab. Passing it was no problem, but then, community college had always been easy for me.

"Then I transferred to the university. I was planning on majoring in accounting. The first semester I took a full load. I took a couple of accounting classes, and they were out-of-control hard. I was also working as an RA. I worked 5 to midnight, 4 days a week. The harder accounting class was the first class I dropped. I got Cs in the other courses. Then I decided I was going to change my major to engineering. I did good in all the math classes, but I had one engineering prof who didn't speak very good English, and that was how I got put on academic probation. I either failed or dropped half of my four courses. At that point, they kicked me out."

The root of the problem was that Samantha was determined to do things her way, using only her old, very basic study skills. "Before the accident I went to all my classes, but I took notes casually, I made no special effort to get everything written down. I didn't read the textbook or study except for cramming, and I was good at cramming. When I went back to school after the injury, I tried to do things the same way. My class notes weren't that well structured—they were all over the place. I'm sure I left out a lot of information. I can't take notes and pay attention to the lecturer. I ended up missing things, not understanding everything they were explaining. That had never happened to me before. I did not go back to tape recording until the end of the second semester, after it was too late. The night before a test, I tried to cram while I was working as an RA and I couldn't finish.

So I would cram some more beginning at midnight. By the time I went in to take the test, I was so tired that I couldn't think. At the end, I tried to read ahead, understand, take notes out of the book, ask questions, see the professor, use flash cards, the whole nine yards, everything the therapists had trained me to do. But by then it was too late."

She identifies failing out of college as the turning point in her recovery. "I had to fail in order to succeed. I learned from it. My attitude had been a barrier to my recovery. I figured I lived through a brush with death—I can do anything. I felt invincible. I went back to partying, driving drunk, not studying, got put on academic probation, and got kicked out of the university.

"At that point, I had moved out of my parents' house. My roommates were party girls. My life was spiraling out of control."

At this point, Samantha began dating a man who was almost 5 years older than she was. A classic "love at first sight" relationship for both of them, she found in him a mature, sensible supporter. When she was with him, she did not drink to excess. He encouraged her to make another run at a university education. She resolved to get her life under control. She got counseling from the junior neuropsychologist in her rehab program for 3 months. "He was the supportive guy. He gave me a hug and talked me into believing that I wasn't the same person I had been before the injury—the same thing I had not been willing to admit in rehab. It was only then that I realized how badly I had needed the rehab. Then I shifted from his support to my boyfriend's. I settled down and backed off of partying. I realized that if I was ever going to get to stay with a guy like that, I would have to get my act together. All of it was a reality check. Six months later I moved in with him, which took me completely out of the partying scene."

5. Accomplishments of Recovery

"When I went back to the community college, I continued applying all my studying strategies. I didn't come home from classes and plunk down on the couch to watch Jerry Springer. I did my studying as I went along, week by week. I partnered up with somebody, too. I borrowed their notes, which gave me two views on things. Then I went back to UCF and went full time. I got straight As from there on out. I finished with a 4.0 after my return.

"I ended up doing an independent study course with two professors. I collected all of the research data myself, and we wrote it up together. It was published in the *Journal of Financial Research*. It compared male and female mutual fund managers. We found out that female managers are more successful at first because they are more careful, but investors prefer to hand their money over to the less successful male managers.

"While I was in school, I also got my real estate license. During the summer, I took a 40-hour course to prepare for the license exam. Again, I used all of my study techniques full force, and the class was no problem. I passed the test the first time I took it.

"I have been accepted to graduate school to study for my master's in math. I would like to be able to teach college courses in math when I get done. That would give me another good option to do the kind of work I enjoy. I have also thought about more advanced study, not in math, but possibly law school. I'm a permanent student—I love going to school, love learning.

"In 2004, one of the kids in my office was having a problem in math, and I helped her out. She took to it immediately. Because of my dyslexia, I've learned different ways to teach math. I had always helped my friends with math, and I also helped a famous athlete who lived in my residence hall. I was known as the person to see for math help. The girl got an A on a test she had failed the last time, and we just went on from there. My name just got around. At one point I was tutoring nine kids per week, sixth grade to college level trig. A school was actually giving out my name to parents. Right now I'm tutoring four kids. A year ago I took on home schooling a kid I had been tutoring. I do that 4 hours a day, 12 hours a week.

"All my life, math had come easy to me. It became a lot harder after the injury, but I'm still successful with it. Now I have to be extra careful with the organization and the problem solving. I did tons of flash cards to make sure I got my old math skills back. I also became more careful in doing math problems than I had ever been before. A problem that someone else would do in half a page took me two pages, because now I never skipped a step. If I screwed up a problem, I needed to figure out where I screwed up so that I wouldn't mess it up again.

"I applied for a few jobs after finishing school. I realized during the interviews that I didn't want to work in a bank. While I was in school, I had been helping my mother to keep the books in her business. When I got done with school, I went to work for her full-time, and we built the business since. It's a graphic design company, specializing in apparel. My mom, myself, and my husband are partners. I am the organizational, financial, methodical person. It's fun for me to work in my own business. In the process, 3 years ago I got my insurance license and so I also started working part-time for the insurance company where my dad works selling policies."

Four jobs would be more than enough for most healthy adults, but Samantha is also able to pack in a few additional free-time activities. "I'm the vice president of the home owners' association. I have done that for the last 3 years. I also take one college course per semester at night whenever I can fit it in." A year ago, she heard that the "big" neuropsychologist she once disliked so much had a community program for head injury. She came to a meeting of GiveBack and told her recovery story, and immediately was offered a role as a trainer, which she accepted. One month later, she began serving as the treasurer. She has just been appointed to the board of directors. Finally, after pursuing medical treatments for infertility, Samantha conceived a child. In her characteristic fashion, she was excited about the challenge, and felt up to meeting it.

6. Methods of Recovery

"You need a family member that will call you out and stay on your ass. In the beginning I had my mom to do that. Even to this day, she will call me out on things every once and a while. It's another reality check.

"Recovery became my issue when I failed out of the university. At that point I called myself out. I knew I was spiraling out of control and I was going to end up back living with my parents, doing nothing. I was on my way to being a failure. I had the tools and everything I needed to cope. I needed to do everything that was humanly possible. I would have felt embarrassed and disgusted if I hadn't taken my best shot. My high school friend was a victim of his injury, and I couldn't handle that. 'I was in an accident and I'm a victim.' So f____ing what! Get off your ass and deal with it! It would drive me insane!

"Now that I'm pregnant, I've lost my mind. I can't remember s____t. I wake up in the middle of the night and remember something, and I reach out and get the note pad off my end table. I'm the 'rememberer' of the couple, so I have to be sure to get *everything* down on paper. The pregnancy makes me more emotional, too. I'm so cautious about impulsivity that I haven't had a problem with that, even with the pregnancy. I do have to be extra careful lately because I get impatient and edgy. I also have to keep a handle on impulsive eating, and I've been successful with that. I was starving for yellow cake with chocolate icing, so I made a cake and gave it away to all the neighbors, leaving only a little bit left for myself.

"You have to organize everything. Daily planners, lists, routines. It's too easy to forget, to get distracted, to lose track of what you are doing. My compulsive organizing can get pretty extreme. Fortunately, my husband and I are both compulsive, both very careful with our credit rating, both neat-freaks, and both happy to help one another with anything. We have a true partnership, and I realize how fortunate I am to have that.

The authors asked Samantha to describe the organizational scheme she created in the business she operates. She offered to sit down with a tablet and lay out the whole system. Here is what she produced about a year later:

1. *Filing system:* vendors filed by name and by date in separate folders in own drawer; utilities by name and date in separate folders in own drawer; files on each client in a separate filing cabinet: one-job clients all go into one file, whose contents are alphabetically organized; as soon as a client orders a second job, he/she gets own folder labeled with the name of the team or organization; the file is labeled with the year, the contact person's name, and number. Each new order is paper clipped to the file until completed, then stapled into the file.
2. *Orders:* When an order is placed, (1) the file folder is pulled, (2) the e-mail is printed, (3) a work order is made out including contact information, type and number of item, type and placement of the design, names of key people involved with the order, the price and invoice mode, and the deposit (if any) with the deposit paperwork. When the order is filled: it is immediately put on the completed order clipboard. The name is also written on the job sheet along with the due date. The file is placed with the person creating the design.

   All orders include a work order that says: the item, the item number, the item color, the design placement, the design color, the design style, the name of the design maker, the sizes and quantities of each, the price per unit, tax exempt or non-exempt status, a check stock box, and notes for special instructions.

When the items arrive: the file is passed from the design maker to the product basket; the basket is placed on the shelf for that day; the job is put into production. Once the job is up for production, the product printer gets the basket and looks over the file.

After the product is printed, it goes to the folding table and the file goes to the invoices inbox.

Once a day, items on the folding table get folded and packed.

Once a day, the invoices inbox is checked and customer is e-mailed or called to pick order up. After the contact, the file is placed in the rack for outstanding bills.

Other record-keeping: Bills are paid on the 1st and 15th day of every month. All credit cards are set to automatic draw. There is a meeting every morning to go over the jobs to be completed for the day and those to be started for the next day.

Any rush jobs are scheduled in.

Vendor orders are placed on Monday and Wednesday before 3 pm.

Lists kept at work: (1) daily calendar, (2) weekly calendar, (3) monthly calendar, (4) job sheet, (5) order sheet, (6) designs, (7) a personal "to do" list, prioritized, with each step checked off as it is completed.

She developed the system by pure trial-and-error-analysis over a period of about 2 years.

She also maintains several organizational schemes at home. Here is a general description of the daily schedule she maintained when this book was completed, after her daughter was born:

1. get up at 7:00 a.m. and get her daughter up
2. find something for her daughter to busy herself with so she and husband can get ready
3. shower is not necessary as she always showers the night before
4. get daughter ready for the day
5. unnecessary to pack items for daughter as she packs them the night before
6. review list of items to be taken to the car, and get items and take them to car

7. take daughter to babysitter and leave off daughter items
8. work 9:00 to 5:00, pick up daughter and daughter items
9. go home, start dinner
10. optional free time activities: tutor, or do GiveBack business, or take walk or bike ride
11. feed family
12. bathe daughter and put her to bed at 8:00 p.m.
13. repack diaper bag and pack lunch for tomorrow
14. sit down until 9:00 p.m., then perform evening routine, go to bed and read until 10:00 p.m.

Samantha keeps a number of lists and other organizational procedures at home: (a) a weekend do-list, (b) a long-term do-list, (c) four shopping lists for the four stores where the family does regular business, (d) a daily calendar, (e) a monthly calendar, (f) an options for dinner (menu) list, (g) a coupon collection, (h) an inventory of backup equipment in the car, including baby clothes, diapers, wipes, snacks, drinks, medicine, toys, and spare stroller/high chair.

"Accountability—you have to hold yourself accountable for things you have to do, call yourself out on things I forgot to do, or treating people badly. I have a friend I can do that with, too. I tell her about the things I've done wrong, and what I need to do about it. I even call myself out to people when I mess them up with my mistake—I'm so honest. My way of talking things out is a kind of internal EA, without stopping and writing it down. You need to know what you're doing wrong—to know your limitations, and what you're prone to do wrong. As long as you know what these things are, you can find out a way to fix them—a new routine, a new strategy. It's not hard to come up with a strategy. You think of something you've done before, try it out, adjust it if you have to. Like I forgot to make a call—it depends on where it was, and what it was about. I have a way I'm supposed to keep track of each thing I do—tablets I keep for specific purposes in certain places, sticky notes I put in certain places, order forms. It's a system. If I don't do something I'm supposed to do, it means I didn't use my system—I got side-tracked. I think about what happened to side-track me, and figure out how to keep it from interfering in the future. Maybe I need to tell someone to wait or put the phone on hold while I take time to make a note. I will be sure to do it the next time. And once I figure out what I need to do, I make sure I do it.

"I control my emotions carefully, more so over the years. I can get a bit out of control. When I got upset with a particular situation, I pitched a fit, said a lot of things I probably shouldn't have said. Afterward, I realized that I put myself in that situation before I was ready, and let certain things bother me that I should have thought through. I let myself get angry. I made sure that I would never put myself in a situation like that again. It did come up again, recently, with a different person. This time, I handled it differently. I didn't ask questions leading to answers that would have pissed me off, and I kept control. I felt a lot better about it.

"Some situations, at work, tutoring, and doing schoolwork are things I need to really concentrate on. If I'm tutoring a college student in calculus, I review my notes, I'm careful not to be caught with a question I can't answer.

"I don't think my recovery will ever be done. I have to keep watching myself and do what I have to do. I'm going to have a baby. I'm going to have to restructure my whole life. I'm lucky in that I'm going to be able to bring the baby with me into work. With the help of my mother at work. And my husband and I share a lot of responsibilities. I'm ridiculously organized, a saver and planner. When my sister had her baby 3 years ago, I got the crib and half the stuff. When my friend had a baby last year, I got the other half. I'm going to have to catalogue everything I've got so that I can arrange my registry. I have the baby's room completely planned out. I'd like to have it done already, but I have a plan for when I'm going to do it.

Samantha has suffered from migraine headaches since her injury, a problem she rarely mentions to other people. She has one every other day, on average. Sometimes they are tolerable—painful but not bad enough to stop her from working. At other times, they get so bad that she has to turn off all the lights, kick everyone out of the house, and huddle on the bed waiting for it to pass. Because she is pregnant, she decided to stop using pain medication. It took a talk with her physician for her to allow herself a pain pill when it gets bad. Even when it comes to headaches, she has a system, and even taking a pill is planned out for what it might mean 9 months from now.

"I think I did everything I possibly could to recover from my injury. I didn't take the easy road out at any point. I never played the victim. I don't know what life would be like without a brain injury. It's not something I think about."

The Journalistic Perspective

In the limited amount of time I have known Samantha, she has already made a strong impression. At meetings, she takes copious notes in her little notebook, with a hawk-like, almost predatory awareness of her surroundings. When she speaks directly to you, her eyes remain focused on yours, even when yours occasionally zip up to the scar across her forehead, as if you were talking to Harry Potter. She commands respect, carrying herself with determination. The same way a freight train gets moving again after it stops to take on a load, Sam has gotten going again after her injury. You'd be an idiot to stand in the way of either one.

Her austerity may be necessary in business, but on top of it is a layer of geniality. She is not the kind of person you'd call "fun-loving," but she does know how to put people at ease. And her outgoing manner always contains a subtle hint of, "Don't get on my bad side, y'know?"

The Neuropsychological Perspective

Samantha appeared well recovered from the acute effects of her injury when she took her admission neuropsychological tests at 2 months post-onset, a sign of her phenomenal powers of concentration. She was aware that testing would establish her need for outpatient treatment, and made every effort to prove herself ready to return to school.

A particularly low score was found, as expected, on one of the key indicators of frontal lobe damage, the word fluency test, which was severely impaired. She was also severely impaired on Purdue Pegboard in the nondominant hand condition, reflecting the presence of greater focal damage on the right side of the brain. There was similar, lateralized impairment at the moderate level of severity on Finger Oscillation. She also showed focal impairment on measures of visuospatial perception, as expected, with her copy of a Greek cross rated as severely impaired, and moderate impairment on the Visual Search and Attention Test and Woodcock-Johnson Visual Matching. Her lowest score, at the profound level of impairment, on the Rey-Osterreith Complex Figure copy, showed the combined effects of disorganization and perceptual deficiencies. She also performed in the moderate range of impairment on the long delay memory subtest of the Rey Complex Figure and on Digit Span in the forward condition (whereas the reversed condition was within normal limits). Prominent among many tests eliciting mildly impaired scores were Mazes, Tactual Performance Test (dominant hand condition), the NYU Shape Cancellation Test, WMS Visual Memory (immediate), and TPT Memory. Her narrative self-description was marked by run-on construction and grammatical errors.

Both her premorbid personality inventory and the Rorschach characterized her as highly defensive. Her basic personality was described as dominant and outgoing, with traits of aggressiveness and stimulation seeking that would amplify these characteristics. The Rorschach indicated that she was psychologically overloaded in the present situation, exacerbating her natural tendency to react impulsively. She showed a tendency to set her level of aspiration too high and thus to "bite off more than she could chew." She also appeared to be self-critical.

She masterfully applied the strategies and the approach that conquered her childhood learning disability to recovery from her head injury. Her main recovery tools—determination, preparation, focus, self-monitoring, and problem solving—are old tricks put to a new purpose.

PART III

Exceptional Recoveries as Partnerships With Family

One surprising finding of this investigation is how often an exceptional recovery is the product of a survivor working alone. Many of the survivors whose stories are told above have supportive families. However, they did not invite close involvement of family members in their rehab or recovery, nor did the family members demand it. On both sides, they were accustomed to the survivor functioning autonomously. Most programs view this "lone wolf" approach to rehab as a problem and a last resort, and many require family involvement. However, these recoveries stand as testimony that family participation is not necessary in every case.

On the other hand, in other cases family members were heavily involved with treatment. In two of the three cases below, a family member was an equal partner in the training process, invited by the psychologist, but welcomed by the patient. Family offers the special advantages of another point of view, framed by normal awareness of deficit, and the seamless transfer of therapy from the clinic to home. In these cases, the family participation did not prevent the survivor from learning to function independently.

Chapter 12

The Story of Brooke and Charlotte

This mother-daughter team is part of an accomplished family. Father Paul is the sales manager for an industrial firm. Mother Charlotte is a southern belle with a dash of glamour, a hard-working, modern businesswoman who runs her own firm. As you will see, Charlotte threw herself into the role of therapy supporter, learning the language and the logic of rehabilitation. Brooke's mission in life had been to be a top student—the girl with all the answers. When she suffered a terrible diffuse injury complicated by focal language system damage, she refused to abandon this role. Because she did not see the point of therapy, Brooke rejected her lessons and refused the strategies with an iron will. Mother and daughter ended up clashing like an irresistible force and an immovable object. The resulting impasse, which threatened to ruin Brooke's impressive academic career, was only broken after Brooke returned to real life, when the young woman decided to sacrifice her pride and commit herself to success at any cost.

1. The Old Brooke

Brooke is the middle child, with an older sister and a younger brother. She was always the high achiever of the three. Brooke: "For years before my injury, I had been a dedicated, straight-A student, starting in 5th grade. I had established methods and ways to achieve my goals—they had become second nature to me by the time I was in high school. I have always been a perfectionist—before and after my accident.

I never got into a situation I couldn't handle—I could always come up with a strategy. A psychologist diagnosed me as obsessive-compulsive —my mom took me to him during middle school when I felt over-whelmed by my work. I tried to prove to myself that I could be the best in everything I attempted because I knew it was possible if I tried hard enough. I was one of the stars of the JV soccer team, named both the co-captain and the MVP in my sophomore year. I was also on the varsity tennis team. For my junior year I was elected student body secretary as well as the president of InterAct. I didn't really have a social life—I started studying after I got home, and I sometimes continued until after midnight. I was hoping that I would be able to go to an Ivy League college, though I thought of University of Florida as my fall-back option."

Charlotte: "She left a few things out. The night before her accident she was inducted into the National Honor Society. She won the top prize in the county at the science fair—with a project on micro-biology. Her picture was posted at the front entry of the school for "Student of the Month" when the accident took place, and that was not the first time she achieved that. She was just amazing—academics, sports, anything." A few days before her accident, Brooke wrote this in her diary: "A person can't get anywhere without a brain."

2. The Accident—10 Years Ago

Brooke was 16 when she had her accident: "As I was driving to school, I lost control of my car and slammed into an enormous tree. The driver's side struck the tree. I had a seat belt on, but that didn't help much, obviously. Some bystanders had to pull me out through the passenger's side." She had been struck on the left side of the head.

3. The Injury

The impact caused bleeding above and into her left parietal lobe. Blood also imploded into the pool of fluid inside her brain (left lateral ventricle). She remained in a coma for 17 days. She remembered nothing for the first 60 days after the accident, and about 1 week before the accident (when asked 2 years later).

4. Early Recovery

Charlotte: "We had to fight to get her put on BIRC (the region's specialized inpatient neurorehabilitation program). The insurance case manager wanted to put her in a skilled nursing facility. We didn't have rehab coverage, and they didn't want to pay for the hospital. I wrote the Insurance Commissioner. Then she got MRSA." MRSA is an antibiotic-resistant strain of bacteria that lives in hospitals, dangerous and difficult to treat.

"When she was in a coma she could hear us talking, though she had no sense of where she was. One of the nurses told me that Brooke was not going to wake up. She was playing mind games with me. It's so awful when somebody like that has complete control of your kid. You feel so vulnerable. I had such a sense of urgency then to try to bring her out of her coma—wake up, wake up, wake up! The next day, on the way to the hospital, I would say to my husband, hurry, hurry, we have to get there. Finally, after this went on day after day, I realized that nothing about this is going to be quick.

"After literally living in her hospital room [at the acute hospital] for 30 days, I had become so exhausted that I was cognitively impaired myself. At one point, my hands quit working. I got so I couldn't do math—I couldn't pay the bills. It was because I was never able to rest, never able to stop taking care of Brooke: changing her diapers, washing her hair, and when she was so restless and agitated, and they didn't want to put her in restraints, she would kick and kick and sit up again and again until she started to slide off the end of the bed, and I would have to pull her back, pull her back, again and again, and it took all my strength. It was physically challenging. I was a mess. I prayed harder than I ever have. I concentrated on the little chores. I figured, 'I can take care of her physically. It's the one thing I can do. I can't make the coma go away. I'm just doing the best I can.' She was bleeding from the medicine they gave her for the MRSA, and I'd just be trying to wipe the blood away, and I couldn't, and I got so frantic, wiping and wiping. I remember looking up and all of the nurses were staring at me.

"When she was in the agitation phase, she was talking so quickly, and she was talking about things from her childhood, almost like she was reviewing her life. One day when I was leaving the ward to do a chore for one of my other kids, she begged me to take her home with me, when she was still trached [a tracheostomy tube for breathing through a hole in the throat].

"Meanwhile, she was coming up the Rancho Scale [waking up out of coma]. Finally she got to the point where she could be admitted to BIRC. And then they agreed to trade 4 weeks at BIRC for her SNF [nursing home] coverage.

Brooke: "When I woke up, everything seemed very strange to me. There were so many things I couldn't remember at that time. As a result, I had no foundation with which to connect or compare the things I was seeing around me. The hospital activities just happened to me, and I don't remember much about them."

Charlotte: "She got to BIRC 5 weeks after the accident. The first night she had to ask us to leave, because she had to go to sleep. She would lie down and go right to sleep. She couldn't wait for me to get there the next day. I came every day at 4:30. She could hear my walk, and she would call out, "Mom, mom." I would come and she would usually have some visitors. One day some girlfriends came to see her, and her face had broken out. She got her mirror out and was checking her complexion. She felt uncomfortable because she didn't have any makeup on. A therapist told me that was a sign that she was coming back to herself.

"After the friends left, she and I would visit. First she ate her dinner, and then we would have our spa time. We got our towels and I took her to the bathroom, and I had to wash her everywhere. Little by little I started teaching her how to bathe herself and wash her own hair. Then I'd take her back in time to watch "Xena" (the Warrior Princess). She really liked that show. I would brush and blowdry her hair while the show was on. Then I left. That was every night.

On the BIRC inpatient unit, Brooke asked to telephone her mother so often that it interfered with her therapies. When something upset her or the staff did not cooperate with her requests, she would ask for the phone. She also called frequently during inactive periods in the late afternoon. "She called me all the time. Over and over again, many times every day. One time, she left a message on the answering machine. She went on and on, on the tape—it must have been 15 minutes. It was pitiful, heartbreaking. She just wanted to talk to me."

Brooke: "I remember that my mom and dad left their phone numbers on a post-it note by my bed because I couldn't remember the numbers. I must have called them a lot, because the nurses would take the phone away from me. They would say, 'You called them already!' but I didn't remember making the call. One day, they took the post-it note off my bed rail. They thought it would stop me from making the calls. By that time, I had memorized the number and I called my parents anyway. I do remember the day I got to go home. I was excited, but I don't remember much else about it."

Charlotte: "When I took her home, she said to me, 'Mommy, is this really happening? Am I still here? Is this real—because I can't tell. It seems like a dream. I just don't know what's real anymore. Well, here is what I'm going to do. If it's still like this in 2 days, I'm going to figure that it is real.' She couldn't trust her thoughts because she was totally disoriented at that point."

Brooke: "Two weeks later I started outpatient therapy. I had therapy 4 days a week. On the 5th day I stayed with my grandmother because I was not safe to be left alone."

Charlotte: "At the outpatient, [we got proof of] all the bad news right away—we were devastated—we knew we were in deep trouble then." Although the parents accepted the test results well after asking many questions, Brooke did not. Her basic personality was beginning to reassert itself. Brooke had an aloof, let-me-be-the-judge attitude toward every item of feedback she received, from testing, therapies, and her peers. And, of course, her judgment and insight were so impaired that she was quite certain that there was nothing wrong with her. Brooke: "It was difficult adjusting to my outpatient program—it was hard to accept that there was something wrong with me." She maintained this attitude, even to the point of open argumentation, throughout her therapy stay. Because she has an achievement-oriented, self-confident, and somewhat dominant personality, she not only disagreed with the feedback, but also refused the compensations. Although she was rapidly learning to monitor her own performance and was dissatisfied with any imperfections, she wanted to fix them her own way—which never worked.

Her stubborn insistence on doing things only in the way she saw fit brought her therapy to a standstill. Charlotte: "Not long after [her admission to the program], the therapists told me that I needed to step up my involvement. I had been helping Brooke with some of the homework she had been assigned, but I didn't realize how much they were expecting me to do. They said that if she wasn't making more progress soon, 'We won't be doing this anymore.' That got my attention! Her biggest problem in therapy was the grades she got from the therapists. She was used to getting top grades. It was really hard for her to get lower grades. That was very humbling for her. She had a lot of trouble with writing papers—and she felt she didn't need to outline."

Outlining is a strategy that this program requires in the therapy for expressive language. It compensates for deficits in initiation and organization. "I would tell her, this isn't organized enough—you need to do a brief outline. She didn't want to do that, in the beginning.

"The schedule was a problem. There was a specific way it had to be done, and she didn't want to do it that way. I would tell her, 'If it was me, if somebody gave me a way out of this hellacious life we're in, I'd use it. I can't figure out why you won't use it. [I'd been told] that brain-injured people who don't use this strategy will fail in college.' And she would fight me. 'If there is a way to fix it, why don't you use it?' She also said, 'Why should I have to write down absolutely everything?' and now she perfectly well understands that."

Brooke: "They taught me to do things in different ways than I was used to. That was hard for me. I was used to doing things my way. I didn't deal well with being told to do something. I am a very independent person. I have always felt sure that I can make things work my way if I try hard enough, and it was hard to accept being told that my way wasn't good enough anymore. It was difficult for me to realize that I'm different and *I* need to change when everything around me was the same as it had been, and I felt the same and saw everything the same way. I found myself being put in a new game with new rules and I didn't know how to react."

It seems that Brooke had always been willful, even before her injury. Charlotte: "The week before her accident, we had a knockdown, drag-out fight in the car. 'Why does everything have to be so hard with you? Why do you have to fight me on everything?' A week later she has a car accident, and she [now] needs to listen to everyone." She shrugged at the irony.

Charlotte: "In the very beginning she did most of her studying by herself. I would only try to give her some suggestions about what might need work. I would say this doesn't make sense. And she would come back insisting on her view of things—that's just how she is. She would say, 'Yes, it does make sense!' I could only fight so far. I was able to help her a little bit, but not a lot. She wanted to do it herself whether she succeeded or failed. She insisted that she should be judged for her own work."

Eventually, after exhausting all in-house options, a meeting was held with the entire staff and family. Brooke's deficits and self-imposed obstacles to her progress were reviewed. Everyone in the room came down on one side (acknowledge your deficits and do your program), whereas petite Brooke resolutely refused to budge on the other side. As a last resort, the program director had a counseling session in which he pointed out that her refusal to cooperate was only going to end up delaying her return to school. He advised that if she would play along with the staff and show them that she understood all of their methods, they would probably let her go to school and then she could do things her way. Brooke: "It wasn't easy to get me to use the strategies, but the last month I decided to go along with them just to get out of therapy."

Brooke was persistent in pressing for a return to school at the start of the next school year, and was supported by her family in petitioning for her release from the program to allow her to earn enough credits over the coming year to graduate with her class. The staff was very concerned about her failure to accept any insight, and they knew that she was not committed to using the compensations. However, they had already seen a similar course of therapy in the case of Hillary, another dominant and confident personality, end successfully when she decided to use the compensations on her own. The program director had also seen the same process of "delayed compensation" occur with another dominant personality treated at Robert Wood Johnson Rehabilitation Institute (Schutz, 1989). After providing the family with extensive written and oral instructions and encouraging them to stay in touch, the team reluctantly discharged her.

What did Brooke get from her outpatient therapy? Charlotte: "She got the tools she needed, and she got the information that she needed. She didn't utilize them right away. She was really so impaired when she got out. That next year she improved so much. She improved so much intellectually. Even her eyes—they got brighter over that year. As she became more alert, she was more able to realize about what she needed to do."

She was placed on a driving restriction when she left the hospital. Although she eventually reached the point where she could respond quickly enough to meet our predriving standards, she remains on a driving restriction due to epilepsy-like symptoms of uncertain clinical significance. She experiences "dazes" with reduced concentration, slowed speech, and a fixed gaze, as often as several times per day. Although the frequency has been reduced to several times per week on one medication, the episodes continue. Brooke accepts her driving restriction.

Brooke: "A few weeks after graduating from therapy, I went back to start my senior year of high school." Her neuropsychologist requested that all of her teachers attend the IEP meeting, where he explained about her strategies and the need for weekly family feedback. Most teachers seemed disinterested and all ignored the request for feedback. Later, one told Brooke he knew she was recovered. This response left Brooke and Charlotte on their own. "I took two classes, had a student government class that never assigned any homework, and had a free period to use as a study session. I could also rest my brain during that period. They let me use the conference room in the administration building. I could even take short naps. Later in the year, they worked with me individually, but only after they had seen for themselves how restricted I was."

Charlotte: "I remember being in an absolute panic when she started back to school. At that point, she got tired so easily, but she was also so easily distracted. If the TV was on, she would just sit down and watch the TV, even if she had something to do. I would have to tell her to get to work. Before she had her first test, I was trying to help her organize and study. She didn't want me to do that—she always wanted to do it on her own. But she wasn't doing it—she didn't have her strategies down, and here was the test coming right up!

Brooke: "When I resumed my English class, I tried using my old-Brooke study strategies. I realized that I had been advised not to do this, but I also felt sure that I had to see how my old ways worked before I could consider trying anything else. I quickly realized that my old strategies didn't work. I went back to self-testing as I was trained in rehab. I highlighted my books, which helped. I used every strategy I'd been taught. I made all As."

Charlotte: "I wasn't able to help her much. There was a power struggle between her and me about scheduling. Her organizational skills weren't good enough. Now they are. But in the beginning things were not organized—it was a mess. Sometime during high school she realized how important that daily schedule was for her. She realized that she was going to sink without it. Now, she plans out everything and feels she needs to adhere to her plan. She even has to plan out time to use the bathroom. She's gotten it down to a science by now. Her father calls the schedule book 'her Bible.'"

Brooke: "Social life—I have several friends. I prefer close friendships and I have several of those. I'm not dating anyone currently, although I have recently. I haven't found anybody I would want to date right now. It's not one of my main priorities at this time. I expect that at some time in the future I will devote the time to it that it calls for, but not right now."

Charlotte: "Because of her impairments, she does not read other people well. Sometimes she takes the things they say literally, and she comes off looking naive and awkward. She can act very mature; you'll never find a person who's had to take life so seriously. But when she lets her guard down and tries to act cute and bubbly, she can seem immature. She makes mistakes, socially. She's not stupid—she knows she makes mistakes. She might be too loud, or say the wrong thing. Social life is hard work for her."

Before the injury, Brooke had been like a second mother to her brother, who was 4 years her junior. Afterward, he did not allow her to nurture him, and became critical of her. This deterioration of sibling relationships is very common in TBI families (Lehr, 1990).

Charlotte: "Brooke's impairments today are not as visible as they once were. Her detailed daily schedule and other strategies make her life appear more normal and certainly it now looks easier than it is. In fact, just recently she asked me to sit down so that she could address some issues she had with me and some other family members. She had given careful consideration to what she wanted to say and had written down her points, knowing that it would be an emotional conversation. Basically, she pointed out that because she manages her life so well, I sometimes forget that she still has major impairments and act impatient with her in a way that is hurtful. She was right. This brain injury thing is really hard. With someone like Brooke, who daily expends a tremendous amount of energy to make her life work and appear almost normal, even those closest to her can react unfairly if she forgets something or uses bad judgment.

"One of her current impairments is in impulse control. Her control has improved, but there are still impulses that get through. She can see a McDonald's billboard while she is riding in the car and just starts going on about how she wants a hamburger right now. Of course, she still has the processing speed deficit. The whole picture still eludes her at times. Obviously her memory is not great, though it has improved so much. Her judgment depends on what the subject is. For things outside of the world she lives in, especially new things, she doesn't have good judgment about them. Inside her world—she's got this school thing pretty much down cold."

5. Accomplishments of Recovery

Charlotte: "She said, 'In some ways I'm glad I had my injury.' Before the injury she studied everything. Afterward she couldn't. She realized that it was better that she learned to study selectively. She said that she wished she'd had those strategies before her injury, because it would have made her life so much easier if she had learned how to self-test and isolate what was important. And however awful the brain injury was, it did take her off the fast track that was burning her out."

Brooke: "(My success) came at a price—exhaustion. It was very taxing. A good night's sleep never left me feeling well rested. I woke up and had to get back to the grindstone—it never ended. My second semester back it was the same story. I tried to stay up past midnight almost every night. A month or two of that and I was whipped. I couldn't keep up with that. It changed my perspective. One night my mother walked in and I had been crying. I told her that I don't want to live a life like this, working and tired all the time, and no matter how much work I put into this, I'm not getting the results I wanted. I reduced my work load and expectations and got put on low-dosage antidepressants. I couldn't study everything—I would have to pick and choose. My new outlook became more positive—I didn't demand my best work on everything. It was hard for me to compromise on my principles, but I did. And I still made straight As." Brooke finished high school with a 4.0, a better grade point average than before her injury.

Charlotte: "She started to figure out where she needed to get guidance from user-friendly teachers. She would ask them pointed questions about what she needed to know. Now she pretty much knows what she needs to learn, but at first she needed guidance from the teachers. She self-taught herself quite a lot. She took the strategies from therapy and streamlined them—for example, figuring out how often to do her self-tests. She didn't want my help. She didn't want her success to be due to my input."

Brooke: "I did get offered admission to UF as well as some private colleges. But my mom and I decided that Rollins (located adjacent to Orlando) would be the best choice, since I would need more attention and help from my parents in my first year."

Charlotte: "Rollins was the right choice. There were so many things she needed my help with those first couple of years. I don't see how we could have managed it in Gainesville or Jacksonville, let alone someplace farther away."

Brooke: "The first year was very, very hard. I enrolled in three classes, realized that I had overloaded myself, but I stuck it out. For spring, I dropped down to two courses. It was much better—I wasn't stressed out as badly. In summer school, I took two classes. I was in the habit of studying all the time. I tape recorded nearly all my lectures and used the tapes to review and study for the first 2 years." Charlotte: "She would listen to the tapes as we drove home in the car. I finally got her a headphone so I didn't have to listen, too." Brooke: "After that, I gradually reduced my use of the tapes. Sometimes I was able to rely on notes I took in class—it depended on how good my notes were. But I continued to make the tapes. It was like a safety net. If I didn't get it all, I could turn to the tapes. Over time, I got better at knowing what I need to write down. I stopped making the tapes about a year and half ago. I can take fully effective notes now because I know what the instructor is emphasizing, so tape is no longer necessary. I take notes in outline form, as I did in high school. I still bring my recorder and tapes to every class, though, in case I need them for some unforeseen reason. After all, you never know."

Charlotte: "She doesn't want a period of inactivity. She needs the stimulation—she's sharper when she gets it. She's gone up from 9 hours to 12 per term. She doesn't want too much idle time."

Brooke: "My GPA at Rollins is a 3.95. I've gotten two B's in 5 years."

Charlotte: "They corrected a grading error, which turned one of her Bs into an A, so she has only one B on her record, now. She also has two A-minuses. I rarely need to help her with her academics. I went to a meeting with an academic counselor to discuss her prospects for the future. That's about all I've had to do recently. She's very self-reliant in that way.

"Since she wasn't dating prior to her accident, she doesn't have experience to fall back on. School has taken all of her energy, focus, and time. She went through periods where she wanted to make something out of her dating life. She sees guys looking at her. At first, I think she was attracted to the wrong guys—the frat boy/bad boy type. Now she has adjusted her standards—she just wants somebody who's nice, smart, and going somewhere in life—but not Mr. Perfect. She was not successful with the dating at first. She is constantly looking at her social interaction, to see what she has said or done that was wrong. She doesn't know how to initiate. She tries to be very careful about what she says and does, but it doesn't always work and she doesn't always know why. She wants some kind of rules to go by. For a period of time, she dated a boy and he said, 'I don't know if I can be with somebody like you. I mean, that schedule that you keep.' She chose the schedule over the boy.

"Brooke wants to be independent, now. She keeps a perfect bank book. She plans her groceries, cooks her meals, now she wants to take on more and more. She's always ready to try more. She was able to go to Europe last year. She explored London all by herself, and she didn't get into any trouble, so we know she can handle some things entirely on her own. She would like to move away from home and thinks she can manage that on her own. Right now, she's talking about maybe finding a job that she could live near, so that she could get to work and do her errands by riding her bicycle. I don't know that I can agree with that idea.

"Planning her future is one of our biggest challenges at this point. Right now she's very concerned about her career future. She has been thinking about it for several years, and is having a hard time settling on a choice. Brooke has worked very hard and achieved much, not the least being her academic excellence, and wants to do something really great with her life. Finding a career that balances her strengths and allows for her impairments and yet still gives Brooke the meaningful career that she has worked so hard for is elusive just now. When she tries to picture herself in a career, the picture she gets is not always realistic. But she has gotten every book on careers, we have talked over one career after another, and we have tried to figure out what she would be interested in and what she would have difficulty in doing."

Brooke: "There are a lot of things I'd like to do. It's been hard to choose a career. I had to give up my interest in microbiology. I'd like to become an author, and I enjoy photography. I'm also interested in protecting the environment. My major is advertising/public relations."

Charlotte: "I'm still her best friend. She's disappointed with me right now because I don't have the kind of time she needs. Until recently she would still call me every day. 'Mommy, I still need your help. You have to help me.' I used to think, 'What would she do without me?' I knew that my role was critical. I know now that she'll be OK if I get on a plane and it crashes. But I know we have this much to do—we need to find what she needs to do with herself in terms of a career. I have not completely taken care of this because I'm not sure exactly what to do. I can see clearly that my daughter needs to do something not too far beneath her expectations of herself—it needs to be big enough and important enough. She's always wanted to contribute to the brain injury field. She's concerned about the environment. She wants to do something to make the world better."

Finally, she settled on a career. "My current plan is to become an English teacher. I've been debating what age to teach. I'm going to minor in English and take courses in the summer and fall. I know I'll be a good teacher." She tested out the idea by serving as a classroom aide, and took a semester to prepare for the Graduate Record Exam. She got 1160, an excellent score for an education career, and was admitted to the master's program. And she continues to earn top grades, of course.

Charlotte: "Life is so hard. I'm so blessed. It gets easier but it's always hard. Especially depending on the temperament of your child. Somewhere along the line you have to find your peace with it. People ask you, 'Is she all recovered yet?' You have to know this is your life and your child's life and you have to accept it. Every new thing that comes up, your kid will have to figure out a way to deal with it, a strategy. You're going to worry about the future, and all the things that will come up, and now I just don't allow myself to think about it. My husband is so worried about this kid right now. 'What's going to happen?' It's hard. For me, I say it's gonna be what it's gonna be. It's always going to be hard for Brooke. That is heartbreaking. But there's only so much you can do about that. You go along and all you can deal with is what's going on day to day. You can't fix it. I did a lot of crying in my car at the beginning. Sometimes now when all of this is going on what I think is, 'What would Brooke be doing now? She'd be finishing graduate school.' My life could have been very different. I'd have more of a life. But it is what it is and I'm grateful to have it. And I mourn for the losses—I'm not through yet.

"Mourning the losses is a long process. In the beginning, you don't know what you've lost—you don't know for sure what parts of her are gone forever and what parts will come back. It was horrible for me. When I was alone, almost like saying a prayer, I'd talk to the spirit of the part of her that was dead, and I'd say, 'I'm so sorry, Brooke. I'll always remember who you were.'" At this point, Charlotte was in tears. "It's like I got her back but I lost her, too. I'm so lucky to have her, but it's tough, and no one, no one, no one understands.

"I think I've done a good job so far, with the social thing left to deal with. If I can help her with that, then she would have peace and I would have real peace, knowing that she had conquered what she needs to conquer."

6. Methods of Recovery

Brooke: "At this point I wouldn't say there is anything wrong with me. I just function in a different way. I had to learn how to adapt. It's like having been born a second time. Now I have to learn how to exist. To begin with, I process information slower and in a different way than before. My memory is challenged—it takes me longer to learn things than it used to. I have to use new methods of memorizing and learning. But not only that—I learn in a different way. In my first 2 years of college, when I took a class in an unfamiliar subject, I sometimes struggled to understand the concepts. I needed to track down the instructor and get those ideas explained to me in another way. I only have that problem now when I am learning a brand new kind of information, so I haven't had any difficulty with comprehension in the last year plus. It was very hard to admit to myself that I had to learn in a different way, but I do."

Here are Brooke's principles of recovery: "Topmost is the recognition that you are different. You have to learn to adjust to different needs and limitations than you used to have. I had to lower my expectations of what a success was. For a while, it seemed to me like I'd made myself settle for a mediocre level, but that was just because I was comparing myself to the person I used to be. I had to see myself as a different person and pointedly adjust my expectations. I still expect to excel—I still demand that I do the best that can—now I just realize that my best is not the same as it was. I am now a different person with different capabilities, so obviously my expectations have to be reset to a different level.

"Because of the injury, I have to work twice as hard as the average person to get what I want. If I had to credit my recovery to a single strategy, that's it. Do the amount of work that's necessary to get good results.

"In therapy I had learned quickly that I had to curb my tendency to rush. I forced myself to develop real patience. Only if I slowed down could I be accurate. In college, it was no problem for me because I accepted my need to go slowly and be extra careful.

"Emotions—I was used to having control—complete control. After the accident, I lost so much control in so many different things, and my emotions developed a will of their own. Once I became emotional, I could never think clearly. Anger, frustration, fear, these emotions all took hold of me and I couldn't just stop myself from feeling that way. I soon realized that losing my temper and subjecting myself to my emotions only made me weaker. When I grew excited, I lost control in a different way. I lost my powers of reason. In time, I figured out how to change my expectations so that the things that used to frustrate me were no surprise. No surprise—no emotional reaction.

"If I try an interaction and it doesn't go exactly the way I wanted it to, the first thing I do is self-analysis—I break down all of my actions, kind of like outlining material I read—and the reactions each thing has gotten from the other person. When the reaction I got was less than what I was hoping for, I think about other ways I could have expressed myself that would have been more effective. The next time I find myself in a similar situation, I try to use the better approach. You see—it's a learning process. Recently I analyzed one important interaction in writing.

"I can't just stick with the strategies I've developed up to this point. My recovery is an unending thing. I need to keep changing how I do things. It's a pain in the ass. It's hard. But I have to accept it, if I'm going to be a success. You will be adjusting to things all your life—better not fight it. Just try to understand it. I couldn't do that right off the bat. It took time.

"I don't regret my injury happening. I don't regret having it because it has taught me a new way to thrive, to be myself. I didn't lose anything I needed. I just took a different path. My life is no less fabulous than it would have been. My life is harder but more fulfilling than it was before. I've been told I'm heroic. I don't know if I'd use that term. Doing what I've done takes a lot of personal strength. I've sustained a severe head injury, and I've recovered very well, thanks to my determination and therapy. The ability to be great lies within each of us. I guess if I did something exceptional it was in wanting it so much."

The Journalistic Perspective

A small, slender student, Brooke came across as a subtly authoritative person; not someone who screamed and bit and kicked her way into the center ring, but rather one who commanded respect through style and dignity. The first impression was of a high-octane intellect—not just a smart kid, but one of the smartest, not just a hard worker, but a demon with her face in the fire all the time, not just well-educated, but a petite expert. She seemed ready to answer any question at any time. With the brain injury weighing her thinking down, it wasn't always easy for her to put her answers into words, but she always wrapped her mind around the question. She looked away slightly and composed herself before speaking. The words were always strong and confident, though her tone didn't always match them. Her voice was halting, and kept breaking into unnaturally low tones. And she always took that extra second to make sure she had perfect diction, like she was on stage at the national spelling bee. From behind her wire-rimmed glasses, her dark eyes betrayed a false sense of security, making her appear more hurt by the injury than she wanted to let on.

She had been a straight-A student before her accident and she is still a straight-A student. That has to be enough for her. It might be easy to reassure herself, as some of her fellow students and professors do, that she came out of the injury as the same old Brooke, because she still performs at such a high level. But a glance at her day planner shows that it has taken over for a part of her brain that doesn't work anymore, the part that once focused her mind like a laser.

The Neuropsychological Perspective

Brooke was assessed at Glasgow Coma Scale level 8 by paramedics at the site. Her level declined to 7 at admission and continued to decline to level 3 later in the first day. She sustained cardiac and pulmonary contusions, with respiratory compromise in the field, requiring intubation prior to transport; thus, a hypoxic insult was also possible. Her CT scan at 3 days post-onset revealed a burst left parietal lobe (subdural and intracerebral hematomas), with an underlying zone of encephalomalacia. At her outpatient intake interview at 10 weeks post-onset, she had no recollection of the first 60 days. At that time, she stated that she was "still kind of thinking that things aren't real." Her last clearly defined retrograde memory was an event 5½ months prior to the accident. Interview revealed imprecise articulation, excessively rapid speech, poor breath control, dysprosodia, and concrete cognition.

Her test performance was marked by easy distractibility, gaps in working memory, and off-task verbalizations. Even at this early stage in her recovery, testing was emotionally taxing. She demonstrated signs of tension and anxiety, frequently apologized for her errors and gaps in knowledge, and withdrew effort readily when she ran into difficulties. At one point, she was able to spot an answer on the inverted test form the examiner was marking, and she warned: "I sort of cheated —you might want to move it." Her performance on the Tactual Performance Test was interrupted by complaints of upper extremity pain. Brooke also became confused easily during spatial tasks, spending an extended period of time on Trail Making Part A searching for a circle she had already marked. Overshoot and undershoot errors were made on this task. She demonstrated errors in following test instructions, particularly instructions that required inhibiting movements or refraining from giving certain kinds of answers. Recall for newly learned information elicited confabulation on all trials. Recall for prose passages failed to preserve the gist of the story. Quantitatively, she showed mild to moderate impairment of focal attention, suggesting that her acute recovery had not progressed far enough for full participation in her rehabilitation. Measures of executive function (word fluency, mazes), new learning bimodally, and Gates-McGinitie Reading Comprehension were profoundly impaired. Scores on tests of complex cognitive function ranged from severe (Halstead Category Test) to profound impairment (Tactual Performance Test [TPT]). Problems in receptive language were also suggested by empty speech in response to a narrative task, and incorrect interpretation of figurative and complex language. These executive, mnestic, and expressive and receptive language problems figured prominently in her performance in her speech and cognitive therapies.

The neuropsychological treatment strategy was framed by the insistent expectations of this powerful family. They were seeking a complete educational recovery that would allow Brooke to attend a prestigious university and pursue graduate education, and they wanted her to become a distinguished student again if at all possible. However, they also insisted that she return to school at the start of the new term and take a course load sufficient to allow her to graduate with her class. The risks inherent in these mutually antagonistic desires were discussed, but there was no room for compromise. This meant that Brooke would need to learn all of the necessary compensation strategies in just beyond 3 months, despite her comprehension deficits. It also meant that the refinement of her strategies would need to take place after discharge, through a combination of self-therapy and family-mediated training. Because Brooke had very poor insight in the context of posterior damage (an added obstacle to insight) as well as a dominant and somewhat narcissistic personality, the self-therapy would be unlikely to be fully developed at discharge. Hence, every effort was made to educate and involve Charlotte. This was easy to do, as this mother was extremely bright, heavily involved, and curious by nature.

As noted in the body of her story, her therapy required constant supervisory management because she was so willful and unwilling to accept or attempt the compensations. Because Brooke ultimately kept her own counsel on these matters, immediate education was not effective irrespective of who presented the information. Instead, she was taught under a conditional approach: "Here are things you will want to know just in case you run into these impairments later." Because of her perfectionism, Brooke learned and later implemented what she was taught.

By the time she completed therapy, she was able to demonstrate fully effective attention to task most of the time, and her impulse regulation and quality control were excellent on tasks she acknowledged as therapy related. However, if the task was not one she had mastered in training sessions, for example, in social behavior, her behavior was highly impulsive, poorly planned, and often disorganized or inappropriate. This indicated that she understood how to develop adequate cognitive control of behavior given structured practice, but that she could not yet use anticipatory or spontaneous methods of symptom prevention.

When tested for her proposed return to school at 8½ months post-onset, she showed excellent attention to task and consistent motivation, but still demonstrated profound impairments on TPT, mazes, delayed verbal recall, and Trail Making Part B. She improved on the Category Test to the moderate range of impairment, and on measures of recall for nonverbal information to mildly impaired. As expected, focal attention had returned to the normal range.

She was tested by another neuropsychologist at 2 years and 1 month post-onset. At this time, she demonstrated severely impaired delayed verbal recall, moderately-to-severely impaired delayed recall for complex nonverbal information and performance on Trail Making Part B, and mildly-to-moderately impaired word fluency. A late MRI, performed at 16 months post-onset, found evidence of bilateral deep parietal atrophy attributed to her chronic TBI. Thus, the entire body of clinical evidence reveals enduring deficits in learning ability, language processing ability, executive functioning, and the adaptively critical set of nondominant perceptual functions (Schutz, 2005a), which would ordinarily preclude mainstream instruction in high school or progression to college. From a neuropsychological perspective, this is a badly broken brain that would not be expected to support the academic accomplishments she has made. Clearly, Brooke's development and use of compensations has been both persistent and masterful.

The dynamics of Brooke's personal adjustment are confusing seen through the traditional psychometric lens. The neuropsychologist who performed her final evaluation recommended medication and supportive counseling for her "anxiety" and "depression" as indicated by standardized testing, despite the denial of these symptoms by his subject. He suggested that medication might also have been beneficial for her obsessive-compulsive condition. In a more realistic appraisal, life after a head injury is hard and life for an exceptional achiever is much harder. Her recognition of the difficulties is indicative of her superior adjustment rather than a disorder. Patients like Brooke have also taught us to reconceptualize compulsive traits as adaptive assets in successful recovery (Schutz & Micucci, 1984).

Chapter 13

The Story of Tom and Dawn

Tom and Dawn come from a small, rural town in Ohio. They both have a high school education and worked in blue-collar vocations. They describe themselves as "laid-back rednecks." Dawn: "Tom is just your Average Joe, and I just follow along behind him." Tom: "We met when she moved in across the street from me." Dawn: "My daddy died in 1972. The next year, we moved in across the street from him. We went to 6th grade together, 32 years ago. We were just buds—we used to hang out together all the time. I just always knew Tom was the guy for me." Tom: "I just got tired of being chased."

1. The Old Tom

When Tom was 5 or 6 years old, he was hit from behind by a bicycle rider. "He knocked me over and fell on top of me. I had to have 48 stitches. I was knocked out, probably a good half hour to an hour. I woke up in the hospital." Tom's CT scan 30 years later showed an old scar on his left frontoparietal brain that appeared to be the result of this accident. "I always had trouble with reading. I hate reading. Spelling was a problem, too. School was always hard for me, especially high school. I had no clue why until now. Even when I worked, making mistakes bothered me. I hated making mistakes. It still bothers me."

Tom was a serious baseball player in Little League. He was chosen as an all-star second baseman in Babe Ruth League. He played injured, with a cast on his arm, or with new stitches. He was fast, and he played a very aggressive game. Dawn: "He would kick your ass."

Tom: "I was a hard worker. I liked to hunt and fish—I could live off the land if I had to—it would be no problem. The old Tom was never scared of nothin'. He could do anything he wanted and not give it a second thought.

"I'm a recovering alcoholic: I had my last drink June 25th of 1995. I checked myself into a rehab the next day. When I got out of rehab, they told me to go to AA meetings every day for 30 days. After that, I went for 2 years." Tom believes strongly in the principles of AA, and tries to live by them. He knows he could resume drinking at any time, but because he got through the worst parts of his injury without doing so, he figures drinking is probably going to remain a part of his past.

Tom worked as a derrick hand in an oil-well drilling operation. He was being trained as a driller. Previously, he supervised a crew that cut concrete, so thorough a worker that the contracting agent (Miami International Airport) sent him a letter of commendation and refused to hire anyone else. Dawn worked as the credentialing coordinator for a medical practice. With only a 19-year-old son who was soon to be married, they were on their way to becoming empty nesters at the time of Tom's accident.

2. The Accident—9 Years Ago

Tom: "I don't remember anything about the accident. I was working on a rig, getting it ready to be moved. One of the drillers called down and asked for an adjustment. We worked on pairs of drilling pipes. I separated the pipes and was working on one of them, while the other one was held off to one side by a chain. The rig jerked just enough to pull the chain off that pipe, and it came swinging. It weighed in at 2500 pounds. Pipe hit me on the right side of the head, knocked the back of my head off the collar on the other pipe, then my head bounced back off the first collar.

A bone was pushed in at the right temple (depressed skull fracture), and the whole skull had taken the worst kind of damage, sometimes called an eggshell fracture. "A lot of my skull was gone." Dawn: "The bones in his face and sinus were all shattered. That's why he can't smell anything. Dr. Robert said it was like somebody took a hammer and hit a windshield. There were all kinds of tiny cracks all through those bones. They gave him a craniotomy [open-skull surgery] in an attempt to lower his intracranial pressure. He had a lot of spinal fluid coming out of his nose and ears. The pressure kept going up, got to 18, very close to the critical level they said could kill him, which was 20. They tried three times to do a ventriculostomy [drilling a hole into the fluid-filled hole in the center of the brain]. Finally they were able to get the shunt installed." Tom: "I also had a hematoma they had to drain out on the top of my head."

3. The Injury

Tom lost consciousness in the ambulance and remained in a coma. He was given sedatives to keep him in coma for 13 days as a way to hold down the brain swelling. He could mouth words when they removed the medications, so his true coma duration is less than 13 days. His CT scan showed damage all across his right brain: a large right frontal contusion, another in the parietal lobe, and a third in the frontotemporal area. His left side was completely paralyzed.

Dawn: "In his first (medical) hospital, they told me he might not make it, and if he did, he could have a lot of problems and wouldn't be able to do very much. They said he would be 'very limited.' I was gearing up to prepare my home for an invalid who I'd have to take care of for the rest of our lives." Tom: "I'd rather have been put under."

4. Early Recovery

After he got a trach and a PEG (a stomach tube for feeding), he was transferred to BIRC for acute rehab, 3 weeks after the accident. Dawn: "Dr. Rosenberg was taking me on a tour of the unit, telling me how safe the staff was going to keep Tom. We walked into his room. Tom wasn't in his bed. He was on the floor on the far side. Dr. Rosenberg said, 'What the hell are you doing on the floor?' Tom said he had to go to the bathroom." Tom: "That's when I found out I couldn't walk. I recognized that there was something seriously wrong with me, but I didn't know what or why. I asked myself how I could have screwed up so damn bad." Dawn: "At that point, I hadn't told him what happened.

When I told him, he cried real bad. What is that called—lability? Yeah. He totally lost it when he was told that his son (who was also working on the job site) saw him being taken away in the ambulance."

With such a severe injury to the right side of the brain, Tom had no ability to be aware of the left side of his body or of the world. Dawn: "When he would eat, he wouldn't eat or drink anything to the left. I didn't understand about left neglect until [it was explained] in the family group. You had to turn his plate around. Then he would finish off the meal. Shaving—he would only shave one side of his face."

Toward the end of his inpatient stay, Tom met his neuropsychologist for the first time. "I looked at him and had one question: 'Will I ever get back to what I was before?' He looked at me and said, 'Do you want it sugar-coated or do you want the truth?' I said, 'If you lie to me one time, I'll never trust you again.' I don't care much for doctors, and after some bad experiences when I was younger, I expected them all to lie. But he didn't even talk around the truth. 'You'll never be the same.' Of course, I still didn't believe him at that point. It took about 3 weeks, until the time I left the hospital. Then I was starting to see that he was right. It was important to know that he wouldn't lie to me. Did I like the answer then? No. Do I still like it to this day? No. But I can live with it."

Dawn: "The social worker came into Tom's room and told me they were about to hold a family meeting." At the meeting, Dawn also, reluctantly, asked to hear the truth about Tom's condition and his prospects. "I cried, of course. I remember being told all of these things about his injury, and what the right side of the brain was for, and that his whole right side was damaged. I kept telling myself that what the doctor was saying about his permanent deficits was bulls____. I said to myself, my husband is tough, he's mean. Even if some of the others have problems, my husband's the one that's going to be fine. It took me a couple, three sessions to get it through my head that the doctor knew what he was talking about. Some of the things he was saying, like about the left neglect, and about his frontal lobe injury, I would see the things he said in what Tom was having trouble with, and I realized that I needed to listen to him.

"The week before he got released, he came home for a 2-day trial, and that didn't go very well at all. The ride home was a little rough on him with his double vision, and he got nauseous. Of course everybody wanted to see him. There was a house full of people. He got a little overwhelmed. I had him go back to the bedroom and lay down. Then his brother called and told him he was going to get back to normal. From that point on until Sunday evening, he was curled up in a ball on the sofa and wanted nothing to do with anybody or anything. He finally said, 'I just want to get back to the hospital where I'll feel better.'" Tom: "It still seems hard to believe, me wanting to get back to a hospital." Dawn: "He said it was a safety net for him. A good week after he came home, he hadn't had even one good night's sleep. He would wake me up at 3:00 a.m. determined to take a shower right then. He was on a cane for a good 2 weeks. They gave us a wheelchair, but he wouldn't use it. He had me up before daybreak to cook his breakfast. Very impulsive, very disorganized, disoriented to day or night." Tom: "I didn't know what was what." Dawn: "At night, he walked like a drunken sailor."

Unexpected problems provided important learning experiences. Dawn: "We went to K-Mart, not long after we got home from the hospital. We were going up the main aisle. I told him, 'Stand right here— I'll be right back.' I grabbed the bag, came right back, no Tom. I'm freaking out. I go to the front of the aisle, no Tom. The front of the store, no Tom. All of a sudden I see his head bobbing. He's over in the pharmacy section." Tom: "I needed a toothbrush." Dawn: "I told you to stand right there." Tom: "I got chastised worse than my damn grandson." Dawn: "I was so ready to kill him." Tom: "I couldn't be trusted to stay in one spot. I don't think I ever did that again."

"I remember hearing from Dawn about my left neglect. I guess I might have noticed missing quite a bit on my left side when I shaved. I remember her turning my tray around. But believing it—I guess not. The shaving—I tried to shave on both sides, just missed some spots. And I didn't know I had double vision until a week or two after I got out of the hospital, from my speech therapist. When they put the patch on I said, 'Wow—I can see now!' I don't remember my therapists saying anything about neglect. I remember [hearing] about my neglect as an outpatient, when I still didn't believe it. They said, 'You see it but it don't register in your brain.' I just couldn't understand that. I thought it was bulls____. That didn't convince me of anything. I didn't completely reject the idea, but I was having a hard time believing it, and I didn't want to believe it. I thought about it after therapy, and I started to notice some things at home when I was by myself. I would carry the portable phone with me and set it down on the left side. When the phone rang, I would stand up, walk around the couch, come around the other side, and there it would be, right next to where I was sitting. I thought, 'I guess [it was] the truth.' First I tried to explain it to myself as just a short-term memory loss problem. After the third or fourth time it happened, I said, 'I guess there is something to this. I guess I should start listening.' Then one day in rehab we broke for lunch, and coming out of the elevator some little old lady was standing right there and I almost ran her [expletive] down, and she was smaller than my granny. That's when I said I'd better pay attention to left neglect. I started doing what my neuropsychologist said, moving my head from left to right. When I did that, I felt about two inches tall for not believing what I'd been told—since I'd said I would believe him and I didn't. I noticed a lot of difference once I started doing that—I could find everything where I put it—I didn't have to get up off the couch so often. I also developed the habit of putting my drinks down on the right side after that. I don't think I ever put a drink down on the left side anymore."

Tom did have continuing problems with left neglect into the second half of his first year post-onset. Dawn: "One day he was looking for the chip dip. I told him it was in the refrigerator, on the second shelf. He said, 'It isn't—I just looked in there.' I pointed it out to him, and he still said it's not there. I had to actually pull the dip out and throw it on the table, and he said, 'Oh. Yeah, there it is.'" He wrote this problem up as an Error Analysis for his cognitive therapy. The group discussed the steps he would need to take to prevent the problem from happening again. He wrote the corrective plan, which involved searching the refrigerator by fixing his gaze on the left side wall and then slowly looking back to the right. That procedure puts his entire search into his intact right field of vision, which is sufficient to allow him to find anything he is looking for. That strategy, if he used it, would solve the problem completely.

However, he didn't use it. Instead, he overlooked another item on the left side of his refrigerator, and wrote that problem up as another Error Analysis 2 weeks later. The group got all over him about not using his corrective plan from 2 weeks earlier. He admitted that he made his second mistake while he was rushing. Faith pointed an accusing finger. "Fishbrain!" This was our group's pet term for brain overload, produced by rushing, excitement, and other kinds of sensory/emotional overload. Tom acknowledged the truth of it. It was suggested that he needed to make himself a hat with a fish hanging down over the bill into his right field of vision. The fish would remind him both of his tendency to rush and the need to compensate for his left neglect. It was recommended that he wear it at all times. Tom: "I wore it for about 2 months. It taught me to look from left to right."

After he quit wearing the hat, he had one more dramatic run-in with left neglect and fishbrain. Tom: "We were cooking fish on a weekend, and I had a bunch of Lake Erie perch in the deep freezer in my garage. I went out to get the fish, was in so big of a hurry that I just turned and walked right back into the house, shut the garage door, didn't go back there all day. When I finally did, I saw that I left the freezer door open. And of course, the door was on my left as I walk toward the freezer. That was two or three thousand dollars worth of fish I almost thawed out. How did I correct that problem? Now, every time I close my garage door, I turn my head and check the freezer door just to make sure it's shut."

"I still ran into door frames on the left side. Finally I worked my way out of that. I decided to start walking to my right so I could judge the door frame better. I used the right side as my guide. It's a wonder I never dislocated my left shoulder."

Dawn: "When Tom is looking for me, and I'm in my craft room, which puts me on his left, he goes right by the room to look for me in the bedroom. He still does that."

Tom: "I have some other problems from my right brain injury. I don't notice things as well as some other people. I guess it's a lot of small things that I should notice and don't. And it doesn't matter as much to me as it should that I don't notice it. I don't see dangers— they don't slap in the face the way they used to. And I can't read Dawn's moods and feelings like I once could. There are also some things I've had to give up. My pride—you can get it back eventually, but it takes a long time to get it back. I had to give up work. That was all I knew how to do, was work, and work my butt off. For my family. And I had to give up the old me. I'll never be the old me. I'll never be able to do a lot of the things I used to do."

Tom's accident also damaged his spine, resulting in pain and limited movement and ability to carry heavy objects. For the first 2 years, he was medically restricted from doing physical work of any kind. This left him at home with very little that he could do. He walked to a local park and shot a basketball with neighborhood children every day. He took care of the family dog and three cats. And he worried about what he could possibly do to earn a living. In his 3rd year, his orthopedic surgeon proposed implanting a device that would block his pain electrically. A trial attempt went well. He finally received the surgery in his 4th year, and became fully able to perform physical tasks for the first time.

Another unexpected experience taught Tom how much of a problem his temper could still be. "Going to my daughter-in-law's house, some young kid passed me on a double yellow line on a construction site, cut my ass off, so I chased him down the road and rear-ended him. I got out of my truck, walked up, poked my hand in his chest, and asked him what the hell he was thinking. If he hadn't been on his cell phone, I probably would have whipped his ass. He was on the phone with the police. The cop showed up, said, 'I heard there was an altercation.' I told the cop what I had done and said. The kid agreed to what he had done. The cop didn't write no tickets. I told the cop I learned my lesson. Don't let your emotions control your temper. I felt like the s___ on the bottom of someone's shoe, because I put myself and other people in danger. If there had been anyone else on the road, I could have killed them. I didn't know if anyone was there, and I didn't care. If he hadn't have hit his brakes, I would have kept following him until I got him to stop. Since that time, I had a very close call on I-4. Some guy yakking on his cell phone cut right into my lane, almost ran me into a barrier wall. I flipped him off, told him to get the [expletive] off the cell phone, and kept right on driving. But I have learned from my mistake. I didn't just blow it off the way I would have done before. It wouldn't have even been a thought process. I would have chalked it up as a bad day. I learned that I have to keep my emotions under control, and I know if I let 'em out of control what kind of trouble I can get into."

5. Accomplishments of Recovery

Tom: "When I was in the hospital a minister came to visit me and helped me to find God. I never had much faith in God before. I never went to church growing up—I never knew what church was. I figured the only person who could have spared my life was Him. That meant to me that He cares about me, so I guess I gave my soul to Him. I keep asking Him to show me what He spared it for, but people tell me I have to wait and see for that. I'm a better person—I do know that. I look at people totally differently than I did before. I used to be an SOB. Now I look at people with an open heart. I don't judge them —I look deeper."

The couple has been able to keep their marriage vital. Dawn: "He's still breathing. I haven't killed him yet." Tom: "I've had to step down from being the head of the household. I used to make all the decisions—any major decisions, now, I have my say but I no longer have the final say. My input ain't as great as what it used to be. Before what I said went no matter what. Now, sometimes it seems like why should I even say anything, and stick my foot in my mouth. I work harder on my marriage, now. Before I'd never have cooked or cleaned. It's a way I can help out my wife. I look at it as we're in this 50-50, and my 50 is the cleaning and the cooking, paying the bills, taking the animals to the vet. I don't always feel like I'm holding up my end, not all of the time. I should cook more often. I do my own laundry. Don't do hers."

What is Tom like as a husband? "I can be a pain in her ass, more so than before. One of the biggest things we had to adapt to was being around one another 24/7, because I used to be away working quite a bit. I've learned to give her her space, and she gives me mine. If I walk into the room when she's on the computer, and she looks at me a certain way, I know to get out of there." Dawn: "I think it's just a matter of toleration. The caring and the love makes the tolerating a little easier. We fight sometimes, but I get over it. There's times I feel that instead of being a partner he acts like my child. I feel I have to reprimand him, set rules and boundaries, like you would for your child. That part has gotten better over time. I've become more accustomed to it, he doesn't get as hyper as he used to, but I also don't have to criticize him as often—he has gotten better at things. There's times I feel he's like my roommate. We're just kind of here together. Then there's those times when we're intimate and I feel he's still my husband. I know he's in it for the long haul with me."

Tom: "For the first 3 years after the injury, we had sex once a month." Dawn: "And *then* I had to beg—and I hate begging. Not only was sex pretty much nonexistent, but closeness. Cuddling on the couch. Having a little kissing-fest, sitting on the floor, or standing in front of the sink, has gone down to a little peck here and there. As far as Tom taking a shower, shaving, sprucing up, putting on some cologne, and us going out for a nice dinner, that doesn't happen anymore. The little gestures are missing. When I'm drying my hair, coming by and giving me a little squeeze and a kiss—that doesn't happen anymore. That just sucks. I guess I just don't feel attractive or loved or wanted. I just feel like a caretaker, and to me, that's sad." Tom: "The romance side took a big hit." But Tom has not lost his romantic streak altogether—for their last wedding anniversary, he had a box of roses delivered (by Faith) to Dawn in the group meeting. This very common problem with sex and romance seems to stem from several causes. For one thing, Tom takes an antidepressant medication, which reduces sex drive and performance. Because he is not depressed, we are trying to get the psychiatrist to wean him off the drug. For another, Dawn has trouble understanding that Tom's sexuality is no longer triggered by looking at her. It can be jump-started by touch, or it can be activated with words. In group, any comment that they should be doing better than they were prompted them to work on bringing both the frequency and satisfaction up to higher levels. This is still an area in which they are making adjustments.

One part of the problem stems from the deficit in noticing changes in Dawn that comes with right posterior focal damage. "Until I found the hair in the trash can, I didn't realize that she had cut her hair. Right now, I didn't realize she had no eye makeup on until we started talking about it." Dawn: "It bothers me that I don't ever get feedback from him unless I ask for it. I'm starting to realize and accept that."

Tom reported feeling depressed about losing his career, though when we investigated it, it seemed more like self-pity than true depression. Dawn: "I know that he was supposed to jump up and do something with his life, to get motivated, to stop being a couch potato. And I knew he didn't feel motivated enough, and I still don't think he's totally motivated. But I just couldn't do push it. I knew that if he got off his ass, he would want to go back into construction work, because that's what he really knows." Tom: "To a certain extent, that's true. Because I would make a hell of a supervisor." Dawn: "Instead of pushing him, I try to make sure as much as possible that I can control Tom being safe. I don't want to lose him. I will do whatever I have to do to keep him safe. I know that's the wrong attitude. I know he has to do things on his own, and he has to make his own mistakes. But I'm afraid if I don't take these precautions, if something were to happen with him again, the guilt would be more than I could take. Because I let him get hit in the head once. I know it's not my fault, but there's still the feeling that if things had just been a little different, he wouldn't have gotten hit. This time I have to make sure."

"We did a lot of talking about him keeping busy. He worked on cleaning up the garage. He became motivated to help more around the house." Tom: "I built a TV stand for our new widescreen TV, and I built a computer desk into one of our closets. I built an entertainment center for her TV set. I've refinished all the floors in the house. I put up a hood range cabinet, and kitchen cabinets. It's not fancy, but it gets the job done. I do the oil changes on my car and all the family cars. I also fix my power lawnmower." Later in that year, Tom installed a new roof on their home by himself, without any difficulties, and without having to redo any of the work. He explained that he simply took the job step by step. "I wouldn't ever try that again" because it was so difficult. He also retiled both of the bathrooms in his home, and he and Dawn are happy with the way these jobs turned out. "My plan is to get my house here ready to sell, and when I sell it, buy a piece of land up near where we grew up, about 100 acres. I worked on a farm for 7 years, so I know that life like the back of my hand. There'll be enough to do on my own place to keep me busy until I'm old and crabby."

Dawn: "He started talking about volunteering in a veterinary clinic. Then he talked to our vet. And then he found a spot to volunteer at the animal clinic." Tom: "I clean the inside and outside of the kennels. I take the dogs out to play, interact with them to get them less aggressive. I spray for weeds, mow the yard, do other things to clean up."

Dawn: "And then he started babysitting our grandson." Tom: "My kid and his wife let my grandson get away with murder, and we don't. He pushes every button, tries to play us like strings on a banjo. I get a little cranky with him. Last Friday I had him for 12½ hours. He's usually here for about 8 hours. I don't ever spank him. I raise my voice to him, though. I take good care of him, though it would be better if I were more patient with him. Sometimes Dawn will tell me that— that I needed to be more patient with him, and I don't see it. If I do see it, I don't recognize it. When she tells me that I take it to heart and I work on it."

Tom took up bowling. "I had to relearn how to bowl after 40 years, because I couldn't remember how I threw my ball. I used to be a 187-average bowler, went down to 154 when I started back bowling about 2½ years ago (i.e., at 2.5 years post-onset). I mainly had to relearn by trial and error. I got some tips from a good bowler I know, but the advice he gave me, but I couldn't picture what he was telling me to do so I couldn't do it. I explained to him, 'There's no more film in the camera.' He got more specific, and it's helped. I've rolled a 300 in 2004 and a 299 in 2005. Both of those games were in league play. I'm averaging a 199. I put blinders on, so I don't see anybody else. That way I can keep my concentration." Since that time, Tom has rolled a second 300 game.

"My biggest struggle that came from the injury was not going back to drinking. I'd been dry 5 years at the time I got hurt. I've been able to stay completely sober. I did that for me, myself, and I, and nobody else. I thought it was going to be harder this time than it was the first time."

Tom returned to a full-time (and heavy overtime) job cutting concrete for road construction in the middle of year 7, so he has been working for a year and a half at last contact. Asked to explain this major step to the readers of this book, Tom said that the process began when the veterinary clinic at which he volunteered was closed. Although he continued to help the owners keep their animals, he felt an urge to look for a full-time job. "It had to be in construction. That's the only thing I really know how to do." He said that he is doing well on the job, and is serving as the senior member of his work crew. "I still make head-injured screwups all of the time, of course." He explained that he can function in this high-hazard environment without mishaps because he concentrates so hard on what he is doing.

He was still getting full disability benefits when he chose to end them by taking a job. He said that he never really felt right about being on disability, and was pleased and relieved to rejoin the work force. "I don't really know if I can fully explain why I did it. There are just some things you have to do only when you're good and ready. I was ready to go back to work."

6. Methods of Recovery

Tom: "A person needs to care about what their life is going to end up being like. I don't want to be a f____-up my entire life. I still screw up, but if I do screw up I try at least to fix it and to learn from my mistakes. I have to learn from my mistakes so I don't make 'em again. Little mistakes are just as important as the big ones. If you don't learn from the little ones, they keep getting bigger and bigger until you're not in control of your life. Until I pay attention to my mistakes, I can make 'em over and over again. People say to me, 'I do that.' I don't care if they do that. I shouldn't do it. I know I can't ever stop myself from making all mistakes. You can't see all of the things that might go wrong, so I have to learn from what does go wrong. If I take a hard look at it, I can prevent it from happening again. I might figure out that I have to double-check myself two or three times.

"I think what helped me is being a recovering alcoholic—because outpatient to a certain extent felt like AA. Different programs, not just 12 steps, but what they had in common was that if you don't do it, nobody is going to do it for me. It has to be one day at a time. Work through each day. It made life harder to get sober, and it made my life harder to have a brain injury. It took about the same amount of time to learn what I had to do to handle them. People look at me and don't think anything is wrong with me. They don't realize the emotion I have, the back-steps I've had to take to go forward again.

"Some people want an instant fix, but there's no instant fix for a brain injury. That's where the 12 steps come in. I know I can't go back to my old job, because of my health and I don't want to be responsible for other people's safety. I always try to make time for myself—if I didn't I'd go nuts. I have to have my down time, like when I go to the bowling alley. I go on a night when the league is not held, so there is no pressure on me. I accept feedback—I think you can learn from it. If other people have gone through what you're going through, they're talking from their heart. I guess I learned that strategy from AA also. Feedback helps you out a lot. Psychologically, AA helped me also. It's just another demon you have to fight. My grandson brought me out of it, also. He brought out the kid in me, when I went to the park and played with him. I think it's helped me, because I want to be there for him, and because I've learned to enjoy my life more."

Dawn: "I don't let him get away with anything. We try to structure things—like putting hooks on his car keys and his watch, so they are always hooked onto his belt loops. His meds are always sitting in a plastic container on his dresser top. His phone numbers and information are always written in a book. We try to keep to a routine, because he always does well with that. The dog is always fed at the same time in the same place, and the dog food is always in the same place. It helps to keep him organized. We used to have a dry-erase board that did that for him.

"[I was told] I'm going to have to let him make mistakes, I'm going to have to let him fall down, and that was a very hard pill for me to swallow. It was not too long after that when I gave up on being the home therapist. I felt that it would be too hard to follow that role, being as fearful as I was. [Eventually], I discovered that I could handle letting him make mistakes, with the help of Christ. He has to learn to make his own choices and decisions. When he makes mistakes, he works hard to correct them, to not do them again, and that's what matters. As for me, I'm totally committed to our marriage, to us being a couple, to Tom's recovery."

Tom: "In my old life, if I had problems on the job I left them on the job when I went home. In my new life, I can't do that. I have to take them home and think about them, because otherwise they will follow me."

The Journalistic Perspective

Every time I see Tom, I hear that George Thorogood song: "Buh-buh-buh-buh-buh-bad! Bad to the bone!" He leans back in his chair with a detached smirk under his camouflage-green fishing hat and wrap-around sunglasses, styling himself as a cross between "the Fonz" and a Duke of Hazzard. At first it came off as self-righteous defiance: "I'm proud to be the only country boy in a room full of city slickers." Maybe there's some truth to that, but after getting to know him better, it feels more like he's protecting himself behind a psychological barricade. He doesn't step outside of his fortress very often, rarely speaking above a terse mumble unless someone prods him pretty sharply, in a way that suggests he might be ashamed of himself in some way. Stories Dawn shared about how he'd spent all day and nearly started a fire struggling to make peanut butter fudge reveal how he copes with his life. After losing his career, his tough-guy self-sufficiency, his emotional trunk line to a wife he's known all his life, and the old self he still feels he ought to be, he pushes past his feelings of hopelessness and impotence and simply goes on doing what he has decided to do in the best way that he can.

Dawn is a different story. Although Tom feels incapacitated, she is overwhelmed. I'll never forget her words: "[I] have to be the alpha and the omega to the family." Tom's injury took away not only his ability to work, but his emotional investment in family activities. Dawn had to take over his responsibility to stay involved on top of her own. I know that survivors' relationships sometimes go into the toilet, but these two have such a huge investment in each other that they can't afford to let that happen. They have fought to stay together, to make this strange new relationship work. Dawn isn't looking to get the old Tom back, and is doing her best to accept him as a new person. But after many years of access to the inside of Tom's fortress, the injury has booted her out and now she pleads for him to find a way to let her back in.

The Neuropsychological Perspective

Tom was admitted, air evacuated, to the level one trauma center and admitted at Glasgow Coma Scale level 3. He suffered multiple episodes of respiratory failure in the field and at the hospital, and his resuscitation in the field was delayed for several minutes, raising the possibility of additional cerebral anoxia from heart-lung failure. His admission CT scan revealed a basilar skull fracture, eggshell fracture of the cranium, a right parietal contusion with epidural hematoma and sulcal effacement (the flattening effect of massive swelling), and right frontotemporal and frontoparietal contusions with subdural hematoma and sulcal effacement. This open head injury also resulted in an infection in the cerebrospinal fluid. His brain injury was so massive that he was immediately medicated to sustain the coma and reduce swelling. Medication was discontinued on day 15, and he did not emerge from coma until day 18; however, anterograde memory resumed on that day, suggesting that the 18-day interval probably overestimates the true overall severity of the diffuse injury.

Because of his medical complications, he was not discharged to outpatient status and seen for his cognitive rehabilitation program intake evaluation until the 11th week post-onset. Due to fatigue, his testing required 2 weeks to complete. He was a fully cooperative subject, but showed unusual emotional and behavioral reactions to being tested. No patient evaluated for this program ever made more self-deprecating remarks or predictions of failure before attempting a test. He predicted failure on every test that involved verbal or academic skills or any form of problem solving. He freely used foul language when frustrated by tasks. He also made a variety of excuses for the actual or imagined inadequacies in his performance, including references to his pain and physical disablement. He complained about a number of the tests. His most unique test-taking behavior involved striking himself with his dominant hand in conjunction with self-critical statements, observed on several occasions. He also showed difficulty in keeping his mind on the task at hand, and frequently made off-task comments of all kinds. This kind of a display of elaborate, dysfunctional behavior is usually a poor prognosis indicator.

In his test performance, executive symptoms were prominent. Key diagnostic measures elicited scores in the moderate-to-severe range. Qualitative evidence was extensive, including impulsive errors, perseveration, violations of prohibitions, and reduced efficiency on two-handed conditions of manual tasks. Measures of complex problem solving were consistently impaired at the severe level. There was also considerable evidence of nonverbal perceptual impairment, including profound impairment on the nondominant and both hands conditions of the key measure of tactile problem solving. Qualitatively, there was evidence of left neglect, defective learning of spatial locations and orientations, dysstereognosis, constructional errors, gross errors of visuospatial tracking, figure-ground reversals, and inattention to object contours.

Measures of focal attention and working memory were within normal limits. Processing speed varied from the normal range to the mild-to-moderate level of impairment. There was no evidence of any impairment of verbal learning, suggesting that the diffuse aspect of injury was relatively minor. For memory for nonverbal stimuli, only the key measure of incidental memory was more than mildly impaired, and that score reached the severe level.

Confirming the earlier interpretation of the behavioral observations, the MMPI-2 indicated extremely high concern about health matters, in a configuration that is often associated with symptom magnification. There was also evidence of limited self-esteem, presumably a chronic problem.

In therapy, Tom formed good working relationships with all of his therapists. He demonstrated a deep aversion to paper-pencil tasks, which Dawn assured the team was a lifelong characteristic, so he never became adept at the written compensation behaviors. He also showed a relatively rapid improvement in his left neglect, but his carryover to home was unusually poor, in part because Dawn refused to intervene.

A reevaluation was performed at 9 months post-onset, after his discharge from intensive rehabilitation. Somatic complaints were prominent at this time. He spent extended periods of time inactive and preoccupied with self-pity. The unusual, self-deprecating behavior and qualitative dysexecutive symptoms were largely absent at this time, whereas the perceptual symptoms remained prominent. However, he did not show frank left neglect, but rather occasional inattention to left hemispace.

Scores on key tests of executive function improved to the mild level of impairment. On the other hand, his performance on the most complex measure of perceptual integration (the Tactual Performance Test) actually declined in comparison with his intake scores, demonstrating increased emotional interference on spatial processing tasks. All measures of learning and recall were now found within normal limits. Complex problem solving on the Category Test improved to the borderline level. His MMPI-2 profile had normalized substantially, although his scores still suggested mild symptom preoccupation.

Overall, Tom's alcoholism history, preexisting brain disorder, somewhat advanced age, massive brain tissue loss, right parietal focus, and poor initial psychological reaction made a poor prognosis seem like a virtual certainty. To accept such a base-rate prognosis would have been to radically underestimate this man's rehabilitation potential. Although his recovery course was certainly uneven, it was apparent even in acute hospital that Tom was a stubborn and determined man who had overcome addiction through these traits. In such cases, the ultimate prognosis is determined by these personal qualities, and by the individual's decision to prioritize recovery.

Chapter 14

The Story of Jomo and Wengari

Jomo and Wengari are two strikingly intelligent and accomplished Kenyan immigrants. Both earned bachelor's degrees in computer engineering in England. They returned to Kenya to marry and then came to the United States to pursue their careers. Both were early employees of a major software company who rose to higher management as the company's fortunes blossomed. Both were supervisors, though they worked in different divisions. As important, long-time employees, they were on a first-name basis with the company's celebrated founder.

They had two children, an infant boy and a girl in elementary school at the time of Jomo's accident, 4 years prior to this writing. Though their speech is accented, both were second-language speakers of English from early childhood, with no difficulty in expressing themselves eloquently. They are both committed to spend their lives in this country.

1. The Old Jomo

Jomo was a brilliant student, so bright that even the most technical and challenging courses in college came easily to him. Like Abdullah, he confessed that he had never needed to work hard, nor had he ever been required to develop any particular mental discipline. Wengari, on the other hand, had been the devoted student, a methodical thinker who stayed organized "because I had to." When I asked whether Jomo ever made a daily schedule for himself before his injury, they both laughed. Although somewhat reserved by nature, Jomo had excellent social skills and was adept at making small talk, enlisting cooperation, and discussing business concerns with his superiors, colleagues, and subordinates alike. He had a "laid-back" and "easygoing" manner, managing by guiding others to come up with Jomo's ideas as their own. He was a senior director, which meant that a number of managers, each with his or her own technical staff, reported to him. The workforce under his direct management varied from year to year, but usually exceeded 100 professional workers. He acknowledged that he was a key operative for his company, working in a highly sensitive position and responsible for relationships with major corporate customers. An ongoing reorganization effort required him to use great diplomacy, as he was removing and redistributing authority, while trying to influence other wings of the firm with interacting responsibilities to cooperate with his plan. He explained that the overall reorganization plan would probably fail for several reasons, and that a new and possibly very different plan directly affecting his area was likely to be drawn up eventually. Jomo made so many urgent policy decisions on a daily basis that there were problems if he needed to take even one day off for illness.

Although Jomo was clearly devoted to his work and ambitious to rise higher in the company, he was also very much a "family man." He was concerned about the education of his daughter, and played an active role in parenting both children. In the region and culture in which both of them grew up, the husband was the unquestioned head of the household, with the wife deferring to him in all matters. Despite their education and American acculturation, they followed this tradition until the accident happened.

2. The Accident—6 Years Ago

Jomo had driven to Atlanta to attend a high-level symposium representing his company. His rental car was T-boned, putting him into a coma for 15 days. He also suffered a tonic-clonic seizure at the scene of the accident. His MRI scan revealed large, bifrontal contusions as well as scattered foci along the tentorium bilaterally. It was not possible to establish the date of his emergence from post-traumatic amnesia, but he did report scattered, vague recollections from his hospitalization.

His neurosurgeon and neurologist, well-established senior specialists in head trauma, agreed that his prognosis was limited; that is, they felt sure that he would not return to work.

3. Early Recovery

Jomo has essentially no recall of his acute hospitalization. Wengari was contacted by the medical center 2 hours after the crash, and was allowed in to see him at 11 hours post-onset. Wengari: "It was very confusing to go in and see him like that. Physically, he looked OK—he didn't have any lacerations. But he was hooked up to every machine imaginable. The neurologist looked worried. He said that my husband was not responding. I asked him what we could expect, and he responded, 'We'll have to see.' He told me the same thing for many, many days. When Jomo began to respond to questions and commands, his responses didn't make any sense for quite a long time. I would hold up two fingers and he would say say four. I would show him a triangle and he would call it a circle. He said that he had four kids. He didn't start to respond sensibly for about 3 weeks. The doctor told me that he had contusions of the grey matter and diffuse axonal shearing."

When Jomo was released to return to his home in Orlando, Wengari rode in the ambulance. Wengari: "He seemed like a happy little kid to be going home. He was still in a daze, and he wasn't talking a lot, but he was able to recognize some things. He could walk, but the way he looked so weak, I worried that he might fall. He didn't fall, though." He was transferred to BIRC for his inpatient rehab. Because he had no medical complications or physical disabilities, he was judged to be ready to go home in less than the facility's average length of stay, which at that time was just under 4 weeks.

Jomo was referred to the outpatient center for his neurorehab. He was still experiencing extreme fatigue and other early symptoms. "He slept and rested quite a bit. People would come over to visit him, and I would tell them that he was sleeping. He wouldn't get up to socialize."

At this point, the holistic cognitive rehabilitation program had closed, and only single-discipline outpatient services remained. He was assigned to the occupational therapist from the holistic program. There was no neuropsychologist on staff. He received treatments for fine manipulative dexterity, processing speed, impulse control, and note taking to aid recent recall. His occupational therapy treatment continued for approximately 2 months, supported by workers' compensation. As the treatment was coming to a close, the therapist referred him to the senior author's private practice for the treatment of his higher cognitive and prevocational skills.

Although his therapists had given him considerable feedback concerning his cognitive deficits, at our first session, he reported only minor difficulties with memory, and waxed optimistic about his readiness to return to driving and work immediately. He admitted that his occupational therapist did not agree with his idea of resuming work right away, but he dismissed her opinion. When the couple was told that an injury producing 15 days of coma and bifrontal contusions would be expected not only to leave him too disabled to work at the present time, but at any time, his first response was optimistic and even jaunty. "He wasn't completely convinced—he didn't realize it because of the state he was in."

Jomo had actually been aware of being impaired for some time, though he kept this knowledge to himself: "I realized something was not right when I was going for therapy sessions and asked to do multiple, simple tasks. I was doing them comparatively well for the group to which I was assigned, but had the realization that with this level of competition the bar is set so low that I must be really impaired. Realizing this made me feel sad, and gave me the realization that I needed to prove myself all over if I want to lead a credible life."

In contrast, Wengari responded to the discussion of his condition with a look of studious concern. She took extensive notes, and cast a number of worried glances in the direction of her smiling husband. She had "no reason to doubt the accuracy" of the assessment of her husband. She had been with him since the first day of hospitalization and had seen many of the problems that were described to her.

In this session, his follow-through on his daily planner was discussed. His compliance with the recommended procedures was limited and his attitude was lax. It was explained why full compliance was important, and Wengari was deputized to make sure to monitor his follow-through. This turned out to be sufficient to get him back on track.

He completed his neuropsychological testing during the following week. When the test results confirmed deficits that would stop him from functioning on the job, Jomo lost his smile and stopped taking notes. He was cued to write down the results of the evaluation, and he wrote a few more words here and there. The sketchy notes made it clear how much trouble he was having in accepting guidance.

Jomo: "Coming to the neuropsychological evaluation was not to see if I was impaired or no. I took the evaluation to see how much damage there was. Anything I did not believe, I considered to be a challenge that I needed to prove it to myself and the other person."

Wengari: "I was a little more serious about his problems than he was at first. I was ready to give them their due attention. He was not convinced that things were as bad as the testing indicated, but he was afraid, and that made him take the possibility seriously."

Jomo: "Not being able to do some of the jigsaw puzzles and recognize the patterns (Block Design and Object Assembly from the Wechsler Intelligence test) during the evaluation helped me to see the point."

After receiving the recommendation that he refrain from returning to work for the present because the errors he was likely to make might cost him the job, he pleaded for a chance to try going back immediately. When Wengari responded that the risk was not worth taking, he backed off and uneasily accepted the recommendation for continued therapy. It was recommended that they come for therapy as a couple. Time was clearly limited, as was his awareness of deficit. Family participation seemed to be the best approach to pursue rapid results.

The next session introduced the Error Analysis, assigning him to complete a minimum of one EA per day. The patient and caregiver roles were explained. After some reinforcement and correction in the next session, both were able to follow up the homework effectively. Jomo needed Wengari's help in noticing his errors, but when challenged to do so on his own a week later, he became able to do it without her help.

We then discussed the use of a planning algorithm, and established a menu of community, couple, and parenting activities that would call for making a detailed plan. Wengari was recruited to monitor his accuracy in planning and execution, and working in tandem they quickly reported good success. It also became obvious that the wife had been urging the husband to become more realistic and committed: "'We can't ignore this! Our whole future is at stake!' I would never had said anything like that to him before his accident. But it registered and he realized that this was extremely important. Then he gave recovery his full attention." Now, Jomo began to approach his work with a serious demeanor and to take detailed notes without being prompted.

Jomo: "I realized that I was able to do some mathematical tasks easily using a calculator, but I could not do the same thing manually. I used to take pride in not using a calculator for most of my common daily activities. Now, not being able to do these things was a sad revelation."

Still, his level of effort was not sufficient to get him back to work, and we were running out of time. It became necessary to break through his self-assured shell, and it appeared that only direct feedback would be strong enough to do that. He was told that the kind of recovery he was hoping to make was unprecedented. His job was simply too difficult and demanding. Patients with severe TBI never returned to such high-level management responsibilities. If the employer was willing to cut back on his job duties, a return to work might become more practical. But Jomo felt sure that his employer would not waste time on a manager with limited capabilities—if he asked for any accommodations, he would be summarily fired. Reluctantly, Wengari had to agree. It was all or nothing. The neuropsychologist was willing to try for a record-setting recovery, but it would be pointless unless he made a maximum effort, and he was not doing that. A unique recovery requires a level of extreme motivation that only comes with terror of failure, and it was clear that Jomo was not terrified. He was sent home to think about it, and to consider what his next plan would be if the job did not work out. At the next session, 2 days later, Jomo raised the issue immediately. "I'm terrified now. I thought you ought to know." "Good, now perhaps you have a chance of keeping your job." At that point, an exceptional recovery became the explicit objective of our treatment plan.

Jomo now accepted his compensations without hesitation. "All of them (slowing down, being careful, avoiding pressure, taking notes for recall, analyzing errors) helped me a lot. In meetings, I always listened carefully and took notes of what I will do or not do. I also had to change my habit of multitasking when talking to somebody. Instead, I had to just actively listen to the person I was talking to. That made it easier to concentrate on what they were saying."

By the end of the second month, Jomo had become adept enough in using these strategies to go back to work. A protocol for gradual increase in work hours was put in place, beginning at 40%. His extreme initial fatigue verified that the conservative protocol was warranted. It was recommended that his immediate supervisor provide him with regular, written feedback concerning his performance, a protocol that was not implemented due to the reluctance of the supervisor to commit feedback to paper.

They were advised to hold warm-up and wrap-up conferences before and after each work day to anticipate areas of potential difficulty, prepare appropriate strategies, plan the use of daily scheduling, note taking, and rest breaks, and evaluate the effects of the day's events. These conferences proved to be both valuable and necessary, as the couple was able to set up effective preventative strategies. Jomo continued to report occasional impulsive errors, but he was diligent in analyzing and correcting them, and they became less frequent week by week.

Wengari: "Later on, we had only one conference each day, whether it was in the morning or in the evening. If he was going to undertake a particularly difficult task that day, or write something important, he would always make sure to discuss it with me ahead of time."

Jomo: "Luckily, one of my trusted friends was there in the workplace to help me. I had always protected his interests and supported him whenever possible, and he repaid me by helping me when I needed it, upon coming back to work."

The feedback from Jomo's supervisor was glowing. "He said I was even better in some ways than I had been before. He found me more serious, and more focused."

Jomo continued to receive follow-up sessions with his neuropsychologist on a weekly and eventually a monthly basis after he returned to work. However, he reported fewer and fewer mistakes, and ultimately had no errors to report over the span of a full month. At 6 months following his return to work, he was discharged from therapy.

4. Accomplishments of Recovery

He continued to receive excellent reviews from his supervisor even after going back to a full-time schedule. Then in his 2nd year post-onset, his position was completely reorganized, with different duties and new subordinates and supervisor. Although he remained at the level of a senior department director and continued to be a "key contributor," he shifted to providing customer service on a completely different aspect of the product. Such radical changes in job description and setting represent the most challenging possible circumstance for vocational adjustment. By continuing to employ his strategies, Jomo was able to weather the transition and continues to receive excellent performance reviews on his new job right up to the present day.

Wengari: "His supervisor relies upon him heavily. You could say he is back to normal—almost. Although he was fearful for a long time, his confidence has come back. He's confident again—and that's his nature. But now he's confident but cautious—a kind of informed confidence, not arrogant or overconfident."

In the past year, Wengari has contracted a life-threatening illness and is undergoing treatment. She has become disabled, and Jomo has taken over her role as well as keeping up his own. "He is both Mom and Dad. He is doing everything he did before for the children and much more, and he is doing it well."

She feels that his social life had pretty much recovered when she fell ill. Because of her illness, they lack the energy and desire to socialize at present, but she feels he can manage a full social life now whenever he chooses.

5. Methods of Recovery

Wengari: "We rely on using all of the strategies [the doctors and the therapists] helped us to learn. We follow all of the steps—taking notes, putting things down on paper to get organized, and being extra alert about how he goes about doing things. Jomo is very good about writing things down now. He makes up a 'to do' list, which was never his style. When we have a lot to do together, he will make up the list on his own if I don't do it first. It has become a part of him, now. If he forgets something, it is important not to take it lightly, and we wouldn't do that. We take time and figure out, what should he do?"

Jomo: "The strategy of 'being humble' really helped me at work. When you are being polite and humble and accommodating of others, they work with you and try to support you instead of fighting or challenging you. For example, in a meeting I would let others address the subject while I sat and listened. They did not know that I had brought in a list of all the things we needed to accomplish. If they did not get to one of the points, I would frame my input this way: 'I'm just thinking out loud, here. Let us explore if this idea will potentially help us' . . . never offering the solution as my own idea or the best idea, but just as ideas for us to explore."

Although they worked intensively on his impulsivity, "He still does it to some extent. He takes a more simplistic view of things when he comes up with an idea or a plan. He thinks to himself, 'Oh, this will be easy and we can do it.' I'll say, 'No,' and he'll get mad about it for a minute, but then he'll end up laughing at himself and accept my point of view. He's open to listening, and he often seeks out my opinion. Once we've talked about something, he doesn't do it—that's how he controls his impulsivity." Jomo: "It is better and safer to ask for a few minutes to think about a problem and address it carefully than it is to respond quickly and make a mistake. Being correct has become more important than being the first one with an answer."

Wengari: "We have changed our outlook about things in general. We try to take one day at a time. We value things a lot that we once took for granted. Basically, both of us have become more careful. In a way, we are more scared than we were before, but it is scared in a good way, to prevent trouble. It is useful to be well prepared the way we are now. It even extends to our kids—we are more cautious to protect and take care of them. And when we get in the car, the kids tell us, 'Be sure to fasten your seatbelt!'"

Jomo: "I feel that I am a better person now than I was before the injury. I appreciate life more. I realize my responsibilities more, and I recognize that focusing on them is the most important thing in life, and not just chasing after the short-term materialistic goals. I have become more caring about others' feelings, as well. Paying attention to people helps you to build camaraderie and support with them. By always being positive and happy when interacting with others; my attitude brings out the same in them."

The Journalistic Perspective

Jomo is a tall, slender, neatly dressed man with a tuft of dark hair above his eyes and an engaging, boyish smile. He is soft spoken by nature, but you can see the gears shift when the topic turns serious. He is very careful about how he presents himself, and he gives no evidence of his impairment most of the time. On rare occasions, he is caught unprepared, and at those times he stammers and struggles to get organized just as any survivor might. It is obvious that he is intent on keeping those occasions to a minimum, and impressive how well he does so.

The Neuropsychological Perspective

Jomo was assessed at Glasgow Coma Scale level 8 on the scene. He suffered a tonic-clonic seizure in the field. His admitting level was not included in his records, but the level had dropped to 3 by the day's end.

Intake testing was performed at 6 weeks post-onset, just after Jomo had returned to Central Florida from the trauma hospital in Atlanta. In interview, his speech was dysfluent, and punctuated by long pauses as he gathered his thoughts. Problems with the syntax and organization of his speech were prominent. On testing, his greatest deficits were elicited by the Trail Making Test, where his scores were profoundly impaired on Part A and severely impaired on Part B. Dynamometer grip strength was also profoundly impaired for the dominant right hand and severely impaired for the nondominant hand. Complex problem solving on the Category Test was also severely impaired. Word fluency was moderately impaired, as were immediate and delayed word-list learning. On the Tactual Performance Test, scores ranged from moderate impairment on the dominant hand condition and mild impairment on the both hands condition to normal on the nondominant hand condition. Incidental memory for the TPT task was borderline impaired. Other measures of nonverbal memory from the WMS-III ranged from mild-to-moderate impairment on Family Pictures to normal on Figural Memory. On measures from the WASI, Block Design and Vocabulary were moderately impaired, Similarities was mildly impaired, and Matrix Reasoning was within normal limits.

Here is his autobiographical narrative: "I am Jomo Soyinka (perseverated), 36 years old (perseverated) with a wife & 2 lovely kids a 5 yr. boy & 2 yr. girl. My son will be starting pre-K this Sept. My daughter will Start going to day care in August. I work at Microsoft & so does my wife. I have been married since 1995. I & my wife we went to School together for B.S. I am very hard working professional & work very diligently my wife also does a very good job. She is always thinking of kids and trying to come up with Good way to enrich them and there [sic] development. Both my kids are very cute & keep my busy. I want to work hard to maintain the lifestyle I have got me and my family accustomed to. I'm originally from Kenya & visit home every 2 yr. My parents are very keen of kids & asking about them & want to pamper them & spoil them as much as possible" This tendency to run-on construction was also apparent in his spoken speech. Although the transcript gives the impression that he is not completely fluent in

English, that was not the case. Instead, he was inconsistent in following the rules of sentence construction in English at this point in his recovery. His speech regained almost complete fluency by the time of his discharge.

Chapter 15

The Story of Ernie and Helga

When a traumatic brain injury occurs at age 58 and produces serious focal damage and coma measured in weeks, little recovery is expected. The nervous system does not spring back from injury very well at that age, and individuals tend to be more accepting of disability and a retirement lifestyle. Ernie is an exception to every rule.

1. The Old Ernie

A quiet and shy individual born and brought up on a farm, Ernie came out of his shell in college to become a guitar player in a rock band. Always athletic, he also cultivated an interest in fast cars and motorcycles. He had a knack for math and science, and he used those smarts to earn a BA degree in chemical engineering. He went to work for foreign companies, married a Dutch beauty, and ended up in Brazil as the chief operating officer of a huge metal products manufacturing plant with more than 5000 employees under his supervision. "Prior to the accident, I was the construction manager and then the operations manager of a plant which produces in Argentina and is oriented toward steel-making. They ship all of their product to steel mills. I had completed the 6-month training of a new operations manager, was coming into the plant, and that went from February until September of 2005, and I came back here at that point in time, thinking that the future work would be part-time down there, and I'd be up here part-time. I really wanted to spend more time in Florida and less time overseas." He is described as having been a friendly boss, easy to get along with as long as you did your job. He was something of a company star, having developed several other successful plants for his German corporation.

In his spare time he was a true techno nerd, designing and marketing computer programs to run metal products manufacturing equipment. "At that time I was also working on the development of the SCREP optimizer computer model, which is used in steel-making, and that was with the partnership I had with two other partners, who worked with me on these models."

His wife, Helga, ran their home and set up their social schedule in Florida, while he worked in South America. He was getting tired of the job routine, which limited him to short visits to Florida. He had arranged to step down in favor of his assistant, while remaining at the plant 2 to 3 weeks per month as a consultant. Just before the change of jobs was to take effect, he was in Florida when a motorcycle accident damaged his brain.

2. The Accident—4 Years Ago

"I was going on my Harley Davidson motorcycle to a bike shop which is located up on US 19 in Tavares, Florida, and just going to pick up a battery. Just as simple as dropping a motorcycle to pick up a battery when this occurred. I was wearing a helmet. I was traveling about 55 mph on US 19, heading north, and a man pulled out of a side road where he had a stop sign and should not have pulled onto the highway. He pulled in front of me, of course, not moving, and I'm going 55 mph on the motorcycle and hit the car. My wife, Helga, had been at a bridge tournament very close to that, and just by accident came by just after my accident. So she saw me on the highway after falling off the motorcycle. She said that they said—and I don't remember this—that I was being combative upon falling off the motorcycle, and I was in shock, I think, at that time." In this high-speed crash, Ernie bounced down the highway on his head, shattering his safety helmet.

3. The Injury

He remained in a coma for 21 days, and was in post-traumatic amnesia for another month. "I had three brain lesions. The first was in the left temporal lobe on my head, the second was the right frontal lobe, and the third one, which did not show up on my CT scans but is measured on my neuropsychological testing, was in the right parietal lobe." The most serious damage was found in the left temporal area. There was a fracture of the temporal bone, extensive bleeding in and around the brain (subdural and intracerebral hemorrhages), and an explosive rupture of a blood clot into the fluid-filled cavity under the damaged area (intraventricular hemorrhage). These injuries reveal devastating damage to the language brain, almost certain to produce permanent aphasia, and gravely concerning in a man of Ernie's advanced years.

4. Early Recovery

"I was hooked up to a breathing machine as well as a feeding tube for several weeks. So you can imagine, if you're not eating and you're not breathing, you have to be hooked up to machines to live through that situation. I was in a coma for 3 weeks, and I lost 30 pounds of weight, from 175 to 145, during that period.

"After 3 weeks in intensive care and another 2 weeks on a medical floor, I was accepted at a local rehabilitation hospital. I went into intensive rehabilitation for 3 weeks, and I had to relearn to walk and talk. At that point I wasn't walking and talking, and so I had to relearn how to do that part of my life. I have no memory of the first 2 months in the hospital, so the whole period I was in the hospital, I have no memory of it. I had to write everything down from my wife telling me, but I have no memory of this occurring. I vaguely remember going home on the 28th of November. I have no memory whatsoever of how the accident occurred or of the accident itself."

As expected, Ernie emerged from coma with severe language impairment (aphasia). He remembers being unable to talk, and having difficulty understanding what others were saying to him. Right away, he became concerned about how this might affect him in going back to work. The medical staff was surprised at how quickly he recovered his energy and vitality. Ernie attributes this to his motivation and also to the exercise routine he faithfully followed to keep himself in top physical condition. He gradually recovered his physical abilities and eventually became able not only to walk but to resume his home exercise program full force.

Because Helga was not working at the time of the accident and was healthy and willing to take care of him, the hospital discharged him a bit earlier than the average patient with a head injury. "When I came out of the hospital, I was not well. I was speaking like a child. I was incapable to write, repetitive in talking, and my ability to think was not good. My judgment was not good. The logic I use for judgment was not good." Thus, he went home with considerable cognitive deficit, and returned for outpatient therapy. Again, he worked hard in outpatient therapy. "I went through the physical and occupational therapies quite fast, that was over very early in this treatment. And I stayed with my speech therapist for 58 sessions, twice a week." Although he still had fairly serious problems in language, his speech therapist was more concerned about his cognitive deficits, and referred him to the neuropsychologist who had supervised the local cognitive rehabilitation program. At the time of referral, Ernie's language was largely functional, although his conversation would grind to a halt when he could not think of a word (dysnomia). His grammar was impaired, but he was usually able to get his ideas across. He responded appropriately to simple conversation, but had great difficulty in understanding new or complex ideas. His physical recovery was surprising, but a stiff, rigid quality about his postures and movements remained.

Like many patients who have language disorder, he realized that he had these problems, although he underestimated their seriousness. He also realized that he was quite forgetful. However, he was unaware of his remaining cognitive problems and barely willing to consider that there might be problems he did not know about. "Mentally, I just wasn't prepared to understand the kind of damage I had. I needed to take these problems seriously, and I'd been avoiding it. I mean, I just didn't think I was as bad as I was." Given his viewpoint, it seemed perfectly reasonable to him that he should go back to work in a week or two, flying to Argentina and resuming living alone in his apartment. He was surprised and somewhat annoyed to find that the neuropsychologist thought he would probably need more therapy. After receiving the test results, like most engineers, he realized that repair work would be needed and asked only that it be completed as quickly as possible.

He was further surprised to hear that his prognosis for vocational recovery was poor. It was explained to him that the extensive damage to critical brain systems at his age simply did not allow for a return to work at a white-collar level, let alone at a top supervisory level. The neuropsychologist echoed appreciation for the unusually good physical recovery he had shown, and went on to state: "You would need to have the best cognitive recovery in the history of rehabilitation to be able to go back to work in the capacity you desire. From what I have learned about you, I don't rule out that possibility. If you want to strive for the goal of getting back to work, I am willing to help you. But you must be aware that it will take maximum effort for you to even have a long-shot chance of success." Ernie was satisfied with this arrangement, and gave an assurance that he would work as hard as possible.

Helga was also surprised to be confronted at the third session. She had elected to miss the first two sessions, and had implemented Ernie's home program in a compliant but halfhearted manner. It was reiterated to her that he could not possibly recover vocationally without making unprecedented progress, and if she did not play her initial role of taskmistress and strict monitor, the effort would be pointless. It was acknowledged that Helga had never been a stern overseer, and that the role was foreign to her unassuming and playful manner. It was also foreign to their relationship for her to give orders and impose judgments on Ernie. Nevertheless, she agreed to try. Over a span of 3 weeks, she took on the prescribed role more and more until she was implementing it fully. At this point, Ernie sometimes became irritated because Helga would identify one of his errors and would not back off despite his vigorous protests and arguments. It soon became clear that she was going to give Ernie's recovery all she had to give, and that she also took a kind of devilish pleasure in getting him to recognize his deficits. In the end, she became one of the most effective home therapists in the program's history.

Because the testing indicated that Ernie's greatest weaknesses were in high-level attention skills and executive functions, a heavy emphasis was placed in his initial program on recruiting and maintaining high levels of mental effort for controlled processing and decision making. He began with hour-long, timed search for strings of numbers embedded in a large matrix of numbers, and with similar word search puzzles. He spent an hour searching through the newspaper for every instance of a particular word. These word searches graduated to watching videos to identify every time a particular word was used, and reading novels searching for every instance of two different words. He also performed timed puzzles that required him to find tiny differences between two complex pictures. He spent 1-hour periods playing the video game, Breakout, which had been a staple in several hospital-based cognitive rehabilitation programs.

He completed a large jigsaw puzzle, but for the therapy, the task was modified in a way that greatly increased the requirement for effortful self-control. He was not allowed to touch any pieces that did not fit together. He had to align them from a distance, bringing them together only when he was sure he had a perfect fit. "The puzzle had 732 parts to it. And it took me 32 hours to put it together correctly. I only made three errors in fitting up, because I had to be watching very carefully what I did with the pieces, to not make errors with them. So it took me 32 hours to put together a puzzle, which to many people might seem extremely long." Thus his score was 99.5% correct impulse control.

"I studied 10 hours a day for 7 days a week; in addition to that, because of my body shape, I did 1 to 2 hours of exercise every day, so I had an 11- to 12-hour schedule daily for the whole year, essentially, until the end of the year when I got out. So I spent many months working like that in order to deal with the situation I was in. Some of the things I was told to do, if you listen to it, you say, 'What in the dickens were you doing with this?' But it really helped, and it made a lot of sense at the time."

Another heavy emphasis in Ernie's home program was on impulse control exercises, which require thoughtful decision making under increasingly difficult conditions. "It was 20 questions, and a thing called Boggle, which you may have heard of. I worked with slapjack, sudoku, and the tower of Hanoi, just to improve my capability." As most patients in well-developed cognitive rehabilitation programs are asked to do, Ernie kept a daily schedule that he typed into his computer every evening and followed the next day. The requirement was stringent— he was expected to schedule each specific activity separately, to fill his entire day, and to keep his schedule 7 days a week. Although he was not accustomed to this much regimentation, the organized way of doing things appealed to him, and he quickly became faithful and proficient in scheduling himself. "I have daily plans every half hour, from 6:00 in the morning until 9:00 at night." He also discovered quickly that his used daily schedules were an invaluable memory aid in case he forgot what he had done on a previous day.

He was taught to rely on making written, taped, or computerized notes to support his memory for information. He used this procedure to keep track of the contents of important phone calls, and also to make minutes from his therapy sessions. He was taught to use the Error Analysis procedure to self-correct the effects of his cognitive deficit. These procedures worked well together. Thus, when he realized that he was forgetting to bring everything he needed to therapy, after filling out an EA form, he decided to write a checklist that would prevent leaving anything he needed to take with him. And when he failed to use the checklist and ended up forgetting to bring the check he needed to pay for his therapy, he recognized that he had allowed himself to run late and forced himself to rush, which resulted in the flawed execution of his self-corrective plan. Ernie is still in therapy, but at the last session his records indicated that he has completed 150 Error Analyses. "My improvement in decision making has come from learning from my mistakes. After I study my errors, I might make one again once or twice, but then I don't make it after that. I remember what I had done improperly before, and prevent doing it again. Now that I am back at work at the plant in Argentina, I find that I make very few errors."

As another executive task, he was charged with developing an agenda for the therapy meetings. He took this responsibility quite seriously, including a copy of the previous week's agenda as a kind of meeting minutes in the packet he presented to his neuropsychologist at the beginning of each session. The packet also contained summaries and graphs of his performance on each of his home therapies, a table he designed to show the results of his EAs, and any other materials he anticipated might be needed to complete the agenda for that week. He never failed to prepare and bring a packet, and they were always neatly and professionally done. He occasionally made errors in some of his entries, and for each of these he completed an EA.

The most cognitively complex aspect of his training was Targeted Situation Recognition. His EAs were systematically analyzed to identify the circumstances under which he made errors, so that he could be vigilant to prevent them in the future. For example, it quickly became obvious that he tended to make errors in the kitchen, because he did not take the tasks seriously and did not make the same level of effort to ensure his correctness. It also became obvious that he made mistakes when he was preparing to leave home because of his tendency to rush at those times. And he tended to make his most serious language errors when talking to his wife, again in association with reduced effort toward quality control. Like most engineers, Ernie had difficulty in identifying the emotional states in which he tended to make errors, although he gradually became aware of the importance of emotionality.

"The other thing I want to mention is, since we lived over an hour from the therapy offices, Helga and I didn't want to waste time traveling, because to get down here is an hour each way. So she would ask me questions as we were riding, to name 10 vegetables, 10 fruits, 10 countries in different locations and their capitals. So as we rode, I'm thinking all the time about naming fruit, which you think maybe is easy, but it isn't. So I'm trying to think, 'What the devil did I have in the salad?' And I can't remember exactly what I had in the salad, or what did we eat, in order to get the 10 vegetables together, so it really was time consuming for me, and it still is, I have to admit. To remember that, it's not easy."

5. Accomplishments of Recovery

"My vocational recovery was something I'd really been striving for. During that year, from the time of the accident and recuperation and treatment in the hospital, that was the only thing I dedicated myself to. So a year later I was ready to go back to work, and I went to Argentina to work for Orinoco Iron, starting November the 1st of last year. I was there in November, December, and January for 3 weeks out of each month. So in other words, I was back fairly close to where I wanted to be, not working full-time down there, but being in Argentina and working at the plant.

"In addition, in the months of November and December, I prepared the papers and the presentations that I had in two conferences. One was in Dusseldorf, Germany, and one was in Charlotte, North Carolina, and I made those presentations. I did not present in Germany; we had another guy to do that, but I did present the paper in Charlotte, North Carolina, for the company in Argentina." Ernie has been quite successful as a technical speaker at international conferences, and currently presents almost once a month either as a representative for his former employer or as the owner of his software firm. He has been diligent about preparing formal outlines well in advance of the due date, and videotaping a dress rehearsal for self-critique. He also reports that this level of preparation has allowed him to handle questions more effectively.

"I just want to mention, in Argentina, the work I'm doing now is technical assistance to the CEO. It's not being the direct manager of the plant, or of the production or of the construction of anything. I'm also working on the study of CO_2 admissions that we're trying to attack with the plant in Argentina, to lower the CO_2 emissions worldwide.

It's becoming more of an event and a problem here in the United States, but it's a much larger, I guarantee you, in Europe. The European community is very concerned about the carbon dioxide release from either living, or from plants, and they're now undertaking reduction of CO_2 in Europe over the next 2 years, and they'll continue that over the next 20 years at least. So we're working on that as well. I'm also working again on computer programs, with two people I work with here in the United States, Chicago and up in Pittsburgh. So I'm actually back to working on the computer models like I did previously. Initially, I could not do that, so I have improved in those areas. I'm working two locations, in the US as well as in Argentina.

The authors of this book solicited a letter describing his capabilities and limitations during his return to work from the corporate Vice President of Operations. This letter stated that before his injury Ernie

> . . . was responsible for all project related aspects such as engineering, procurement, construction, and project management including contract management. The plant TIC was $900 million, and involved resources that gathered over 18 million man hours of work and employed approximately 5,200 workers. The project resulted in a world-class safety record. . . . [Following his accident, Ernie] returned as Technical Advisor from November 2006 to December 2007. He assessed the plant production increase and was involved in the preparation of [technical] process performance results presentations for international conferences in Europe and the U.S. He led activities for corporate training in [his specialty] and was also involved in corporate Market Research activities and strategic planning activities. As he returned to work, he showed a positive and enthusiastic attitude, ready to recover from the consequences of the accident. He progressively recovered, following his re-learning exercises and treatments up to the point that the differences between "before and after" were almost unnoticeable . . . we only noticed a few high blood pressure events and occasional difficulties in long term memory.

6. Methods of Recovery

"What about my recovery? If you get recovery, it's because you work at it. What I'm finding is that many people around me, not here, but in other locations, feel that I have completely recovered from the accident. They don't see any problems, either with my body, because they heard I was crippled initially and they don't see that, and they feel like I'm thinking like I used to. But I don't, and I know that. It's very clear to me that I don't have that capability, and I have to continue to deal with it. The people that are talking to me and looking at me don't see it. They see me down there they come and they hug me and they say I'm just wonderful, but I'm not, and I have to continue to work with that, and that's very important.

"I am a brain-injured person, I am not a normal person. I'm different—I'm not the old Ernie. I would like to be my old self—I just see that I can't. I hate that my cognitive problems will always be there, but since I'm aware of this, I will continue to study and try to improve myself for the rest of my life. I know how bad I was initially. It's not something that's going to grind to a halt here; I have to keep after it. I've worked on getting better and dealing with my impairments, with using techniques. I always look at my deficiencies. When I am less than totally adequate, that is not what I want to be. So I try to learn how to compensate for my inabilities. I hope to further improve. Originally, as I said, I gave myself 1 year to have this work out, and it has improved me, but I have a ways to go to get better, and I intend to do that.

"My wife gave me all the assistance she could during this period. She was with me every day in the hospital, and took decisions because either I was in a coma or I wasn't capable of doing that, so I really appreciate all the help that I got from her.

"The company I work with in Argentina has also supported me, and allowed me to go back to work for them. So that's quite a change that one doesn't expect from a company, and I really find it's more than I was expecting out of Argentina. When I was getting prepared to go back to work, I was clear with the people I work with about what I expected from them and what they could expect from me.

"When I am on the job at the plant in Argentina, I am careful to make sure that I am well prepared for everything I have to do. Each day begins with a meeting with all of the supervisors, reviewing the events of the past 24 hours and planning for the next day. A secretary prepares minutes for the meeting, and I study them in advance. Then as the meeting is taking place, I take notes on a tablet to try to get as much of the information written down as I can. I certainly pay more attention, listen much more intensely to what a person says. I have to focus, focus, focus on what the person is saying. You have to be totally concentrated on listening. Sometimes I will e-mail one of the others to ask about some of the details I could not write because they were speaking too quickly.

"I have to try harder than I ever did before because I don't think as well as I did. I have to think harder. I have to be totally devoted to that. People who see me at the plant can see that I am working harder than I ever did. I devote every second to figuring out what I need to be doing and to making sure that I do it correctly. I'm at the plant 12 hours a day right now, and I probably get done about what I used to do in 5 to 6 hours, and I don't waste a second. To have to be doing something productive every second—I would have hated the ordeal before—but now, I want to do it, man. I want to make things work out.

I have a full, written schedule of each meeting I will have, and each place I am going to visit. Before I go to a particular part of the plant, I always sit down and reread the old operating manuals to make sure I remember how things are done in that area. When I am planning, I write things down step by step to aid in thinking them through, or if I can, I put the steps on the computer in the form of equations.

"I still have trouble with is remembering people's names. These can be people I just met, or people I did business with for years. When this happens, I try to search through my memory and write their name down on my tablet. If I cannot remember, I write down a description of them so that when I get their name I can put it in my notebook, in a section for names I have to relearn.

"Some of the computer programs I work with, and some of the ones I have designed, are very complicated. They are much harder to use now. It takes more time, and the work is more difficult. I have trouble thinking of what step needs to be done next, and to remember what other cells the cell I am working on is connected with. Sometimes a cell can be linked to 10 or 50 other cells by equations entered in another part of the program. When you change one cell, you have to go through and change all the equations. This very hard for me to do now, where it was once very simple. I have to work through the connections one at a time. When I write conversions or make simulations, I have to be sure to write into the program a lot of explanation of what I am doing, both to stay on track and also to be able to use it later.

"I think I've demonstrated recovery is possible. I mean, you don't get all of it out that you want to, but you can recover, and as you know, I'm much better looking than I was when I started here. In fact, some months ago, and I hadn't recovered even at that point, I wasn't as good as I am now, and I realize what I'm saying is really the case, but you have to keep after it. I've only had a little bit over a year now, but I do see the ability to recover from my injury. I'm glad to be here, and even though I'm a young fella, I'll keep after it."

The Journalistic Perspective

Ernie is a "just the facts, ma'am" kind of guy with a strong Midwestern accent and a no-nonsense delivery. His fluffy hair and short-cropped moustache would not look out of place on the farm where he grew up. But unlike the stereotyped farmer, he stands up straight with good posture, and looks like he is in the physical condition of a man 20 years younger. He faces you squarely and looks you in the eye, the look of command. He thinks carefully about what he is about to say. Then he stumbles over the third word out of his mouth and bears down trying to explain himself out of the hole he just dug by his slightly jumbled sentence. You can tell that Ernie hates to be so clumsy in explaining himself, but he shows extraordinary patience and persistence in finding ways to get his point across. In 5 minutes, you can see that this guy is totally dedicated to recovery, and that he will not be denied.

The Neuropsychological Perspective

The accident was a motorcycle versus automobile accident with helmet applied. He was found at Glasgow Coma Scale level 7 and required intubation in the field. On admission, he was found to have a left fronto-temporal subdural hematoma, which was surgically evacuated. CT also revealed a right frontotemporal contusion, a right frontal subarachnoid hemorrhage, a right parietal laceration, and scattered parenchymal hemorrhages, as well as spinal and rib fractures. His mental status then declined (level unspecified) and a second craniotomy discovered a left inferotemporal hemorrhagic contusion, which was also treated surgically. Subsequent respiratory distress secondary to MRSA pneumonia required mechanical ventilation. Although cleared to take food by mouth in mid-hospitalization, his intake was limited and he developed anemia and electrolyte imbalance. Speech therapists on the acute unit also observed expressive aphasia. Repeat CT at 4½ months post-onset found left frontotemporal encephalomalacia, dilation of the temporal horn of the left lateral ventricle, and a new potential lesion on the left parietal lobe. The duration of post-traumatic amnesia was difficult to establish, and is estimated at 5 to 7 weeks.

Referral for neuropsychological evaluation was made at the end of the hospital-based outpatient rehabilitation, at 5½ months post-onset. At this point, the only cognitive symptoms he reported consisted of inefficiency in using and modifying his computer programs.

Profound impairment was elicited by almost all measures focusing on the executive functions as well as verbal learning and recall. Gates-McGinitie reading comprehension elicited a moderately-to-severely impaired score. WASI Verbal subtests showed moderate impairment. The Tactual Performance Test was severely impaired on both one handed conditions and moderately impaired on the both hands condition. Incidental recall from TPT, mazes, the Visual Search and Attention Test, and Trail Making Part A were all moderately impaired. Purdue Pegboard scores were inconsistent, ranging from moderately to profoundly impaired. His strongest performance was found on measures of learning and recall for nonverbal stimuli, which were within normal limits, and the Category Test and WRAT-3 Arithmetic, which were in the borderline range. It was also noted that he made impulsive errors on many procedures, but corrected them, usually with full effectiveness, after a single instruction.

Here is his written narrative self-description: "Ernie Sedner. Age 58. Has a history of working overseas in Argentina as plant constructor and in the part of operation. As of February, 2005, the operation responsibility of the 2,000,000 ton/year iron plant was passed on to the new operation manager in San Felipe. [paragraph break] Ernie Sedner can travel to work full time for Meadowlark Iron in Argentina until Sept [sic] 2006. The plan was to reduce to part-time after September 2005. [paragraph break] Ernie came to DeLand at the end of Sept [sic] 2005 for a week. Towards the end of the week stay at home, Ernie was hit on his motorcycle by mistake by the driver of the car. [paragraph break] He was in the hospital for almost 2 months."

His MMPI-2, of questionable descriptive validity due to his reading comprehension problems, produced a floating profile in which demoralization and dysphoric affect were prominent problems. He also indicated concern about his cognitive capabilities.

In view of the global cognitive impairment at this late point, a hierarchical approach to treatment was felt to be indicated. Initial emphasis was placed on self-monitoring, concentration, and other aspects of mental effort, including planning. His implementation of this program, with the assistance of Helga, was so consistent and time intensive that he made strong progress, and was advanced to include Targeted Situation Recognition in the 2nd month. Ernie also readily accepted the suggestion that he take charge of his own program. He prepared color-coded diagrams charting his progress in every self-therapy and composed a detailed outline for every neuropsychological therapy session, even at the follow-up sessions held 3 years later.

Ernie was administered a neuropsychological reevaluation at a private clinic at 3½ years post-onset, documenting that he continues to experience neurocognitive symptoms. His full-scale Wechsler IQ was found in the moderately impaired range. Confrontation naming and word fluency were severely impaired. Word-list learning was severely impaired in the immediate condition, improving to the moderately impaired level at the delay condition, but with five intrusion errors. Recall of visual information was moderately impaired in the immediate condition and profoundly impaired on delay. His digit span was five forward and five backward. Design fluency was severely impaired. His best performances were on the Wisconsin Card Sorting Test (mildly impaired) and Block Design (normal). Thus his recovery was based on becoming adept at using his still-impaired brain.

PART IV
Conclusion

Chapter 16

Brief Sketches of Three More Great Recoveries

Here are brief descriptions of recoveries made by former patients who were not available to interview during the writing of this book. Juwan's accomplishments are as impressive as any survivor's, occurring in the context of a very serious injury. Adam and Mandy have also built impressive new lives, accomplished while coping with less diffuse injury than most of the others whose stories are told in this book.

Mandy

Mandy was a college graduate with honors who planned to go to law school. Her Geo was broadsided by a van pulling a trailer, resulting in a coma of 2 days' duration, post-traumatic amnesia of 10 days, and swelling of the right side of her brain. She contracted meningitis in the hospital. Mandy was a hard-working trainee who preferred to do things her own way but learned to use the program's strategies. Although she made few comments, she obviously felt it to be urgent to get done with therapy and back to school as soon as possible. She dealt with this urge by working hard, and she completed a 6-month program in 4 months. She then enrolled in graduate school, earned a master's degree in counseling, and is now working as a high school counselor. She remains a bright, confident, poised individual from a successful family. A telephone conversation at approximately 5 years post-discharge found her in good standing in her 2nd year working at a local high school and recently married to a man she met after her injury. She voiced satisfaction with her progress and her new life.

Juwan

Juwan was a college senior who sustained a coma of almost 4 weeks and left temporal, right frontal and right frontoparietal focal injuries. His left-sided focal injury was massive, swelling up enough to push his whole brain to the right. It left him with serious language and memory deficits. He was not ready for advanced rehabilitation training while he was in the program; he had completed the more basic half of the curriculum at the time of his discharge. However, he persisted in his goal and was able to get his bachelor's degree in education. He was then hired as a middle school teacher. When he had difficulty passing his qualifying exams, he called the program and got a cognitive booster shot. After a strategy session, he passed his tests. At that time, he was also engaged to marry a young woman he had met after his injury. His formula for success included hard work, persistence, strong religious faith, and unwavering family support. He continued to hold this job at 5 years post-discharge.

Adam

Adam had graduated from a fine law school less than a year before his injury. He met his wife at college, and they were still enjoying the romance in their marriage. They moved to Orlando so that he could accept a job in a lucrative legal specialization with one of the finest firms in the area. He was a young man on the way up. His main indulgence was going motorbike riding on the weekends with a group of friends. One day, he dumped the bike and struck his head against the pavement at high speed. He sustained a small contusion in the right parietal region. Vigorous and in excellent health, he emerged from his coma after only 3 days. However, he wandered the hospital unit for 59 days in disorientation and post-traumatic amnesia, restless and trying to get home. At times, he became so fixated on trying to get away that he would hurry off with his wife dragging behind him, her arms locked around his neck, saying anything that might calm him down. When he went to the outpatient program, he understood that he had been in an accident, but had difficulty accepting that he was cognitively impaired. Although he worried about the possibility of deficit, he did not translate his worry into working consistently on his recovery. He finished the program in 4 months, but this was not a fully satisfactory discharge.

His employer was willing to take him back, and met with his neuropsychologist to develop a plan for gradual return to his duties. It was recommended that the employer give him written, explicit feedback on his errors to give him the best opportunity to process it. The employer did not provide the feedback as recommended, but Adam's failure to write down the information he later forgot, his failure to prepare adequately for meetings, and his passive willingness to make errors convinced the law firm to discharge him. The neuropsychologist urged the supervisor to review Adam's shortcomings and mistakes in a meeting, and the three of them sat down for an hour. The supervisor gave a running account of what Adam had done wrong, finally not pulling any punches. After the meeting, Adam summarized it by saying it had gone well and that he felt sure he would now get off probation. He was stunned to hear that he had been discharged.

After several months of inactivity, Adam got a volunteer job helping prisoners to prepare their legal cases for appeal. More than a year later, a family friend convinced the partners of his prestigious firm to give Adam a job similar to the one he had lost. In preparation for the job, a meeting was held with Adam, his wife, his mother, his stepfather, and the neuropsychologist. Asked about his game plan, Adam explained that he was going to conceal his head injury, as he had come to the conclusion that his first job was lost due to prejudice. One by one, each of the others in the meeting recommended against his plan, but Adam was adamant.

Three and one half years later, Adam contacted the neuropsychologist on the GiveBack Web site. He reported that he was still holding the job because he decided to change his game plan dramatically. He admitted his injury and put in "endless hard work" to correct his deficits. He stated that he was still impaired, did not yet fully understand his deficits, but was working at coping with his injury. He now expected to be working at it for the rest of his life.

Chapter 17

Lessons Learned From 30 Recoveries

The 15 top recoveries were chosen from almost 250 former patients given routine follow-up interviews after discharge from therapy, a subgroup of more than 1600 working-age TBI patients who were treated across a period of 19 years. As such, they represent the top 5% of the follow-up group. The 15 poor recoveries were also chosen from the follow-up sample, representing the unsuccessful cases with the longest follow-up interval. The length of both the successful and the unsuccessful recoveries ranges from more than 2 years to 16 years. This is one of the longest-duration follow-up studies published to date. The successful survivors have been working in their present jobs for years (with the exception of Ernie, whose job tenure is slightly more than 1 year), and the unsuccessful survivors have likewise been unemployed (or briefly employed) for at least 2 years. These are well-stabilized patterns of long-term recovery.

In this chapter, we will present our conclusions from this project, interpreted in the context of our rehabilitation knowledge base. As scientific data, these interpretations are only educated guesses (hypotheses) about how recovery works, and until they have been formally validated, each reader will have to judge how much sense they make or don't make.

1. Exceptional Recovery Is Possible.

Some survivors lead consistently impressive, full, productive lives in which they compete at the highest levels. It is not a fluke. A substantial group of people is described in this book. Great recovery may be rare but it is real. Severe injury does not prevent every patient from achieving a truly comprehensive functional recovery, competing on even terms with people whose brains are intact, and winning.

2. Anatomy Is Not Destiny, At Least within Broad Limits.

Terrible brain injuries do not prevent exceptional recovery. Survivors can cope with a remarkable amount of brain damage. Coma as long as 1 month is not a recovery killer, although we have not seen great recoveries beyond 1 month, nor good ones beyond 2 months (Schutz, Barry, Gross, & Tupper, 1984). Massive destruction of the frontal lobes can lead to permanent and total disability (in the case of Jericho) but it can also be handled in a manner that restores a full, complex, demanding life (Samantha and Rachel), and we saw another patient with the injury that Jericho sustained (bilateral anterior cerebral artery transection) achieve a good recovery with active family help. Right posterior association cortex damage poses the most serious obstacle to recovery (as seen in eight of the unsuccessful cases), but even significant injury in this part of the brain was managed by Faith and Tom. We have also seen three relatively recent patients with right posterior CVA achieve good recoveries.

3. Recovery Is up to the Person.

No exceptional recoveries were created by the therapy staff. To the best of our knowledge, no brains were repaired: Every patient left rehabilitation with the usual impairments of executive function, new learning, and high-level attention. When the senior author asked the task force how many of them had gotten over their injuries, all reported that the injury was still there, and only Stephanie (who had the mildest injury) felt that her brain function might be better now than earlier in her recovery. In no case did a family force a successful outcome on an uncooperative survivor. Every exceptional outcome was created by the survivor, through a deliberate, determined effort to make his or her behavior work better. Every recovery required active effort and self-correction, and every one still requires the activities today. These survivors decided to listen and learn, used their brain injury education to set their strategies, and made follow-through a top personal priority. Each one was unwilling to accept less than success. It is hard to imagine an exceptional recovery without this kind of total personal commitment.

4. Recovery Is Adaptation.

In essence, exceptional recovery undoes the natural relationship between the amount of impairment and the amount of ability limitation. It is a process of forced adaptation to disability: learning to use the impaired brain in the ways that make functioning effective in real-life situations, and learning to avoid the ways that no longer work properly.

Is there some fundamental difference between these recoveries and the less successful ones that were described in Chapter Two and Chapter Three? In comparison to survivors who did not receive intensive TBI rehabilitation, these individuals accepted the challenge to face their deficits. The knowledge gap created by the short-circuited executive system was breached by high-impact therapy feedback. And unlike those who beheld their deficits and then denied them, turned to substance abuse to feel better, gave up, or responded with indifference, these people chose to deal with the unpleasant reality. Clearly it was necessary to think negatively until the injury was accepted and understood, to skeptically examine how the self functioned, and to discard the old self-concept. Acceptance of the impairments came in different phases of recovery for different individuals, but it was followed by problem-focused coping (Lazarus & Folkman, 1996). Based on what they discovered, they forced themselves to look ahead, anticipate trouble, and prepare for difficult tasks more thoroughly than they had prepared in the past. Once compensation became effective, they went back to positive thinking with a kind of "conditional confidence" that says, "I will be successful, but only as long as I use my strategies properly."

The process of self-examination can never stop, and they report that they are still learning valuable lessons about the injury even in the second decade. They not only have to watch what they do and how they do it, but they also must watch how they function as self-therapists. Whatever they try, they continue to examine and evaluate their own methods, and when those methods are inadequate, they tinker until they work properly. Carver and Scheier (2001) refer to this behavior as meta-monitoring. How good am I at self-therapy? How thoroughly and honestly am I studying myself? How do I need to tighten up my self-therapy program? Deloris and Ernie both went through their own, spontaneous meta-monitoring assessment when they retired from their primary jobs, and both discovered that they had slacked off of continuing their programs. Brooke and Charlotte reevaluate their goals each time another milestone is reached.

The recoverers have come to value their adaptive processes as essential to their overall success. Many of the stories detail a step-by-step process of working out solutions to challenges, for example, Riley's mastery of maintaining a household with one hand and learning to run on one leg, Faith's crusade to improve her difficult social and romantic relationships, Brooke's evolving study techniques, Rachel's new tricks for doing psychotherapy, and Abdullah's arduous trial-and-error construction of the techniques that let him pass his bar exam.

5. Exceptional Recovery Is Self-Therapy.

Each story describes recovery as a strategy-driven, "top-down" process in which the mind fixes the brain. The strategies shared by all of the exceptional recoverers include all of the elements of their formal therapy: vigilance to watch for errors, classify the errors into types based on their causes, select an appropriate compensation behavior (or corrective plan), and evaluate the effectiveness of the compensation. In essence, they are doing for themselves what their therapists would be doing for them if the treatment team had gone home with them after graduation.

All 12 describe relying on pretty much the same basic set of tactics. All acknowledge the importance of quality control through increased *effort*. Other strategies also mentioned by every recoverer include being *cautious* or careful to avoid making errors, preparing ahead of time for important or difficult tasks, working out a systematic plan, and trying to anticipate obstacles before encountering them. Most use a day planner or do-list to organize their time. Only Tom did not keep his own planner; Dawn wrote a "honey-do list" on their dry-erase board. Tom remains allergic to paper and pen, which he agrees to be a holdover from his struggles with education in elementary school.

Ten mention seeking or accepting *advice* from trusted others, and we have seen three others do so as well. Ten report *downsizing* their personal *goals* to make them more realistic, the exceptions being the dauntless Stephanie and Samantha. Ten report using *compensations* for their *memory* deficits, written notes, tape recordings, or a combination as they were trained in rehab. These techniques represent the core tool kit for adaptation to the disabilities of TBI.

Nine note that they try to avoid dividing their attention to keep up the quality of their thinking. Six remark on their susceptibility to fatigue and/or their need to be careful about getting enough sleep, and two others program rest breaks into their days. Social skills are also a common concern: Nine indicate a need to work harder on their relationships, and six report making extra efforts to read people accurately. Six also explicitly comment on using the 12-step strategy of taking one day at a time, and four others comment that they are careful about making sure that they choose achievable goals to keep up their morale. Ten state, and two more imply, that their self-therapy is still going on, and we have never heard an exceptional recoverer disagree.

It is important to recognize that these presentations could be biased. The interviews were conducted by the designer of the training program, and the recoverers all essentially told him that they are still doing some variation of what he and his staff taught them. It could have been a case of telling him what he wanted to hear. However, they described their strategies in great detail, differing in many specific features from the ones taught in the program, and obviously contributing to the accomplishments in each person's life. Moreover, the variations were not always program-approved modifications. For example, most recoverers shifted from written analyses of their head-injured moments to mental work-ups, a shift the program director instructed them not to make when they were in his cognitive therapy group. If there is bias in the stories, it does not seem to account for the descriptions of the recovery processes.

It is interesting to revisit each story asking, "Who was in charge of this recovery?" In each case, it appears to be the recoverer. No family member or community-based counselor took charge. Note the authoritative way in which each recoverer described his methods. There was no uncertainty when spelling out what they needed to do and how they did it. They not only presented the knowledge of an expert, but showed their expertise in their manner of presentation.

The reader should be aware that some scholars and therapists who do not teach self-therapy (e.g., Ylvisaker, Hanks, & Johnson-Greene, 2002) are convinced that it does not and cannot work (Schutz & Trainor, 2007). They believe that survivors of severe TBI cannot transfer lessons from the setting in which they were trained to some other setting (Ylvisaker, 2005). By this logic, they assume that any training performed entirely in the clinic will be used only in the clinic. Most clinicians who perform cognitive rehabilitation are convinced that such transfer of training occurs, sometimes at the initiative and under the self-management of the survivor (e.g., Hart & Hayden, 1986; Wood, 1990). The 12 recovery stories all describe this kind of self-managed transfer, as none of these individuals received any professional treatment in their real-world situations.

The "situated learning" theorists propose that all training should take place in real-world settings (see Sohlberg & Mateer, 1989), and that patients should only be expected to use the functional skills and compensations they are taught in the settings in which they were trained (Guercio & Fralish, 1998). The situated-learning approach may be more effective for patients with extreme deficits and very little independent function (Schutz & Trainor, 2007), particularly in countries that allow unlimited therapy for such cases (see Wilson, 1999, and Alderman, 2003, for examples of these long-term intervention options). The patients in this group also tend to have relatively little geographic mobility (Roberts, 1979), so a carefully designed environmental niche may provide lasting benefits. However, patients whose recoveries allow fully independent functioning in the community are not likely to remain in a single real-world setting long enough to receive lasting benefit from situated training (Schutz & Trainor, 2007).

Consider the environmental mobility that the exceptional recoverers enjoyed. Under a situated learning approach, Brooke would have been trained for high school, but within 2 years she was attending college, dealing with very different environmental, social, and academic challenges. Brooke now attends graduate school and is planning to teach high school English beginning next year. Hillary and Samantha have undergone equally dramatic relocations in moving from college, for which they would have been trained, to new careers, new communities, and new personal responsibilities as wife and mother. Abdullah would have been trained to resume his job in the county jail, whereas he has since relocated to California, completed his legal studies, and started a new career as a public defender. Stephanie would have been trained for middle management, whereas she has progressed to a sequence of top administrative jobs managing cutting-edge technologies. The job to which Jomo returned was eliminated by a corporate reorganization in his 2nd year, and he has had to take on completely different duties and staff, as well as a larger share of the parenting duties for his growing children. Tom had neither a plan nor a vision of future employment when he was in rehabilitation, yet he ended up returning to his former profession against all odds. Only Faith, Rachel, and Deloris remained in their pre-injury jobs, and each of them experienced significant vocational and personal changes despite the stable employment. Training these individuals for the functions of their immediate post-discharge life would have been irrelevant to their futures. Moreover, their stories indicate that what they learned from their therapy, and what helped them, was not specific suggestions or behaviors, but rather the most general concepts about brain injury and how to compensate for it.

6. Controlling Overload Is Important.

All of the recoverers report cognitive difficulties when overloaded, and each one has strategies to prevent and to fix that problem (Schutz, 2005d). Their lifestyles are also built around situations designed to minimize overload. This calls to mind an earlier recovery by the president of an insurance company who was unwilling to renovate his offices to eliminate distractions, but could not function effectively in that environment. When he finally accepted his limitation, he sold the company and bought a wilderness campground where he could run the new business with no distractions (Schutz, 1989).

Even these proficient copers have broken down under sufficient stress. The meltdown Faith experienced when her seizure disorder emerged is documented in her story. Riley underwent an almost total collapse after an apparent hypoglycemic crisis entering the senior year of his second degree program, and needed the better part of a year to regain his health and confidence before resuming his studies. Ernie retired from his primary job after struggling with the onset of seizure disorder and problems with high blood pressure, as well as growing safety concerns for foreigners in the country in which he was working. Stephanie decided to relocate back to Orlando rather abruptly, after becoming disappointed with her lifestyle in Virginia. Faith experienced a temporary setback after moving into a new home in an unfamiliar neighborhood. Rachel became overloaded by new responsibilities after her wedding. Brooke developed stress symptoms while taking several advanced courses and helping to prepare for her sister's wedding. These incidents provide an additional reminder that these are not physiologically recovered brains but rather broken ones, with stress tolerance that can never be normal. The recoverers understand the need to proactively minimize stress because they operate effectively only in a fairly narrow range of stress. Under most conditions, their lifestyle keeps them within that range.

7. Effort May Be the Primary Curative Factor.

It is a truism of rehabilitation that the patients who work hardest have the best outcomes. That same truism, applied to the whole panorama of normal life activities, is known in our culture as the Protestant work ethic. Perhaps our extreme familiarity with this idea has blinded us to a more specific and powerful relationship between effort and recovery after rehabilitation. The stories presented here are provocative, suggesting a reinterpretation of the traditional perspective (Dixon & Backmun, 1999; Prigatano, 2005; Wood, 1987; Worthington, 2005) articulated by Luria (1948/1963):

> In the overwhelming majority of cases, reorganization of the functional systems takes place in the process of active and conscious activity, directed towards the compensation of this defect. The patient must be aware of the disturbance lying at the basis of this defective function; in accordance with his recognized defect,the patient selects adequate methods of reorganizing the disturbed function; these methods are usually made the object of conscious application . . . this active process . . . demands great will power from the patient, and diligent, steadfast work. It is quite obvious that . . . steadfast and intensive motivation . . . is an essential condition of the successful restoration of the disturbed function. (p. 232)

However, the crucial aspect of this recruitment of motivation and effort to adapt is not what takes place *during* rehabilitation, but rather what takes place *after* rehabilitation, when the insightful and educated graduate moves on to adapt to real life. This observation alters the way in which effort's contribution is understood. Beyond facilitating training to adapt, effort seems to serve most importantly to facilitate adaptation on an ongoing basis. If TBI is a disorder of adaptation, then effort should be seen as a curative factor rather than a catalyst (or moderator variable). If TBI is a disorder in which the brain fully self-activates only when maximum effort is evoked as a deliberate compensation strategy, then extra, compensatory effort is always needed to maintain the gains of recovery.

Is this the process that the recoverers are describing? For Stephanie, the mobilization of exceptional effort clearly began in the clinic: "During my recovery I spent every waking moment doing something constructive toward my rehabilitation. . . . I was never satisfied. I always pushed myself harder, always working to do more than was expected of me. . . . I am a stickler for follow-through. . . . I will not commit to something unless I know that I can follow through and deliver on it. Once I make a commitment, I get it done regardless of how many extra hours it takes me to complete the task."

Rachel emphasizes the process she carried forward on her own after graduation: "I continue to learn more about my injury since getting out of outpatient. I see little quirks, little brain-injury moments that I keep having and that I'm sure will continue. The challenge is there for me to fix each one and fix it right because I'm a perfectionist. Sometimes the first fix I try doesn't work, but I don't quit tinkering with it until I get it right. If it's something I can't fix until the situation comes up again, I write down what I did wrong to remind me when I revisit it to figure out a different way to handle it. I write down the failed actions so I won't repeat them. When I do therapy, I concentrate so hard to keep total control of my thoughts that I'm extremely tired at the end of a session. . . . I put my heart and soul into everything I do."

Brooke remarked, "Because of the injury I have to work twice as hard as the normal person to get the results I want. If I had to credit my recovery to a single strategy, that's it—do the amount of work that's necessary to get good results." In summarizing her philosophy of recovery, Brooke put even greater emphasis on effort: "Because of the injury, I have to work twice as hard as the average person to get what I want. *If I had to credit my recovery to a single strategy, that's it.* Do the amount of work that's necessary to get good results. . . . I can't just stick with the strategies I've developed up to this point. . . . I need to keep changing how I do things. . . . You will be adjusting to things all your life."

Riley concurred: He has become "a perfectionist across the board." He says, "The way to recover—hard work is at the top of the list. I'm a very motivated man. . . . I became capable of a fine-tuned kind of dedication. Also, I try to compete with my peers whenever I can. I'm driven by my desire to overcome my impairments and limitations, by my desire to be a complete person again. It comes down to being tough: motivated, strong, disciplined. Accept small steps in your recovery. . . . You have to learn to do things the best that you can do them, which involves doing them a different way. You have to be willing to try new methods of doing everything until you find a method that fits you."

Hillary offered this: "I have to try harder than ordinary people to get everything done correctly, to be aware of myself and my actions." Each recoverer describes working hard, but they go on to characterize the focus of their effort on supervising the effectiveness of their own thought processes (metacognitive self-management).

In retrospect, effort is a powerful explanatory construct for both the injury and the recovery. Impairment selectively occurs where and when effort is required. The most dramatic head-injured moments represent failures to exert the necessary executive effort. In turn, externally triggered effort corrects symptoms temporarily, whereas devotedly, effectively self-managed effort is the cornerstone of a great recovery.

When preparing this project, the first author watched the exceptional recoverers participate in the task force for 9 months. He was struck by how much effort all of them still put forth to engage in the planning tasks. He also noticed that there were occasional lapses of effort, and that when these happened the survivor often had a "head-injured moment." For example, Deloris allowed herself to rush out of the house to go to the group's Christmas party and ended up spending 2 futile hours driving around Orlando before she headed home, chastising herself for her failure to plan properly. He asked them about this as a group: How much effort goes into their daily lives at the present time? They all agreed that functioning as they did took much more effort than life before the injury. Most (with the exception of Stephanie, who had the least severe injury in this group) stated that they still have to exert what seems like the same level of effort that had been required immediately after therapy ended. How did these exceptional recoverers learn to tame and command their level of mental effort? Surprisingly, emotion seems to have played an important part, particularly negative emotions such as fear, dread, and terror. The stories indicate that insight triggered negative emotions toward ongoing activities. Stephanie and Deloris recounted their fear of making errors, and their sense of urgency to prevent them. Tom admitted that his terror at his road rage episode provided him with an instant impetus to prevent the problem from happening again. Rachel and Samantha discussed their fears of failing in their careers as motivating their efforts to compensate. Jomo began to work hard when he became afraid of his wife, and soon thereafter began to fear losing his career. In other cases, it might be more appropriate to characterize the emotional tone of the recovery process as grim (Ernie) or resolute determination (Faith).

This description of the curative role of effort is presently at the scientific level of an educated guess (or hypothesis). More research support is essential to establish its credibility. However, if it survives these research trials, this idea has tremendous practical benefits in guiding recovery, as everyone knows what effort is and how to apply it.

There are some interesting anecdotal (or non-experimental) data supporting our belief in the importance of effort. Jill Taylor (2006) is an established neuroscientist who underwent a left CVA and then wrote a volume that details her recovery. Her progress, which allowed her to resume teaching at the university level, can be regarded as a great recovery. She realizes that she made an unusually good recovery, but also notes that "I am only partially recovered" (p. 128) after nearly a decade of self-initiated work. Dr. Taylor is familiar with current concepts of plasticity, and used popular terminology of this kind to describe the "re-learning" achieved by her surviving neurons. However, she does not describe her recovery as a fait accompli or a goal that has been completely achieved. Rather, she describes herself as marshalling compensatory effort every day to gain "hard-fought" control over her mental processes. Moreover, she describes the use of effort to optimize her executive processes each time she acts. "By paying attention to the choices my automatic circuitry is making, I own my power and make my choices consciously" (p. 158). She continues,

> To monitor how things are going in my life, I pay close attention to how things are flowing. . . . I am in control of how I think and feel. In order to protect my overall mind, . . . it is necessary for me to tend the garden of my mind and keep (unwelcome or irrelevant) thoughts in check" (p. 160).

These compensatory executive processes, including response suppression, selective attention, output control, and self-monitoring, must be mindfully and deliberately performed "a thousand times a day" (p. 162). Clearly, her brain did not resume the fully automatized processing that would be the expected outcome of plasticity; instead, her recovery depends on active alteration of dysfunctional tendencies and thought patterns. Recovery is an ongoing process, and not an objective to be accomplished and then abandoned. The allocation of extraordinary effort appears to be necessary not only during rehabilitation, but on an ongoing basis.

8. Pre-Injury Accomplishment May Be a Prerequisite.

Because these recoveries are exceptional, it is possible that the survivors were exceptional people before the injury, such that these recoveries stem from their special, personal capabilities. In comparing the exceptional recoverers to those who did not achieve exceptional recoveries, there are few distinguishing characteristics. Age is clearly unimportant, with a range from 16 to 58 represented here. The program has produced very good recoveries in members as old as 65. Again, the issue appears not to be about the state of the hardware as much as it is about how the individual learns to reprogram it. Mature trainees are often more capable of understanding the seriousness of the problem and need to adopt a disciplined approach to recovery. Gender also appears relatively unimportant.

The successful recovery group is mainly hard-working, relatively perfectionistic, fairly successful individuals with college degrees, or working toward college degrees. Those who were working before injury held white-collar jobs in most cases. Most have good relationships with helpful and supportive families. Most did not have to deal with severe health problems, extreme poverty, or major, extended family conflict during recovery. Exceptional recovery does appear to require freedom from extreme psychological or environmental interference. However, Tom comes from a blue-collar background, has only a high-school education, and had to struggle with pain and other orthopedic complications of his injury for years. Riley also comes from a blue-collar background, with a high-school education, no family support, and very limited financial resources. So these factors are not absolute requirements.

Although psychological well-being facilitates recovery, this requirement is also less than absolute. Several exceptional recoverers had (or qualified for) preexisting mental health diagnoses (obsessive-compulsive disorder, post-traumatic stress disorder, childhood abuse, alcohol addiction, polydrug abuse). Most of the recoverers got either recommendations or prescriptions for antidepressant medication during recovery, and Faith narrowly avoided psychiatric hospitalization. However, their recoveries shared two important features: All were abstinent of recreational drugs and alcohol during recovery, and none showed any form of character disorder. Strength of character is necessary for successful adaptation, to realistically process rather than hide from evidence of personal failings (Shapiro, 2000; Vaillant, 1977).

There is a relationship between intellectual assets and exceptional recovery. Again, it is not an absolute one. Several genius-level intellects were treated in the Orlando program, and none of them had good recoveries—they were not open to the opinions of others. In the exceptional group, Abdullah, Brooke, Ernie, and Jomo were tested or gave histories of functioning at the gifted level, and most of the others were above average. But Tom was definitely below average, presumably due to childhood TBI, although his practical intelligence was impressive. We believe that some kind of smarts is important, as long as it is leavened with some humility.

Probably the most distinctive feature was a track record of personal accomplishment before the injury. Faith, Hillary, and Samantha were all successful athletes. Ernie was a holder of many patents and a recognized authority in his field. Abdullah was a self-made success as a prosecuting attorney in his native country. Brooke and Faith were campus celebrities in several respects. Tom conquered alcoholism (a favorable factor in many other good recoveries) and was learning a new trade. Riley worked his way up from poverty to business success. Deloris and Jomo had developed impressive careers while starting families. They all possessed the ability to recruit effort and to commit to working hard for a distant goal.

It is also apparent that most of the recoverers led active spiritual lives, and that their spirituality was intimately involved with their recoveries. In some cases, they derived their faith in the future and their sense of purpose from their system of belief. In others it served as a source of inspiration, support, and comfort. It seems unlikely that these recoveries would have been as exceptional if they had lacked or lost their spiritual connection.

In conclusion, the principles reviewed in Chapter Two seem to hold for these exceptional recoveries. Many adaptive resources aid recovery, including the desire and capability for personal commitment, and few exceptional recoveries face extreme environmental obstacles.

9. Therapy Needs to Have Personal Impact.

The popular idea that the program participant forms an alliance with a therapist based on trust and confidence, and the two together explore pathways to the future, is a lovely ideal, and a process that took place in some of these recoveries (particularly Deloris, Faith, Tom, Riley, and Ernie). Stephanie is unusual in that she decided on her own to commit herself to therapy early in rehabilitation, without needing a fully developed therapeutic alliance to bridge the transition. In Jomo's case, his marriage provided the therapeutic leverage for the recovery. However, the early relationships of Hillary, Rachel, Jomo, Brooke, and Samantha were actually in opposition to key therapists rather than allied with them. In these cases, a member with a relatively dominant personality staunchly defended her or his established ways of doing things, inducing the therapists to challenge that viewpoint. Rachel credits the challenge-oriented therapy strategy with motivating her to make her extraordinary efforts. Samantha still insists that no other approach could have worked for her, although it took her several years to realize how she had been "tricked" into recovering with all her might. The common denominators across all recoveries are the interpersonal intensity of the member-therapist relationship and the way in which its valence motivated the individual toward recovery.

10. Recovery Can Make You Better Than Ever Before.

A popular adage claims that any adversity that doesn't kill a person only makes him or her stronger. Although it may be difficult for many brain-intact individuals and some survivors to imagine feeling glad to have had a head injury, it is clearly the view of the exceptional recoverers. Like the individuals whose positive accomplishments were cited in Chapter Two, the great recoverers feel that the experience of injury and recovery has made them more spiritual, more moral, more empathetic, more grateful for life, and more committed to put basic personal values into practice. Most have stated their belief that they have proven something that merits great respect and pride. Hillary embarked on a new career that was more personally fulfilling, and Brooke is trying to develop a similar career. Faith developed a number of rewarding avocational involvements, and Abdullah and Ernie are presently seeking the same. To the participant-observer, it appears that they came to a better way of living because they needed to do so. Only by living a better life after the injury could they end up feeling that their life was truly successful. In this regard their recoveries remain works in progress, as they search for even deeper meanings for their lives.

Conclusions—For the Survivors

You have the opportunity to take what you read to heart. What would it mean to do that? It would mean accepting that you, like all of your head-injured brothers and sisters, don't fully *understand* your injury, even though you feel *sure* you do. You would hang onto this idea not because you believe that it makes sense about *you*, but because it makes sense about *head injury*. You would recognize that every great recoverer had to learn that the injury was much worse than he realized, and that all of them needed guidance at first, followed by a personal search for the hidden truth. You would say, "I'd better start checking out this idea that my head-injured moments may be more serious and more frequent than I realize, because I wouldn't want my own lack of insight to hold me back from a great recovery. Everything I discover about my deficits will allow me to adapt to them, and doing that should give me back something the injury took from me. As I discover more, I adapt more, and I take charge of my life better and better. These are all things I can do if I decide it's important enough to me."

Can a book really jump-start someone's recovery? The answer to that is "no." What jump-started the 15 successful recoveries was *personal* knowledge. A book cannot give you personal knowledge. But it can tell you where to look for it, and this book has told you where you can look. And if you decide to see if you have the deficits that the great recoverers had, you will find them in yourself and then you can begin to jump-start your own recovery. We assure you that it's not too late. You don't need professional help or a $70,000 program, although it would be wonderful if you could attend one. You can make recovery happen yourself if you start doing the things the great recoverers described doing. It's no more complicated than that. If you prefer to follow step-by-step directions, we wrote a set of those up and you are welcome to get them (Schutz, 2006a) from our Web site (http://www.givebackorlando.com). We invite you to post your own recovery accomplishments there, so that others can find inspiration in what you did.

Conclusions—For the Family

More recovery is possible. It all depends on your survivor. You can't do it yourself. It depends on him or her getting that itch to figure out the hidden truth, and then mobilizing to do something about it. If your survivor does not take to this idea immediately, our Web site offers a whole family handbook full of strategies that you can try (Schutz, 2006b). Please remember that recovery is a lifelong objective, so getting started slowly is no crime.

Conclusions—For the Professionals

Is this how you thought recovery worked? It came as a surprise to us in a number of ways. The senior author's approach to therapy was changed by this project. Now, every intervention beginning with "Hello" is evaluated and selected in terms of its contribution to self-therapy processes. We believe that rehabilitation should be devoted to long-term recovery in real life, simply because we have to assume that we are the last TBI professionals a survivor may see across his or her lifetime. Because that is likely, it is imperative to make our efforts count in enhancing the long-term recovery processes that are most important. We believe that we can teach, and our patients and families can learn, strategies of effective adaptation if only we set the bar high enough for them and for ourselves.

References

Adams, J. H., Doyle, D., Ford, I., Gennarelli, T. A., Graham, D. I., & McLellan, D. R. (1989). Diffuse axonal injury in head injury: Definition, diagnosis and grading. *Histopathology, 15*, 49–59.

Adams, J. H., Graham, D. I., Gennarelli, T. A., & Maxwell, W. L. (1991). Diffuse axonal injury in non-missile head injury. *Journal of Neurology, Neurosurgery and Psychiatry, 54*, 481–483.

Adams, J. H., Graham, D. I., Murray, L. S., & Scott, G. (1982). Diffuse axonal injury due to non-missile head injury in humans: An analysis of 45 cases. *Annals of Neurology, 12*, 557–563.

Adams, J. H., Graham, D. I., Scott, G., Parker, L. S., & Doyle, D. (1980). Brain damage in fatal non-missile head injury. *Journal of Clinical Pathology, 33*, 1132–1145.

Adams, J. H., Mitchell, D. E., Graham, D. I., & Doyle, D. (1977). Diffuse brain damage of intermediate impact type. *Brain, 100*, 489–502

Adams, R. D., Victor, M., & Ropper, A. H. (1997). *Principles of neurology* (6th ed.). New York: McGraw-Hill.

Alderman, N. (2003). Rehabilitation of behaviour disorders. In B. A. Wilson (Ed.), *Neuropsychological rehabilitation: Theory and practice* (pp. 171–196). Lisse, The Netherlands: Swets & Zeitlinger.

Alexander, M. P. (1987). The role of neurobehavioral syndromes in the rehabilitation and outcome of closed head injury. In H. S. Levin, J. Grafman, & H. M. Eisenberg (Eds.), *Neurobehavioral recovery from head injury* (pp. 191–205). New York: Oxford University Press.

Alexander, M. P. (1995). Mild traumatic brain injury: Pathophysiology, natural history, and clinical management. *Neurology, 45*, 1253–1260.

Alexander, M. P. (2003). Aphasia: Clinical and anatomic issues. In T. E. Feinberg & M. J. Farah (Eds.), *Behavioral neurology and neuropsychology* (2nd ed., pp. 147–164). New York: McGraw-Hill.

Alexandre, A., Colombo, F., Nertempi, P., & Benedetti, A. (1983). Cognitive outcome and early indices of severity of head injury. *Journal of Neurosurgery, 59*, 751–761.

Alfano, D. E., Paniak, C. E., & Finlayson, M. (1991). Neuropsychological and long-term psychosocial functioning after traumatic brain injury. *Journal of Clinical and Experimental Neuropsychology, 13*, 23–39.

Anderson, S. W., Damasio, H., Tranel, D., & Damasio, A. R. (2000). Long-term sequelae of prefrontal cortex damage acquired in early childhood. *Developmental Neuropsychology, 18*, 281–296.

Andrews, B. T. (1992). Initial management of head injury. In S. Berrol (Ed.), *Physical medicine and rehabilitation clinics of North America: Traumatic brain injury* (pp. 249–258). Philadelphia: Saunders.

Andrews, B. T., & Pitts, L. J. (1991). *Traumatic transtentorial herniation and its treatment.* Mount Kiska, NY: Futura Publishing.

Archibald, S. J., Mateer, C. A., & Kerns, K. A. (2001). Utilization behavior: Clinical manifestations and neurological mechanisms. *Neuropsychology Review, 11*, 117–130.

Arlinghaus, K. A., Shoaib, A., & Price, T. (2005). Neuropsychiatric assessment. In J. M. Silver, T. W. McAllister, & S. C. Yudofsky (Eds.), *Textbook of traumatic brain injury* (pp. 59–78). Washington DC: American Psychiatric Publishing.

Arnstein, A., & Smith, D. H. (1999). Pharmacological strategies for neuroprotection and rehabilitation. In D. T. Stuss, G. Winocur, & I. H. Robertson (Eds.), *Cognitive neurorehabilitation* (pp. 113–135). New York: Cambridge University Press.

Asch, S. (1952). *Social psychology.* Englewood Cliffs, NJ: Prentice-Hall.

Bach-y-Rita, P. (1989). A conceptual approach to neural recovery. In P. Bach-y-Rita (Ed.), *Traumatic brain injury* (pp. 81–85). New York: Demos.

Baddeley, A. (1990). *Human memory: Theory and practice.* Boston: Allyn & Bacon.

Baddeley, A. D. (1993). A theory of rehabilitation without a model of learning is a vehicle without an engine: A comment on Caramazza and Hillis. *Neuropsychological Rehabilitation, 3*, 235–244.

Baddeley, A. D., & Hitch, G. (1974). Working memory. In G. H. Bower (Ed.), *The psychology of learning and motivation* (Vol. 8, pp. 47–90). New York: Academic Press.

Baddeley, A. D., & Wilson, B. A. (1988). Frontal amnesia and the dysexecutive syndrome. *Brain and Cognition, 7*, 212–230.

Bakay, L., & Glasauer, F. E. (1980). *Head injury.* Boston: Little, Brown and Co.

Banja, J. (1992). Ethics, fraud, and the misallocation of rehabilitation resources. *Journal of Head Trauma Rehabilitation, 7*, 114–116.

Barco, P. P., Crosson, B., Bolesta, M. M., Werts, D., & Stout, R. (1991). Training awareness and compensation in postacute head injury rehabilitation. In J. S. Kreutzer & P. H. Wehman (Eds.), *Cognitive rehabilitation for persons with traumatic brain injury* (pp. 129–146). Bisbee, AZ: Imaginart.

Barrett, A., & Gonzalez-Rothi, L. (2002). Theoretical bases for neuropsychological intervention. In P. J. Eslinger (Ed.), *Neuropsychological intervention* (pp. 16–37). New York: Guilford.

Bazarian, J. J., McClung, J., Shah, M. N., Cheng, Y. T., Flesher, W., & Kraus, J. (2005). Mild traumatic brain injury in the United States, 1998–2000. *Brain Injury, 19,* 85–91.

Bechara, A., Damasio, A. R., Damasio, H., & Anderson, S. W. (1994). Insensitivity to future consequences following damage to human prefrontal cortex. *Cognition, 50,* 7–15.

Bechara, A., Damasio, A. R., Damasio, H., & Lee, G. P. (1999). Differential contributions of the human amygdala and ventromedial prefrontal cortex to decision making. *Journal of Neuroscience, 19,* 5473–5481.

Beck, A. T. (1967). *Depression: Clinical, experimental, and theoretical aspects.* New York: Harper.

Becker, D. P. (1989). Common themes in head injury. In D. Becker & S. K. Gudeman (Eds.), *Textbook of head injury* (pp. 1–22). Philadelphia: Saunders.

Begali, V. (1992). *Head injury in children and adolescents: A resource and review for school and allied professionals* (2nd ed.). Brandon, VT: Clinical Psychology Publishing Co.

Bem, D. (1992). On the uncommon wisdom of lay personality theory. *Psychological Inquiry, 3,* 82–84.

Bender, L. (1949). Psychological problems of children. *American Journal of Orthopsychiatry, 19,* 404–415.

Bennett, T., Dittmar, C., & Ho, M. (1997). The neuropsychology of traumatic brain injury. In A. Horton, D. Wedding, & J. Webster (Eds.), *The neuropsychology handbook* (Vol. 2, 2nd ed., pp. 123–172). New York: Springer.

Benton, A. L. (1968). Differential behavioral effects of frontal lobe disease. *Neuropsychologia, 6,* 53–60.

Benton, A. L. (1987). Thoughts on the application of neuropsychological tests. In H. S. Levin, J. Grafman, & H. M. Eisenberg (Eds.), *Neurobehavioral recovery from head injury* (pp. 111–115). New York: Oxford University Press.

Benton, A., & Tranel, D. (2000). Historical notes on reorganization of function and neuroplasticity. In H. S. Levin & J. Grafman (Eds.), *Cerebral reorganization of function after brain damage* (pp. 3–26). New York: Oxford University Press.

Ben-Yishay, Y. (1980). Rehabilitation of the severely brain injured individual: Plain answers to complicated questions. In Y. Ben-Yishay (Ed.), *Working approaches to remediation of cognitive deficits in brain-damaged persons* (Rehabilitation Monograph #61, pp. 1–55). New York: New York University Medical Center.

Ben-Yishay, Y. (1996). Reflections on the evolution of the therapeutic milieu concept. *Neuropsychological Rehabilitation, 6,* 327–343.

Ben-Yishay, Y., Ben-Nachum, Z., Cohen, A., Gross, Y., Hoofien, D., Rattock, Y., et al. (1978). Digest of a two-year comprehensive clinical rehabilitation research program for outpatient head injured Israeli veterans. In Y. Ben-Yishay (Ed.), *Working approaches to remediation of cognitive deficits in brain-damaged persons* (Rehabilitation Monograph #59, pp. 1–61). New York: New York University Medical Center.

Ben-Yishay, Y., & Diller, L. (1983a). Cognitive deficits. In M. Rosenthal, E. R. Griffith, M. R. Bond, & J. D. Miller (Eds.), *Rehabilitation of the head injured adult* (pp. 167–183). Philadelphia: Davis.

Ben-Yishay, Y., & Diller, L. (1983b). Cognitive remediation. In M. Rosenthal, E. R. Griffith, M. R. Bond, & J. D. Miller (Eds.), *Rehabilitation of the head injured adult* (pp. 367–380). Philadelphia: Davis.

Ben-Yishay, Y., & Gold, J. (1990). Therapeutic milieu approach to cognitive rehabilitation. In R. Ll. (Ed.), *Neurobehavioural sequelae of traumatic brain injury* (pp. 194–215). New York: Taylor and Francis.

Ben-Yishay, Y., Piasetsky, E., & Rattok, J. (1987). A systematic method for ameliorating disorders in basic attention. In M. J. Meier, A. L. Benton, & L. Diller (Eds.), *Neuropsychological rehabilitation* (pp. 165–181). New York: Guilford.

Ben-Yishay, Y., & Prigatano, G. (1990). Cognitive remediation. In M. Rosenthal, E. R. Griffith, M. R. Bond, & J. D. Miller (Eds.), *Rehabilitation of the adult and child with traumatic head injury* (2nd ed., pp. 393–409). Philadelphia: Davis.

Ben-Yishay, Y., Silver, S. M., Piasetsky, E., & Rattok, J. (1987). Relationship between employability and vocational outcome after intensive, holistic cognitive rehabilitation. *Journal of Head Trauma Rehabilitation, 2,* 35–48.

Bergquist, T. F., & Malec, J. F. (2002). Neuropsychological assessment for treatment planning and research. In P. Eslinger (Ed.), *Neuropsychological interventions: Clinical research and practice* (pp. 38–58). New York: The Guilford Press.

Berko, F. G., Berko, M. J., & Thompson, S. C. (1970). *Management of brain damaged children: A parents' and teachers' guide.* Springfield, IL: Charles C. Thomas.

Bernstein, N. (1967). *The co-ordination and regulation of movement.* London: Pergamon.

Berrol, S. (1992). Preface. In S. Berrol (Ed.), *Physical medicine and rehabilitation clinics of North America: Traumatic brain injury* (pp. xv–xvi). Philadelphia: Saunders.

Berrol, S., Cope, N., Cervelli, L., Mackworth, N., Mackworth, J., & Rappaport, M. (1982). *Head injury rehabilitation project final report.* San Jose, CA: Santa Clara Valley Medical Center.

Bigler, E. D. (1990). Introduction. In E. D. Bigler (Ed.), *Traumatic brain injury* (pp. 5–9). Austin, TX: Pro-Ed.

Bigler, E. D. (1990). Neuropathology of traumatic brain injury. In E. D. Bigler (Ed.), *Traumatic brain injury* (pp. 13–49). Austin, TX: Pro-Ed.

Bigler, E. D. (2005). Structural imaging. In J. M. Silver, T. W. McAllister, & S. C. Yudofsky (Eds.), *Textbook of traumatic brain injury* (pp. 79–106). Washington DC: American Psychiatric Publishing.

Bigler, E. D. (2007). Anterior and middle cranial fossa in traumatic brain injury: Relevant neuroanatomy and neurophysiology in the study of neuropsychological outcome. *Neuropsychology, 21,* 515–532.

Binder, L. M. (1986). A review of mild head trauma: Part II. Clinical implications. *Journal of Clinical and Experimental Neuropsychology, 19,* 432–457.

Bisiach, E., & Geminiani, G. (1991). Anosagnosia related to hemiplegia and hemianopsia. In G. P. Prigatano & D. L. Schacter (Eds.), *Awareness of deficit after brain injury* (pp. 17–39). New York: Oxford University Press.

Blanton, S., Porter, L., Smith, D., & Wolf, S. L. (1999). Strategies to enhance mobility in traumatic brain injured patients. In M. Rosenthal, E. R. Griffith, J. S. Kreutzer, & B. Pentland (Eds.), *Rehabilitation of the adult and child with traumatic brain injury* (3rd ed., pp. 219–241). Philadelphia: Davis.

Bleiberg, J., Cope, D. N., & Spector, J. (1989). Cognitive assessment and therapy in traumatic brain injury. In L. J. Horn & D. N. Cope (Eds.), *Physical medicine and rehabilitation state of the art reviews: Traumatic brain injury* (pp. 143–156). Philadelphia: Haley & Belfus.

Blosser, J. L., & DePompei, R. (2003). *Pediatric traumatic brain injury: Proactive intervention* (2nd ed.). Clifton Park, NY: Delmar Thomson Learning.

Blumbergs, P., Jones, H., & North, J. (1989). Diffuse axonal injury in head trauma. *Journal of Neurology, Neurosurgery and Psychiatry, 52,* 838–841.

Boake, C. (1991). History of cognitive rehabilitation following head injury. In J. S. Kreutzer & P. H. Wehman (Eds.), *Cognitive rehabilitation for persons with traumatic brain injury* (pp. 3–12). Bisbee, AZ: Imaginart.

Boake, C., & Diller, L. (2005). History of rehabilitation for traumatic brain injury. In W. M. High, A. M. Sander, M. A. Struchen, & K. A. Hart (Eds.), *Rehabilitation for traumatic brain injury* (pp. 3–13). New York: Oxford University Press.

Bogod, N. M., Mateer, C. A., & MacDonald, S. (2003). Self-awareness after traumatic brain injury: A comparison of measures and their relationship to executive functions. *Journal of the International Neuropsychological Society, 9,* 450–458.

Boll, T. J. (1982). Behavioral sequelae of head injury. In P. Cooper (Ed.), *Head injury* (pp. 363–375). Baltimore: Williams and Wilkins.

Boller, F. C., Albert, M. L., LeMay, M., & Kertesz, A. (1972). Enlargement of the Sylvian aqueduct: A sequel of head injuries. *Journal of Neurology, Neurosurgery and Psychiatry, 35,* 463–467.

Bolles, E. B. (1988). *Remembering and forgetting: Inquiries into the nature of memory.* New York: Walker.

Bond, M. R. (1975). Assessment of psychosocial outcome after severe head injury. In Ciba Foundation Symposium #34, *Outcome of severe damage to the central nervous system.* Amsterdam: Elsevier.

Bond, M. R. (1979). The stages of recovery from severe head injury with special reference to late outcome. *International Rehabilitation Medicine, 1,* 155-159.

Bond, M. R. (1984). The psychiatry of closed head injury. In D. N. Brooks (Ed.), *Closed head injury: Psychological, social, and family consequences* (pp. 148-178). New York: Oxford University Press.

Bond, M. R., & Brooks, D. N. (1976). Understanding the process of recovery as a basis for investigation of rehabilitation for the brain injured. *Scandinavian Journal of Rehabilitation Medicine, 8,* 127-133.

Bontke, C. F. (1990). Medical advances in the treatment of brain injury. In J. Kreutzer & P. Wehman (Eds.), *Community integration following traumatic brain injury* (pp. 3-14). Baltimore: Paul H. Brookes.

Bontke, C. F., & Boake, C. (1991). Traumatic brain injury rehabilitation. *Neurosurgery Clinics of North America, 2,* 473-482.

Bontke, C. F., Brockman, N., Clio, M. P., Robert, V., & Worthington, L. (1998). Acute care and rehabilitation. In K. B. Fralish & M. J. McMorrow (Eds.), *Innovations in head injury rehabilitation* (Chap. 4). White Plains, NY: Ahab Press.

Bouma, G. J., Muizelaar, J. P., Choi, S. C., Newlon, P. G., & Young, H. F.(1991). Cerebral circulation and metabolism after severe traumatic brain injury: The elusive role of ischemia. *Journal of Neurosurgery, 75,* 685-693

Braunling-McMorrow, D. (1998). Promoting effective socialization for persons with brain injury. In K. B. Fralish & M. J. McMorrow (Eds.), *Innovations in head injury rehabilitation* (Chap. 21). White Plains, NY: Ahab Press.

Brink, J. D., Garrett, A. L., Hale, W. R., Nickel, V. L., & Woo-Sam, J. (1970). Recovery of motor and intellectual function in children sustaining severe head injuries. *Developmental Medicine and Child Neurology, 12,* 565-571.

Brismar, B., Engstrom, A., & Rydberg, U. (1983). Head injury and intoxication: A therapeutic dilemma. *Acta Chirugica Scandinavica, 149,* 11-14.

Broadbent, D. E. (1971). *Decision and stress.* London: Academic Press.

Brooks, D. N. (1972). Memory and head injury. *Journal of Nervous and Mental Disease, 155,* 350-355.

Brooks, D. N. (1984a). Cognitive deficits after head injury. In N. Brooks (Ed.), *Closed head injury: Psychological, social, and family consequences* (pp. 44-73). Oxford, England: Oxford University Press.

Brooks, D. N. (1984). Head injury and the family. In N. Brooks (Ed.), *Closed head injury: Psychological, social, and family consequences* (pp. 123-147). Oxford, England: Oxford University Press.

Brooks, D. N. (1987). Measuring neuropsychological and functional recovery. In H. S. Levin, J. Grafman, & H. M. Eisenberg (Eds.), *Neurobehavioral recovery from head injury* (pp. 57–72). New York: Oxford University Press.

Brooks, D. N. (1988). Behavioral abnormalities in head injured patients. *Scandinavian Journal of Rehabilitation Medicine, 17*, 41–46.

Brooks, D. N. (1990). Cognitive deficits. In M. Rosenthal, E. R. Griffith, M. R. Bond, & J. D. Miller (Eds.), *Rehabilitation of the adult and child with traumatic head injury* (2nd ed., pp. 163–178). Philadelphia: Davis.

Brooks, D. N., Aughton, M. E., Bond, M. R., Jones, P., & Risvi, S. (1980). Cognitive sequelae in relationship to early indices of severity of brain damage after severe blunt head injury. *Journal of Neurology, Neurosurgery and Psychiatry, 43*, 529–534.

Brooks, D. N., Campsie, L., Symington, C., & Beattie, A. (1987). The effects of severe head injury upon patient and relative within several years of injury. *Journal of Head Trauma Rehabilitation, 2*, 1–13.

Brooks, D. N., Campsie, L., Symington, C., Beattie, A., & McKinlay, W. (1986). The five year outcome of blunt head injury: The relative's view. *Journal of Neurology, Neurosurgery and Psychiatry, 9*, 764–770.

Brooks, D. N., Deelman, B. G., van Zomeren, A. H., van Dongen, H., van Harskamp, F., & Aughton, M. E. (1984). Problems in measuring cognitive recovery after acute brain injury. *Journal of Clinical Neuropsychology, 6*, 71–85.

Brooks, D. N., & McKinlay, W. (1983). Personality and behavioral change after severe blunt head injury—a relative's view. *Journal of Neurology, Neurosurgery and Psychiatry, 46*, 336–344.

Brooks, D. N., Symington, C., Beattie, A., Campsie, L., Bryden, J., & McKinlay, W. (1989). Alcohol and other predictors of cognitive recovery after severe brain injury. *Brain Injury, 3*, 235–246.

Brouwer, W. H., & Van Wolffelaar, O. A. (1985). Sustained attention and sustained effort after closed head injury. *Cortex, 21*, 111–119.

Brown, J. (1977). *Mind, brain and consciousness: The neuropsychology of cognition*. New York: Academic Press.

Brown, J. (1987). The microstructure of action. In E. Perecman (Ed.), *The frontal lobes revisited* (pp. 301–321). New York: IRBN Press.

Brown, M., & Vandergoot, D. (1998). Quality of life for individuals with traumatic brain injury: Comparison with others living in the community. *Journal of Head Trauma Rehabilitation, 13*, 1–23.

Brunswik, E. (1955). Representative design and probabilistic theory in a functional psychology. *Psychological Review, 62*, 193–217

Bryden, J. (1989). How many head injured? The epidemiology of post-head-injury disability. In R. Ll. Wood & P. Eames (Eds.), *Models of brain injury rehabilitation* (pp. 17–27). Baltimore: The Johns Hopkins University Press.

Buchtel, H. A. (1987). Attention and vigilance after head trauma. In H. S. Levin, J. Grafman, & H. M. Eisenberg (Eds.), *Neurobehavioral recovery from head injury* (pp. 372–378). New York: Oxford University Press.

Burgess, P. (1998). Theory and methodology in executive function research. In P. Rabbitt (Ed.), *Methodology of frontal and executive function* (pp. 81–116). London: Psychology Press.

Burgess, P. W., & Alderman, N. (1990). Rehabilitation of dyscontrol syndromes following frontal lobe damage: A cognitive neuropsychological approach. In R. Ll. Wood & I. Fussey (Eds.), *Cognitive rehabilitation in perspective* (pp. 183–203). London: Taylor and Francis.

Burgess, P. W., Alderman, N., Evans, J., Emslie, H., & Wilson, B. A. (1998). The ecological validity of tests of executive function. *Journal of the International Neuropsychological Society, 4*, 547–558.

Burgess, P. W., & Simons, J. S. (2005). Theories of frontal lobe executive functions: Clinical applications. In P. W. Halligan & D. T. Wade (Eds.), *Effectiveness of rehabilitation for cognitive deficits* (pp. 211–231). New York: Oxford University Press.

Burgess, P. W., & Wood, R. Ll. (1990). Neuropsychology of behaviour disorders following brain injury. In R. Ll. Wood (Ed.), *Neurobehavioural sequelae of traumatic brain injury* (pp. 110–133). New York: Taylor and Francis.

Burke, W. H., Guth, M., Guare, R., & Weslowski, M. D. (1999). *Brain injury rehabilitation: An overview* (2nd ed.). Houston, TX: HDI.

Burke, W. H., Zencius, A. H., Wesolowski, M. D., & Doubleday, F. (1991). Improving executive function disorders in brain-injured clients. *Brain Injury, 5*, 241–252.

Bushara, K. O., Grafman, J., & Hallett, M. (2001). Neural correlates of auditory-visual stimulus onset asynchrony detection. *Journal of Neuroscience, 21*, 300–304.

Butler, R. W., & Namerow, N. S. (1988). Cognitive retraining in brain-injury rehabilitation: A critical review. *Journal of Neurological Rehabilitation, 2*, 97–101.

Calvin, W. H. (1989). *The cerebral symphony: Seashore reflections on the structure of consciousness.* New York: Bantam.

Calvin, W. H. (1996). *How brains think: Evolving intelligence, then and now.* New York: Basic.

Cameron, C. M., Purdie, D. M., Kliewer, E. V., & McClure, R. J. (2008). Ten-year outcomes following traumatic brain injury: A population-based cohort. *Brain Injury, 22*, 437–449.

Campbell, M. (2000). *Rehabilitation for traumatic brain injury: Physical therapy practices in context.* London: Churchill-Livingstone.

Campbell, T. F., & Dollaghan, C. A. (1990). Expressive language recovery in severely brain-injured children and adolescents. *Journal of Speech and Hearing Disorders, 55*, 567–581.

Caramazza, A., & Hillis, A. (1993). For a theory of remediation of cognitive deficits. *Neuropsychological Rehabilitation, 3,* 217–234.

Carlsson, C. A., von Essen, C., & Lofgren, J. (1968). Factors affecting the clinical course of patients with severe head injuries. *Journal of Neurosurgery, 20,* 248–255.

Carney, N., Chesnut, R. M., Maynard, H., Mann, N. C, Patterson, P., & Helfand, M. (1999). Effect of cognitive rehabilitation on outcomes for persons with traumatic brain injury: A systematic review. *Journal of Head Trauma Rehabilitation, 4*(3), 277–307.

Carver, C. S., & Scheier, M. E. (1994). Situational coping and coping dispositions in stressful transaction. *Journal of Personality and Social Psychology, 66,* 184–195.

Carver, C. S., & Scheier, M. E. (2001). *On the self-regulation of behavior.* New York: Cambridge University Press.

Cassidy, J. W. (1990). Pharmacological treatment of post-traumatic behavioral disorders: Aggression and disorders of mood. In R. T. Wood (Ed.), *Neurobehavioural sequelae of traumatic brain injury* (pp. 219–249). New York: Taylor and Francis.

Cassidy, J. W. (1999). Neuropharmacological contributions to the rehabilitation of patients with traumatic brain injury. In D. T. Stuss, G. Winocur, & I. H. Robertson (Eds.), *Cognitive neurorehabilitation* (pp. 136–152). New York: Cambridge University Press.

Centers for Disease Control. (1999). Traumatic brain injury in the United States: A report to Congress. Retrieved November 9, 2009 from http://www.cdc.gov/ncipc/pub-res/tbi.congress.htm

Cermak, L. S. Ferfaellie, M., & Lanzoni, S. (1999). Effect of spaced repetitions on amnesia patient's recall and recognition performance. *Neuropsychology,* 10, 219–227.

Chan, J. C., McDermott, K. B., & Roediger, H. L. (2006). Retrieval-induced facilitation: Initially non-tested material can benefit from prior testing of related material. *Journal of Experimental Psychology (General), 135,* 553–571.

Chapman, L. F., & Wolff, H. G. (1959). The cerebral hemispheres and the highest integrative functions in man. *AMA Archives of Neurology, 1,* 357–424.

Chapman, S. B. (2007). Neurocognitive stall: A paradox in recovery from pediatric traumatic brain injury. *Brain Injury Professional, 3,* 10–13.

Christiansen, A.-L., & Caetano, C. (1999). Neuropsychological rehabilitation in the inter-disciplinary team: The postacute stage. In D. Stuss, G. Winocur, & I. Robertson (Eds.), *Cognitive neurorehabilitation* (pp. 188–200). New York: Cambridge University Press.

Christiansen, A.-L., Caetano, C., & Rasmussen, G. (1996). Psychosocial outcome after an intensive, neuropsychologically oriented day program: Contributing program variables. In B. P. Uzzell & H. H. Stonnington (Eds.), *Recovery after traumatic brain injury* (pp. 235–246). Mahwah, NJ: Erlbaum.

Churchland, P. S. (1998). *Neurophilosophy: Toward a unified science of mind/brain*. Cambridge, MA: MIT Press.

Cicerone , K. D. (2002). The enigma of executive functioning. In P. J. Eslinger (Ed.), *Neuropsychological interventions* (pp. 246–265). New York: The Guilford Press.

Cicerone, K. (2004). Participation as an outcome of traumatic brain injury rehabilitation. *Journal of Head Trauma Rehabilitation, 19,* 494–501.

Cicerone, K. D. (2005). Rehabilitation of executive function impairments. In W. High, A. Sander, M. Struchen, & K. Hart (Eds.), *Rehabilitation for traumatic brain injury* (pp. 71–87). New York: Oxford University Press.

Cicerone, K. D., & Azulay, J. (2007). Perceived self-efficacy and life satisfaction after traumatic brain injury. *Journal of Head Trauma Rehabilitation, 22,* 257–266.

Cicerone, K. D., Dahlberg, C., Kalmar, K., Langenbahn, D. M., Malec, J. F., Bergquist, T., et al. (2000). Evidence-based cognitive rehabilitation: Recommendations for clinical practice. *Archives of Physical Medicine and Rehabilitation, 81,* 1596–1613.

Cicerone, K. D., Dahlberg, C., Malec, J. F., Langenbahn, D. M., Felicetti, T., Kneipp, S., et al. (2005). Evidence-based cognitive rehabilitation: Updated review of the literature from 1998 through 2002. *Archives of Physical Medicine and Rehabilitation, 86,* 1681–1692.

Cicerone, K. D., & Giacino, J. T. (1992). Remediation of executive function deficits after traumatic brain injury. *Neurorehabilitation, 2,* 73–83.

Cicerone, K. D., Levin, H. S., Malec, J., Stuss, D., & Whyte, J. (2006). Cognitive rehabilitation interventions for executive function: Moving from bench to bedside in patients with traumatic brain injury. *Journal of Cognitive Neuroscience, 18,* 1212–1222.

Cicerone, K., Mott, T., Azulay, J., & Friel, J. (2004). Community integration and satisfaction with functioning after intensive cognitive rehabilitation for traumatic brain injury. *Archives of Physical Medicine and Rehabilitation, 85,* 943–950.

Cicerone, K. D., & Wood, J. (1987). Planning disorder after closed head injury. *Archives of Physical Medicine and Rehabilitation, 68,* 111–115.

Clark, G. M. (1968). A summary of the literature on behavior disorders in brain damaged children. In H. C. Haywood (Ed.), *Brain damage in school age children* (pp. 182–210). Washington, DC: Council for Exceptional Children.

Clifton, G. (1989). Advances in management of severe head injury. In P. Bach-y-Rita (Ed.), *Traumatic brain injury rehabilitation* (pp. 3–12). New York: Demos.

Coelho, C. A., Liles, B. Z., & Duffy, R. J. (1992). Communication and swallowing disorders in traumatic brain injury In S. Berrol (Ed.), *Physical medicine and rehabilitation clinics of North America: Traumatic brain injury* (pp. 371–388). Philadelphia: Saunders.

Coelho, C., Ylvisaker, M., & Turkstra, L. (2005). Nonstandardized assessment approaches for individuals with traumatic brain injuries. *Seminars in Speech and Language, 26,* 223-241.

Cole, J. R. (1998). Psychosocial rehabilitation. In K. B. Fralish & M. J. McMorrow (Eds.), *Innovations in head injury rehabilitation* (Chap. 10). White Plains, NY: Ahab Press.

Combs, G., & Freedman, J. (1994). Narrative intentions. In M. F. Hoyt (Ed.), *Constructive therapies* (pp. 67-91). New York: Guilford.

Condeluci, A. (1998). Understanding paradigms. In K. B. Fralish & M. J. McMorrow (Eds.), *Innovations in head injury rehabilitation* (Chap. 19). White Plains, NY: Ahab Press.

Cooley, E. A., Glang, A., & Voss, J. (1997). Making connections: Helping students with ABI build friendships. In A. Glang, G. Singer, & B. Todis (Eds.), *Students with acquired brain injury: The school's response* (pp. 255-275). Baltimore: Brookes.

Cooper, P. (1987). Gunshot wounds of the brain. In P. Cooper (Ed.), *Head injury* (2nd ed., pp. 313-326). Baltimore: Williams and Wilkins.

Cooper, R., & Shallice, T. (2000). Contention scheduling and the control of routine activities. *Cognitive Neuropsychology, 17,* 297-338.

Cope, D. N. (1996). A databased managed care system of catastrophic neurological injury rehabilitation. In B. P. Uzzell & H. H. Stonnington (Eds.), *Recovery after traumatic brain injury* (pp. 295-304). Mahwah, NJ: Erlbaum.

Cope, D. N., Cole, J. R., Hall, K. M., & Barkans, H. (1991). Brain injury: Analysis of outcome in a post-acute rehabilitation system: Part 2. Subanalyses. *Brain Injury, 5,* 127-139.

Cope, D. N., & Reynolds, W. E. (2005). Systems of care. In J. M. Silver, T. W. McAllister, & S. C. Yudofsky (Eds.), *Textbook of traumatic brain injury* (pp. 559-569). Washington, DC: American Psychiatric Publishing.

Corkin, S., Hurt, R., Twitchell, T., Franklin, L., & Yin, R. (1987). Consequences of non-penetrating and penetrating head injury: Retrograde amnesia, post-traumatic amnesia, and lasting effects on cognition. In H. S. Levin, J. Grafman, & H. Eisenberg (Eds.), *Neuro-behavioral recovery from head injury* (pp. 355-371). New York: Oxford University Press.

Corrigan, J. D. (1996). The incidence and impact of substance abuse following traumatic brain injury. In B. P. Uzzell & H. H. Stonnington (Eds.), *Recovery after traumatic brain injury* (pp. 139-148). Mahwah, NJ: Erlbaum.

Corrigan, J. D., Smith-Knapp, K., & Granger, C. V. (1998). Outcomes in the first 5 years after traumatic brain injury. *Archives of Physical Medicine and Rehabilitation, 79,* 298-305.

Corsellis, J., Bruton, C. J., & Freeman-Browne, D. (1973). The aftermath of boxing. *Psychological Medicine, 3,* 270-303.

Courville, C. B. (1945). *Pathology of the nervous system* (2nd ed.). Mountain View, CA: Pacific Press.

Courville, C. B. (1958). Traumatic lesions of the temporal lobe. In M. Baldwin & P. Bailey (Eds.), *Temporal lobe epilepsy* (pp. 220–239). Springfield, IL: Thomas.

Craik, F., & Lockhart, R. (1972). Levels of processing: A framework for memory research. *Journal of Verbal Learning and Verbal Behavior*, *12*, 599–607.

Craine, J. F. (1982). Principles of cognitive rehabilitation. In L. E. Trexler (Ed.), *Cognitive rehabilitation: Conceptualization and intervention* (pp. 83–98). New York: Plenum Press.

Craine, J. F., & Gudeman, H. E. (1981). *The rehabilitation of brain functions: Principles, procedures and techniques of neurotraining*. Springfield, IL: Thomas.

Crawford, J. R., & Henry, J. D. (2005). Assessment of executive deficits. In P. Halligan & N. Wade (Eds.), *The effectiveness of rehabilitation for cognitive deficits* (pp. 233–246). New York: Oxford University Press.

Crepeau, F., & Scherzer, P. (1993). Predictors and indicators of work status after traumatic brain injury: A meta-analysis. *Neuropsychological Rehabilitation*, *3*, 5–35.

Crosson, B. (1987). Treatment of interpersonal deficits for head trauma patients in inpatient rehabilitation settings. *The Clinical Neuropsychologist*, *1*, 335–352.

Crosson, B., Barco, P. P., Velozo, C. A., & Bolesta, M. (1989). Awareness and compensation in post-acute head injury rehabilitation. *Journal of Head Trauma Rehabilitation*, *4*, 46–54.

Damasio, A. (1994). *Descartes' error: Emotion, reason and the human brain*. New York: G. P. Putnam's Sons.

Damasio, H., & Damasio, A. (2003). The lesion method in behavioral neurology and neuropsychology. In T. E. Feinberg & M. J. Farah (Eds.), *Behavioral neurology and neuropsychology* (2nd ed., pp. 71–83). New York: McGraw-Hill.

Davison, K., & Bagley, C. R. (1969). Schizophrenia-like psychosis associated with organic disorders of the central nervous system: A review of the literature. *British Journal of Psychiatry, Special Edition 4*, 113–184.

Dawson, P. A., & Chapman, M. (1995). The disablement experienced by traumatically brain injured adults living in the community. *Brain Injury*, *9*, 339–353.

Dawson, R. E., Webster, J. E., & Gurdjian, E. S. (1951). Serial electroencephalography in acute head injuries. *Journal of Neurosurgery*, *8*, 613–630.

Deaton, A. V. (1986). Denial in the aftermath of traumatic head injury: Its manifestations, measurement and treatment. *Rehabilitation Psychology*, *31*, 231–240.

Deaton, A. V. (1987). Behavioral change strategies for children and adolescents with severe brain injury. *Journal of Learning Disabilities*, *20*, 581–589.

Deaton, A. V. (1987). *Pediatric head trauma: A guide for families*. Austin, TX: Healthcare International.

Deaton, A. (1990). Behavior change strategies for children and adolescents with traumatic brain injury. In E. D. Bigler (Ed.), *Traumatic brain injury* (pp. 231–249). Austin, TX: Pro-Ed.

Deaton, A. V. (1991). Group interventions for cognitive rehabilitation: Increasing the challenges. In J. S. Kreutzer & P. H. Wehman (Eds.), *Cognitive rehabilitation for persons with traumatic brain injury* (pp. 191–200). Bisbee, AZ: Imaginart.

Delis, D. C., Kaplan, E., & Kramer, J. H. (2001). *Delis-Kaplan Executive Function System.* San Antonio, TX: The Psychological Corp.

Dell'acqua, R., Sessa, P., & Pashler, H. (2006). A neuropsychological assessment of dual-task costs in closed-head injury patients using Cohen's effect size estimation method. *Psychological Research, 70,* 553–561.

DePompei, R., Epps, A., Savage, R., Blosser, J., & Castelli, E. (1998). Educational needs of children and adolescents after brain injury: A global perspective. *Neurorehabilitation, 11,* 85–100.

Deutsch, P. M. (1998). Transitional employment. In K. B. Fralish & M. J. McMorrow (Eds.), *Innovations in head injury rehabilitation* (Chap. 18). White Plains, NY: Ahab Press.

Diamond, A. (2002). Normal development of prefrontal cortex from birth to young adulthood: Cognitive functions, anatomy and biochemistry. In D. T. Stuss & R. T. Knight (Eds.), *Principles of frontal lobe function* (pp. 466–503). Oxford, England: Oxford University Press.

Dietrich, W. D. (1996). Light and electron microscope studies of fluid-percussion brain injury in rats: Posttraumatic temperature considerations. In B. P. Uzzell & H. H. Stonnington (Eds.), *Recovery after traumatic brain injury* (pp. 67–83). Mahwah, NJ: Erlbaum.

Dikmen, S., & Reitan, R. M. (1977). MMPI correlates of adaptive ability deficits in patients with brain lesions. *Journal of Nervous and Mental Disease, 165,* 247–254.

Dikmen, S., & Reitan, R. M. (1978). Emotional sequelae of head injury. *Annals of Neurology, 2,* 492–494.

Dikmen, S., Reitan, R. M., & Temkin, N. R. (1983). Neuropsychological recovery in head injury. *Archives of Neurology, 40,* 333–338.

Diller, L. (1987). Neuropsychological rehabilitation. In M. J. Meier, A. L. Benton, & L. Diller (Eds.), *Neuropsychological rehabilitation* (pp. 3–17). New York: Guilford Press.

Diller, L. (1994). Finding the right treatment combinations: Changes in rehabilitation over the past five years. In A.-L. Christensen & B. P. Uzzell (Eds.), *Brain injury and neuropsychological rehabilitation: International perspectives* (pp. 1–15). Mahwah, NJ: Erlbaum.

Diller, L., & Ben-Yishay, Y. (1987). Outcomes and evidence in neuropsychological rehabilitation in closed head injury. In H. S. Levin, J. Grafman, & H. M. Eisenberg (Eds.), *Neurobehavioral recovery from head injury* (pp. 146–165). New York: Oxford University Press.

Diller, L., & Ben-Yishay, Y. (1989). Assessment in traumatic brain injury. In P. Bach-y-Rita (Ed.), *Traumatic brain injury* (pp. 161–174). New York: Demos.

Diller, L., & Gordon, W. (1981). Rehabilitation and clinical neuropsychology. In S. Filskov & T. Boll (Eds.), *Handbook of clinical neuropsychology* (pp. 702–733). New York: John Wiley.

Dixon, R. A., & Backman, L. (1999). Principles of compensation in cognitive neurorehabilitation. In D. T. Stuss, H. Winocur, & I. H. Robertson (Eds.), *Cognitive neurorehabilitation* (pp. 59–72). Cambridge, England: Cambridge University Press.

Donaghy, S., & Williams, W. (1998). A new protocol for training severely impaired patients in the usage of memory journals. *Brain Injury*, *12*, 1061–1076.

Donders, J., & Waurschausky, S. (2007). Neurobehavioral outcomes after early versus late childhood traumatic brain injury. *Journal of Head Trauma Rehabilitation*, *22*, 296–302.

Dowling, J. L., & Dacey, R. G. (1996). Factors affecting brain injury in subarachnoid hemorrhage. In B. P. Uzzell & H. H. Stonnington (Eds.), *Recovery after traumatic brain injury* (pp. 39–50). Mahwah, NJ: Erlbaum.

Draper, K., & Ponsford, J. (2008). Cognitive functioning ten years following traumatic brain injury and rehabilitation. *Neuropsychology*, *22*, 618–625.

Draper, K., Ponsford, J., & Schonberger, M. (2007). Psychosocial and emotional outcomes 10 years following traumatic brain injury. *Journal of Head Trauma Rehabilitation*, *22*, 278–287.

Dresser, A. C. (1973). Work status following head injury: The late effects of head injury. *Psychological Medicine*, *12*, 286–294.

Dumont, C., Gervins, M., Fougeyrollas, P., & Bertrand, R. (2004). Toward an explanatory model of social participation in adults with traumatic brain injury. *Journal of Head Trauma Rehabilitation*, *19*, 431–444.

Duncan, J. (1996). Cooperating brain systems in selective perception and action. In T. Inui & J. L. McClelland (Eds.), *Attention and performance XVI* (pp. 549–578). Cambridge, MA: MIT Press.

Duncan, J., Emslie, H., Williams, P., Johnson, R., & Freer, C. (1996). Intelligence and the frontal lobe: The organization of goal-directed behavior. *Cognitive Psychology*, *30*, 257–303.

Duncan, J., & Miller, E. K. (2002). Cognitive focus through adaptive neural coding in the primate prefrontal cortex. In D. T. Stuss & R. Knight (Eds.), *Principles of frontal lobe function* (pp. 278–291). New York: Oxford University Press.

Dye, O. A., Milby, J. B., & Saxon, J. A. (1979). Effects of early neurological problems following head injury on subsequent neuropsychological performance. *Acta Neurologica Scandinavica*, *59*, 10–14.

Eames, P. (1990). Organic bases of behaviour disorders after traumatic brain injury. In R. Ll. Wood (Ed.), *Neurobehavioural sequelae of traumatic brain injury* (pp. 133–150). New York: Taylor and Francis.

Eames, P., & Wood, R. Ll. (1989). The structure and content of a head injury rehabilitation service. In R. Ll. Wood & P. Eames (Eds.), *Models of brain injury rehabilitation* (pp. 31–47). Baltimore: The Johns Hopkins University Press.

Edelman, G., & Tononi, G. (2000). *A universe of consciousness: How matter becomes imagination*. New York: Basic.

Eisele, J. A., Lust, B., & Aram, D. M. (1998). Presupposition and implication of truth: Linguistic deficits following early brain lesions. *Brain and Language*, *61*, 376–394.

Eisenberg, H. M., & Weiner, R. L. (1987). Input variables: How information from the acute injury can be used to characterize groups of patients for studies of outcome. In H. S. Levin, J. Grafman, & H. M. Eisenberg (Eds.), *Neurobehavioral recovery from head injury* (pp. 13–29). New York: Oxford University Press.

Elhardt, L. A., Sohlberg, M. M., Kennedy, M., Coelho, C., Ylvisaker, M., Turkstra, L., et al. (2008). Evidence-based practice guidelines for instructing individuals with neurogenic memory impairments: What have we learned in the past 20 years? *Neuropsychological Rehabilitation*, *18*(3), 300–342.

Elliott, R., Dolan, R. J., & Frith, C. D. (2000). Dissociable functions in the medial and lateral orbitofrontal cortex: Evidence from human neuroimaging studies. *Cerebral Cortex*, *10*, 308–317.

Elmer, O., & Lim, R. (1985). Influence of acute alcohol intoxication on the outcome of severe nonneurologic trauma. *Acta Chirugica Scandinavica*, *151*, 305–308.

Elsass, L., & Kinsella, G. (1987). Social interaction following severe closed brain injury. *Psychological Medicine*, *17*, 67–78.

Envoldsen, E. M., & Jensen, F. T. (1978). Autoregulation and CO2 responses of cerebral blood flow in patients with acute severe head injury. *Journal of Neurosurgery*, *48*, 689–703.

Epstein, F. M., Ward, J. D., & Becker, D. P. (1987). Medical complications of head injury. In P. R. Cooper (Ed.), *Head injury* (2nd ed., pp. 390–421). Baltimore: Williams and Wilkins.

Erickson, E. (1963). *Childhood and society* (2nd ed.). New York: Norton.

Eslinger, P. (2005, July). *Practicing positive neuropsychology*. Keynote address to the International Neuropsychological Society, Dublin, Ireland. (Notes provided courtesy of the author.)

Evans, J. J. (2001). Rehabilitation of the dysexecutive syndrome. In R. Wood & I. MacMillan (Eds.), *Neurobehavioral disability and social handicap following traumatic brain injury* (pp. 209–227). Hove, UK: Psychology Press.

Evans, J. J. (2003). Rehabilitation of executive deficits. In B. Wilson (Ed.), *Neuropsychological rehabilitation: Theory and practice* (pp. 53–70). Lisse, The Netherlands: Swets & Zeitlinger.

Evans, J. J. (2005). Can executive impairments be effectively treated? In P. W. Halligan & D. T. Wade (Eds.), *The effectiveness of rehabilitation for cognitive deficits* (pp. 247–256). Oxford, England: Oxford University Press.

Evans, R. W., & Preston, B. K. (1990). Day rehabilitation programming: A theoretical model. In J. S. Kreutzer & P. Wehman (Eds.), *Community integration following traumatic brain injury* (pp. 125–138). Baltimore: Paul H. Brookes.

Ewing-Cobbs, L., Levin, H. S., & Fletcher, J. M. (1998). Neuropsychological sequelae after pediatric traumatic brain injury: Advances since 1985. In M. Ylvisaker (Ed.), *Traumatic brain injury rehabilitation: Children and adolescents* (2nd ed., pp. 11–26). Boston: Butterworth-Heinemann.

Ezrachi, O., Ben-Yishay, Y., Kay, T., Diller, L., & Rattok, J. (1991). Predicting employment in traumatic brain injury following neuropsychological rehabilitation. *Journal of Head Trauma Rehabilitation, 6,* 71–84.

Fahy, T., Irving, M., & Millac, P. (1967). Severe head injuries: A six-year follow-up. *Lancet, ii,* 475–479.

Farmer, J. E., & Stucky-Ropp, R. (1996). Family transactions and traumatic brain injury. In B. P. Uzzell & H. H. Stonnington (Eds.), *Recovery after traumatic brain injury* (pp. 275–288). Mahwah, NJ: Erlbaum.

Feinberg, T. E., & Farah, M. J. (2003). The development of modern behavioral neurology and neuropsychology. In T. E. Feinberg & M. J. Farah (Eds.), *Behavioral neurology and neuropsychology* (2nd ed., pp. 3–21). New York: McGraw-Hill.

Feinstein, A. (1999). Mood and motivation in rehabilitation. In D. T. Stuss, G. Winocur, & I. H. Robertson (Eds.), *Cognitive neurorehabilitation* (pp. 230–239). New York: Cambridge University Press.

Fernandez-Duque, D., Baird, J. I., & Posner, M. I. (2000). Executive attention and metacognitive regulation. *Consciousness and Cognition, 9,* 288–307.

Festinger, L. (1957). *A theory of cognitive dissonance.* New York: Holt, Rinehart and Winston.

Filley, C. M. (2001). *The behavioral neurology of white matter.* New York: Oxford University Press.

Filley, C. M., Cranberg, L. D., Alexander, M. P., & Hart, E. J. (1987). Neurobehavioral outcome after closed head injury in childhood and adolescence. *Archives of Neurology, 44,* 194–198.

Finger, S., & Stein, D. G. (1982). *Brain damage and recovery.* New York: Academic Press.

Finklestein, E., Corso, P., & Miller, T. (2006). *The incidence and economic burden of injuries in the United States.* New York: Oxford University Press.

Finlayson, M. A., & Garner, S. H. (1994). Challenges in rehabilitation of individuals with acquired brain injury. In M. A. Finlayson & S. H. Garner (Eds.), *Brain injury rehabilitation: Clinical considerations* (pp. 3–10). Baltimore: Williams and Wilkins.

Fisher, J. M. (1985). Cognitive and behavioral consequences of closed head injury. *Neurology, 5,* 197–204.

Fitts, P. M., & Posner, M. I. (1967). *Human performance.* Belmont, CA: Brooks-Cole.

Fordyce, D. J. (1994). Neuropsychologic assessment and cognitive rehabilitation: Issues of psychologic validity. In M. A. Finlayson & S. H. Garner (Eds.), *Brain injury rehabilitation: Clinical considerations* (pp. 187–211). Baltimore: Williams and Wilkins.

Fordyce, D. J. (2003). Reviews. *Journal of Head Trauma Rehabilitation, 18,* 207–209.

Fordyce, D. J., Roueche, J. R., & Prigatano, G. P. (1983). Enhanced emotional reactions in chronic head trauma patients. *Journal of Neurology, Neurosurgery and Psychiatry, 46,* 620–624.

Fralish, K. B. (1998). Characteristics of persons with head injury. In K. B. Fralish & M. J. McMorrow (Eds.), *Innovations in head injury rehabilitation* (Chap. 1). White Plains, NY: Ahab Press.

Fryer, J., & Fralish, K. B. (1998). Cognitive rehabilitation. In K. B. Fralish & M. J. McMorrow (Eds.), *Innovations in head injury rehabilitation* (Chap. 7). White Plains, NY: Ahab Press.

Fuld, P. A., & Fisher, P. (1977). Recovery of intellectual ability after head injury. *Developmental Medicine and Child Neurology, 19,* 495–502.

Fuster, J. (2002). Physiology of executive functions. In D. T. Stuss & R. T. Knight (Eds.), *Principles of frontal lobe function* (pp. 96–108). New York: Oxford University Press.

Fuster, J. M. (2005). *Cortex and mind.* New York: Oxford University Press.

Gazzaniga, M. S. (1998). *The mind's past.* Berkeley, CA: University of California Press.

Gennarelli, T. A. (1987). Cerebral concussion and diffuse brain injuries. In P. R. Cooper (Ed.), *Head injury* (2nd ed., pp. 108–124). Baltimore: Williams and Wilkins.

Gennarelli, T. A., & Graham, D. I. (1987). Neuropathology. In J. M. Silver, T. W. McAllister, & S. C. Yudofsky (Eds.), *Textbook of traumatic brain injury* (pp. 27–50). Washington DC: American Psychiatric Publishing.

Gennarelli, T. A., & Graham, D. I. (2005). Neuropathology. In J. Silver, T. McAllister, & S. Yudofsky (Eds.). *Textbook of traumatic brain injury* (pp. 27–50). Washington, DC: American Psychiatric Press.

Gennarelli, T. A., Spielman, G. M., Langfitt, T. W., Gildenberg, P. L., Harrington, T., Jane, J. A., et al. (1982). Influence of the type of intra-cranial lesion on outcome from severe head injury. *Journal of Neurosurgery, 56,* 26–32.

Gennarelli, T. A., Thibault, L. E., Adams, J. H., Graham, D. I., Thompson, C. J., & Marcincin, R. P. (1982). Diffuse axonal injury and traumatic coma in the primate. *Annals of Neurology, 12,* 564–574.

Gentleman, D., Dearden, M., Midgley, S., & MacLean, D. (1993). Guidelines for resuscitation and transfer of patients with serious head injury. *British Medical Journal, 292*, 449.

Gentry, L. R. (1991). Head trauma. In S. W. Atlas (Ed.), *Magnetic resonance imaging of the brain and spine* (pp. 439–466). New York: Raven.

Geschwind, N. (1965). Disconnection syndromes in animals and man. *Brain, 88*, 237–294.

Geschwind, N. (1982). Disorders of attention: A frontier in neuropsychology. *Philosophical Transactions of the Royal Society of London, 298*, 173–185.

Gevins, A. S., & Illes, J. (1991). Neurocognitive networks of the human brain. In R. Zappulla, F. LeFever, J. Jaeger, & R. Bilder (Eds.), *Windows of the brain: Neuropsychology's technological frontiers* (pp. 22–44). New York: Annals of the New York Academy of Sciences (Vol. 620).

Giacino, J. (2003). Disorders of consciousness in coma, stupor, and minimally responsive states. In T. E. Feinberg & M. J. Farah (Eds.), *Behavioral neurology and neuropsychology* (2nd ed., pp. 337–344). New York: McGraw-Hill.

Giannotta, S. L., Weiner, J. M., & Karnaze, D. (1987). Prognosis and outcome in severe head injury. In P. R. Cooper (Ed.), *Head injury* (2nd ed., pp. 464–487). Baltimore: Williams and Wilkins.

Gigerenzer, G. (2000). *Adaptive thinking: Rationality in the real world.* New York: Oxford University Press.

Gilchrist, E., & Wilkinson, M. (1979). Some factors determining progress in young people with severe head injuries. *Archives of Neurology, 36*, 355–359.

Giles, G. M. (1994). Functional assessment and intervention. In M. A. Finlayson & S. H. Garner (Eds.), *Brain injury rehabilitation: Clinical considerations* (pp. 124–156). Baltimore: Williams and Wilkins.

Giles, G. M., & Clark-Wilson, J. (1993). *Brain injury rehabilitation: A neurofunctional approach.* San Diego, CA: Singular.

Gilroy, J., & Meyer, R. (1979). *Medical neurology.* New York: Macmillan.

Glang, A., Todis, B., Sohlberg, M., & Reed, P. R. (1996). Helping parents negotiate the system. In G. Slinger, A. Glang, & J. M. Williams (Eds.), *Children with acquired brain injury: Educating and supporting families* (1st ed., pp. 149–165). Baltimore: Brookes.

Glenn, M. B. (2006, March). *Functional neuroimaging and cognition following TBI: Neural activation patterns.* Paper presented at the Second Federal Interagency Conference on Traumatic Brain Injury, Bethesda, MD.

Goffman, E. (1967). *Interaction ritual.* Boston: Aldine.

Goldberg, E. (2001). *The executive brain.* Oxford, England: Oxford University Press.

Goldberg, G. (1985). Supplementary motor area structure and function: Review and hypotheses. *Behavioral and Brain Sciences, 8*, 567–616.

Goldstein, F. C., & Levin, H. A. (1991). Memory disorders after closed-head injury. In T. Yanaghara & R. C. Petersen (Eds.), *Memory disorders: Research and clinical practice* (pp. 256–278). New York: Dekker.

Goldstein, G., & Ruthven, L. (1983). *Rehabilitation of the brain damaged adult*. New York: Plenum Press.

Goldstein, K. (1934, reprinted 2000). *The organism*. New York: Zone Books.

Goldstein, K. (1936). The significance of the frontal lobe for mental performances. *Journal of Neurology and Psychopathology, 17*, 27–40.

Goldstein, K. (1940, reprinted 1963). *Human nature in the light of psychopathology*. New York: Schocken Books.

Goldstein, K. (1942). *After-effects of brain injuries in the war*. London: Heinemann.

Goldstein, K. (1952). The effect of brain damage on the personality. *Psychiatry, 15*, 245–260.

Gollwitzer, P. M., Fujita, K., & Oettingen, G. (2004). Planning and the implantation of goals. In R. F. Baumeister & K. D. Vohs (Eds.), *Handbook of self-regulation: Research, theory, and applications* (pp. 211–228). New York: Guilford.

Goodman, H., & Englander, J. (1992). Traumatic brain injury in elderly individuals. In S. Berrol (Ed.), *Physical medicine and rehabilitation clinics of North America: Traumatic brain injury* (pp. 441–459). Philadelphia: Saunders.

Gordon, W. A., Brown, M., Sliwinski, M., Hibbard, M. R., Patti, N., Weiss, M. J., et al. (1998). The enigma of "hidden" traumatic brain injury. *Journal of Head Trauma Rehabilitation, 13*(6), 39–56.

Gordon, W. A., Cantor, J., Ashman, T., & Brown, M. (2006). Treatment of post-TBI executive dysfunction: Application of theory to clinical practice. *Journal of Head Trauma Rehabilitation, 21*, 156–167.

Gordon, W. A., & Hibbard, M. R. (1991). The theory and practice of cognitive remediation. In J. S. Kreutzer & P. H. Wehman (Eds.), *Cognitive rehabilitation for persons with traumatic brain injury* (pp. 13–22). Bisbee, AZ: Imaginart.

Gordon, W. A., & Hibbard, M. R. (2005). Cognitive rehabilitation. In J. M. Silver, T. W. McAllister, & S. C. Yudofsky (Eds.), *Textbook of traumatic brain injury* (pp. 655–660). Washington, DC: American Psychiatric Publishing.

Gordon, W. A., Hibbard, M. R., Brown, M., Flanagan, S., & Korves, M. C. (1999). Community integration and quality of life of individuals with traumatic brain injury. In M. Rosenthal, E. R. Griffith, J. S. Kreutzer, & B. Pentland (Eds.), *Rehabilitation of the adult and child with traumatic brain injury* (3rd ed., pp. 312–325). Philadelphia: Davis.

Gordon, W. A., Zafonte, R., Cicerone, K. D., Cantor, J., Brown, M., Lombard, L., et al. (2006). Traumatic brain injury: State of the science. *American Journal of Physical Medicine and Rehabilitation, 85*, 343–382.

Gouvier, W. (1986). Quiet victims of the silent epidemic: A comment on Dlugokinski. *American Psychologist, 41*, 483–484.

Government Accounting Office. (1998). *Report to Congress: TBI programs supporting long-term services in selected states*. Washington, DC: Government Printing Office.

Gowland, C., & Gambarotto, C. A. (1994). Assessment and treatment of physical impairments leading to disability after brain injury. In M. A. Finlayson & S. H. Garner (Eds.), *Brain injury rehabilitation: Clinical considerations* (pp. 102–123). Baltimore: Williams and Wilkins.

Grady, C. L., & Kapur, S. (1999). The use of neuroimaging in neurorehabilitation research. In D. Stuss, G. Winocur, & I. Robertson (Eds.), *Cognitive neurorehabilitation* (pp 47–58). New York: Cambridge University Press.

Grafman, J. (2002). The structured event complex and the human prefrontal cortex. In D. T. Stuss & R. Knight (Eds.), *Principles of frontal lobe function* (pp. 292–310). New York: Oxford University Press.

Graham, D. I. (1999). Pathological aspects of injury and mechanisms of recovery. In M. Rosenthal, E. R. Griffith, J. S. Kreutzer, & B. Pentland (Eds.), *Rehabilitation of the adult and child with traumatic brain injury* (3rd ed., pp. 19–41). Philadelphia: Davis.

Graham, D. I., Adams, J. H., & Doyle, D. (1979). Ischemic brain damage in nonfatal missile head injuries. *Journal of Neuroscience, 39*, 213–234.

Graham, D. I., Adams, J. H., & Gennarelli, T. A. (1987). Pathology of brain damage in head injury. In P. R. Cooper (Ed.), *Head injury* (2nd ed., pp. 72–88). Baltimore: Williams and Wilkins.

Grant, I., & Alves, W. (1987). Psychiatric and psychosocial disturbances in head injury. In H. S. Levin, J. Grafman, & H. M. Eisenberg (Eds.), *Neurobehavioral recovery from head injury* (pp. 232–261). New York: Oxford University Press.

Gray, J. A., & McNaughton, N. (2003). *Neuropsychology of anxiety: An enquiry into the functions of the septo-hippocampal system*. New York: Oxford University Press.

Greenspan, A. I., & MacKenzie, E. J. (2000). Use and need for post-acute services following paediatric head injury. *Brain Injury, 14*, 417–429.

Gronwall, D. (1987). Advances in the assessment of attention and information processing after head injury. In H. S. Levin, J. Grafman, & H. M. Eisenberg (Eds.), *Neurobehavioral recovery from head injury* (pp. 355–371). New York: Oxford University Press.

Gronwall, D., & Sampson, H. (1974). *The psychological effects of concussion.* New York: Oxford University Press.

Gronwall, D., & Wrightson, P. (1974). Delayed recovery of intellectual function after minor head injury. *Lancet, 2*, 605–609.

Gronwall, D., & Wrightson, P. (1981). Memory and information processing after closed head injury. *Journal of Neurology, Neurosurgery and Psychiatry, 44*, 889–895.

Gronwall, D., Wrightson, P., & Waddell, P. (1990). *Head injury: The facts.* Oxford, England: Oxford University Press.

Gronwall, D., Wrightson, P., & Waddell, P. (1998). *Head injury: The facts* (2nd ed.). Oxford, England: Oxford University Press.

Gross, Y. (1982). A conceptual framework for interventive cognitive neuropsychology. In L. E. Trexler (Ed.), *Cognitive rehabilitation: Conceptualization and intervention* (pp. 99–114). New York: Plenum Press.

Gross, Y., Ben-Nahum, Z., & Munk, G. (1982). Techniques and application of simultaneous information processing. In L. E. Trexler (Ed.), *Cognitive rehabilitation: Conceptualization and intervention* (pp. 223–238). New York: Plenum Press.

Gross, Y., & Schutz, L. (1984, June). *Theory and method in cognitive rehabilitation: Focus on the continuity of behavior.* Paper presented at the National Head Injury Foundation, Boston, MA.

Gross, Y., & Schutz, L. (1986). Intervention models in neuropsychology. In B. Uzzell & Y. Gross (Eds.), *Clinical neuropsychology of intervention* (pp. 179–204). Boston: Martinus-Nijhoff.

Grosswasser, Z., & Stern, M. J. (1998). A psychodynamic model of behavior after central nervous system damage. *Journal of Head Trauma Rehabilitation, 13,* 69–79.

Guercio, A., & Fralish, K. B. (1998). Integration of cognitive approaches to functional rehabilitation. In K. B. Fralish & M. J. McMorrow (Eds.), *Innovations in head injury rehabilitation* (Chap. 9). White Plains, NY: Ahab Press.

Gurdjian, E. S. (1975). *Impact head injury: Mechanistic, clinical and preventative correlations.* Springfield, IL: Charles C. Thomas.

Gurdjian, E. S., Webster, J. E., & Arnkoff, H. (1943). Acute craniocerebral trauma: Surgical and pathologic considerations based upon 151 consecutive autopsies. *Surgery, 13,* 333–353.

Haas, J., Cope, D. N., & Hall, K. (1987). Premorbid prevalence of poor academic performance in severe head injury. *Journal of Neurology, Neurosurgery and Psychiatry, 50,* 52–56.

Hackler, E., & Tobis, J. S. (1983). Reintegration into the community. In M. Rosenthal, E. R. Griffith, M. R. Bond, & J. D. Miller (Eds.), *Rehabilitation of the head injured adult* (pp. 421–434). Philadelphia: Davis.

Hagen, C. (1982). Language-cognitive disorganization following closed head injury: A conceptualization. In L. E. Trexler (Ed.), *Cognitive rehabilitation: Conceptualization and intervention* (pp. 131–151). New York: Plenum Press.

Hall, K. M., Mann, N., High, W. M., Wright, J., Kreutzer, J. S., & Wood, D. (1996). Functional measurement after traumatic brain injury: Ceiling effects of FIM, FIM+, FAM, DRS, and CIQ. *Journal of Head Trauma Rehabilitation, 11,* 27–39.

Halligan, P., & Wade, D. (2005). Introduction. In P. Halligan & D. Wade (Eds.), *Effectiveness of rehabilitation for cognitive deficits* (pp. xi–xv). New York: Oxford University Press.

Hart, T., Dijkers, M., Fraser, R., Cicerone, K., Bogner, J. A., Whyte, J., et al. (2006). Vocational services for traumatic brain injury: Treatment definition and diversity within model systems of care. *Journal of Head Trauma Rehabilitation, 21*, 467–482.

Hart, T., & Evans, J. (2006). Self-regulation and goal theories in brain injury rehabilitation. *Journal of Head Trauma Rehabilitation, 21*, 142–155.

Hart, T., Giovannetti, T., Montgomery, M. W., & Schwartz, M. F. (1998). Awareness of errors in naturalistic action after traumatic brain injury. *Journal of Head Trauma Rehabilitation, 13*, 16–28.

Hart, T., & Hayden, M. E. (1986). The ecological validity of neuropsychological assessment and remediation. In B. Uzzell & Y. Gross (Eds.), *Clinical neuropsychology of intervention* (pp. 2–50). Boston: Martinus-Nijhoff.

Harti, R., & Ghajar, J. (2005). Neurosurgical interventions. In J. M. Silver, T. W. McAllister, & S. C. Yudofsky (Eds.), *Textbook of traumatic brain injury* (pp. 51–58). Washington DC: American Psychiatric Publishing.

Hartley, L. R., Morrison, D., & Arnold, P. (1989). Stress and skill. In A. M. Colley & J. R. Beech (Eds.), *Acquisition and performance of cognitive skills* (pp. 265–300). New York: Wiley.

Hartmann, H. (1939). *Ego psychology and the problem of adaptation.* New York: International Universities Press.

Hasher, L., & Zacks, R. T. (1979). Automatic and effortful processes in memory. *Journal of Experimental Psychology: General, 108*, 356–388.

Head, H. (1926). *Aphasia and kindred disorders of speech.* Cambridge, England: Cambridge University Press.

Heilman, K. (1991). Anosagnosia: Possible neuropsychological mechanisms. In G. P. Prigatano & D. L. Schacter (Eds.), *Awareness of deficit after brain injury* (pp. 53–62). New York: Oxford University Press.

Heilman, K., Bowers, D., & Valenstein, E. (1993). Emotional disorders associated with neurological diseases. In K. Heilman & E. Valenstein, E. (Eds.), *Clinical neuropsychology* (3rd ed., pp. 377–402). New York: Oxford University Press.

Hein, G., Schubert, T., & von Cramon, D. Y. (2005). Closed-head injury and perceptual processing in dual-task situations. *Experimental Brain Research, 160*, 223–234.

Heiskanen, O., & Kaste, M. (1974). Late prognosis of severe brain injury in children. *Developmental Medicine and Child Neurology, 16*, 11–14.

Hockey, G. R. (1993). Cognitive and energetical control mechanisms in the management of work demands and psychological health. In A. Baddeley & L. Weiskrantz (Eds.), *Attention: awareness, selection and control: A tribute to Donald Broadbent* (pp. 328–345). New York: Oxford University Press.

Hoegh, S. M. (1994). Working together: Reflections on fostering an integrated service network for individuals with brain injury. In M. A. Finlayson & S. H. Garner (Eds.), *Brain injury rehabilitation: Clinical considerations* (pp. 393–421). Baltimore: Williams and Wilkins.

Holbourne, A. (1943). Mechanics of head injuries. *Lancet, 2*, 438–441.

Holmes, C. B. (1988). *The head injured college student*. Springfield, IL: Charles C. Thomas.

Hoofien, D., Gilboa, A., Vakil, E., & Donovik, P. (2001). Traumatic brain injury 10–20 years later: A comprehensive outcome study of psychiatric symptomatology, cognitive abilities and psychosocial functioning. *Brain Injury*, *15*, 189–209.

Horn, L. (1992). Systems of care for the person with traumatic brain injury In S. Berrol (Ed.), *Physical medicine and rehabilitation clinics of North America: Traumatic brain injury* (pp. 475–492). Philadelphia: Saunders.

Horton, A. M. (1997). Human neuropsychology: Current status. In A. M. Horton, D. Wedding, & J. Webster (Eds.), *The neuropsychology handbook* (Vol. 1, 2nd ed., pp. 3–30). New York: Springer.

Howard, S. (2004). Conflicts and controversies after brain injury: Struggling to be me. *Brain Injury Professional*, *1*, 28–31.

Humphrey, M., & Oddy, M. (1981). Return to work after head injury: A review of post-war studies. *Injury*, *12* 107–114.

Hux, K., Schram, C. D., & Goeken, T. (2006). Misconceptions about brain injury: A survey replication study. *Brain Injury*, *20*, 547–553.

Ishige, N., Pitts, L. H., Hashimoto, T., Nishimura, M. C., & Bartkowski, H. M. (1987). Effect of hypoxia on traumatic brain injury in rats: Part 1. Changes in neurological function, electroencephalograms, and histopathology. *Neurosurgery*, *20*, 848–858.

Jackson, J. H. (1882/1998). *Evolution and dissolution of the nervous system*. London, UK: Thoemmes Press.

Jacobs, H. E. (1987). *Final report of the Los Angeles Head Injury Survey*. Los Angeles: National Institute of Handicapped Research.

Jacobs, H. E. (1988). The Los Angeles head injury survey: Procedures and preliminary findings. *Archives of Physical Medicine and Rehabilitation*, *69*, 425–431.

Jacobs, H. E. (1989). Adult community integration. In P. Bach-y-Rita (Ed.), *Traumatic brain injury* (pp. 287–318). New York: Demos.

Jacobs, H. E. (1990). Identifying post-traumatic behavior problems: Data from psychosocial follow-up studies. In R. Ll. Wood (Ed.), *Neurobehavioural sequelae of traumatic brain injury* (pp. 37–51). New York: Taylor and Francis.

Jahanshahi, M., & Frith, C. (1998). Willed action and its impairments. *Cognitive Neuropsychology*, *15*, 483–533.

Jamieson, K. G., & Kelly, D. (1973). Crash helmets reduce head injuries. *The Medical Journal of Australia*, *2*, 806–809.

Jamieson, K. G., & Yelland. J. D. (1972). Surgically treated traumatic subdural hematoma. *Journal of Neurosurgery*, *37*, 137–149.

Janus, P. L. (1996). Advocacy and the parent-centered partnership. In A. Goldberg (Ed.), *Acquired brain injury in childhood and adolescence: A team and family guide to educational program development and implementation*. Springfield, IL: Charles C. Thomas.

Jarho, L. (1973). Korsakoff-like amnesic syndrome in penetrating brain injury: A study of Finnish war veterans. *Acta Neurologica Scandinavica, 54,* 1–156.

Jennett, B. (1990). Scale and scope of the problem. In M. Rosenthal, E. R. Griffith, M. R. Bond, & J. D. Miller (Eds.), *Rehabilitation of the adult and child with traumatic head injury* (2nd ed., pp. 3–7). Philadelphia: Davis.

Jennett, B. (1997). Outcome after severe head injury. In P. Reilly & R. Bullock (Eds.). *Head injury* (pp. 439–461). London: Chapman & Hall.

Jennett, B., Snoek, J., Bond, M. R., & Brooks, D. N. (1981). Disability after severe head injury: Observations on the use of the Glasgow Outcome Scale. *Journal of Neurology, Neurosurgery and Psychiatry, 44,* 285–293.

Jennett, B., & Teasdale, G. (1981). *Management of head injuries.* Philadelphia: Davis.

Johnson, D. A., & Newton, A. (1987). Social adjustment and interaction after severe brain injury: 2. Rationale and bases for intervention. *British Journal of Clinical Psychology, 26,* 289–298.

Johnson, P., Thomas-Stonell, N., Rumney, P., & Oddson, B. (2006). Long-term outcomes of pediatric acquired brain injury. *Brain and Cognition, 60,* 205–206.

Johnstone, B., & Callahan, T. S. (1996). Neuropsychological evaluation of traumatic brain injury in the United States: A critical analysis. In B. P. Uzzell & H. H. Stonnington (Eds.), *Recovery after traumatic brain injury* (pp. 115–128). Mahwah, NJ: Erlbaum.

Jongbloed, L. (1986). Prediction of function after stroke: A critical review. *Stroke, 17,* 765–776.

Joseph, R. (1997). *Neuropsychiatry, neuropsychology and clinical neuroscience: Emotion, evolution, cognition, language, memory, brain damage and abnormal behavior* (2nd ed.). Baltimore: Williams and Wilkins.

Jurkovich, G. J., Rivara, F. P., Gurney, J. G., Fligner, C., Ries, R., Mueller, B. A., et al. (1993). The effects of acute alcohol intoxication and chronic alcohol abuse on outcome from trauma. *Journal of the American Medical Association, 270,* 51–56.

Kahneman, D. (1973). *Attention and effort.* Englewood Cliffs, NJ: Prentice-Hall.

Kaila, K., & Ransom, B. R. (1998). Concept of pH and its importance in neurobiology. In K. Kaila & B. R. Ransom (Eds.), *pH and brain function* (pp. 3–10). New York: Wiley-Liss.

Kauppinen, R. A., & Williams, S. R. (1998). Use of NMR spectroscopy in monitoring cerebral pH and metabolism during systemic and focal acid-base disturbances. In K. Kaila & B. R. Ransom (Eds.), *pH and brain function* (pp. 605–619). New York: Wiley-Liss.

Katayama, Y., Yoshino, A., Kawamata, T., & Tsubokawa, T. (1996). Role of excitatory amino acids in neuronal and glial responses to traumatic brain injury. In B. P. Uzzell & H. H. Stonnington (Eds.), *Recovery after traumatic brain injury* (pp. 51–65). Mahwah, NJ: Erlbaum.

Katz, D. I., Ashley, M. J., O'Shanick, G. J., & Connors, S. H. (2006). *Cognitive rehabilitation: The evidence, funding, and case for advocacy in brain injury*. McLean, VA: Brain Injury Association of America.

Katz, D. I., & Mills, V. M. (1999). Traumatic brain injury: Natural history and efficacy of cognitive rehabilitation. In D. T. Stuss, G. Winocur, & I. H. Robertson (Eds.), *Cognitive neurorehabilitation* (pp. 279–301). Cambridge, England: Cambridge University Press.

Kay, T., & Cavallo, M. (1994). The family system: Impact, assessment, and intervention. In J. M. Silver, S. C. Yudofsky, & R. E. Hales (Eds.), *Neuropsychiatry of traumatic brain injury* (pp. 533–567). Washington, DC: American Psychiatric Press.

Kelly, G. (1955). *The psychology of personal constructs*. New York: Norton.

Kennard, M. (1940). Relation of age to motor impairment in man and in subhuman primates. *Archives of Neurology and Psychiatry, 44*, 377–397.

Kennedy, M., & Coelho, C. (2006). Self-regulation after traumatic brain injury: A framework for intervention of memory and problem solving. *Seminars in Speech and Language, 26*, 242–255.

Kennedy, M. R., Coelho, C., Turkstra, L., Ylvisaker, M., Moore Sohlberg, M., Yorkston, K., . . . Kan, P. F. (2008). Intervention for executive functions after traumatic brain injury: A systematic review, meta-analysis and clinical recommendations. *Neuropsychological Rehabilitation, 18*(3), 257–299.

Kennedy, M. R., & Yorkston, K. M. (2000). Accuracy of metamemory after traumatic brain injury: Predictions during verbal learning. *Journal of Speech, Language, and Hearing Research, 43*, 1072–1086.

Kiefer, M., Ahlegian, M., & Spitzer, M. (2005). Working memory capacity, indirect semantic priming, and Stroop interference: Pattern of interindividual prefrontal performance differences in healthy volunteers. *Neuropsychology, 19*, 332–344.

Kim, E., Lauterbach, E. C., Reeve, A., Arciniegas, D. B., Coburn, K. L., Mendez, M. F., et al. (2007). Neuropsychiatric complications of traumatic brain injury: A critical review of the literature (a report by the ANPA Committee on Research). *Journal of Neuropsychiatry and Clinical Neurosciences, 19*, 106–127.

Kingston, W. J. (1985). Head injury. *Seminars in Neurology, 5*, 197–270.

Klonoff, H. (1971). Head injuries in children: Predisposing factors, accident conditions, accident proneness and sequelae. *American Journal of Public Health, 61*, 2405–2417.

Klonoff, P. S., Lamb, D. G., & Henderson, S. W. (2001). Outcomes from milieu-based neurorehabilitation at up to 11 years post-discharge. *Brain Injury, 15*, 413–428.

Kolb, B., & Gibb, R. (1999). Neuroplasticity and recovery of function after brain injury. In D. T. Stuss, G. Winocur, & I. Robertson (Eds.), *Cognitive neurorehabilitation* (pp. 9–25). Cambridge, MA: Cambridge University Press.

Kolb, B., & Whishaw, I. (2003). *Fundamentals of human neuropsychology* (5th ed.). New York: Worth.

Kosslyn, S., & Koenig, O. (1992). *Wet mind: The new cognitive neuroscience*. New York: Free Press.

Kowalske, K., Plenger, P. M., Lusby, B., & Hayden, M. A. (2000). Vocational re-entry following traumatic brain injury: An enablement model. *Journal of Head Trauma Rehabilitation*, *15*, 989–999.

Kozloff, P. (1987). Networks of social support and outcome from severe brain injury. *Journal of Head Trauma Rehabilitation*, *2*, 14–23.

Kozol, H. L. (1946). Pretraumatic personality and psychiatric sequelae of head injury. *Archives of Neurology and Psychiatry*, *56*, 245–275.

Kraus, J. F. (1987). Epidemiology of head injury. In P. R. Cooper (Ed.), *Head injury* (2nd ed., pp. 1–19). Baltimore: Williams and Wilkins.

Kraus, J. F., & Chu, L. D. (2005). Epidemiology. In J. M. Silver, T. W. McAllister, & S. C. Yudofsky (Eds.), *Textbook of traumatic brain injury* (pp. 3–26). Washington DC: American Psychiatric Publishing.

Kraus, J. F., & McArthur, D. L. (1999). Incidence and prevalence of, and costs associated with, traumatic brain injury. In M. Rosenthal, E. R. Griffith, J. S. Kreutzer, & B. Pentland (Eds.), *Rehabilitation of the adult and child with traumatic brain injury* (3rd ed., pp. 3–18). Philadelphia: Davis.

Kreutzer, J. S., Gordon, W. A., & Wehman, P. (1989). Cognitive remediation following traumatic brain injury. *Rehabilitation Psychology*, *34*, 117–130.

Kreutzer, J. S., Leininger, B. E., & Harris, J. A. (1990). The evolving role of neuropsychology in community integration. In J. S. Kreutzer & P. Wehman (Eds.), *Community integration following traumatic brain injury* (pp. 49–66). Baltimore: Paul H. Brookes.

Kreutzer, J. S., Zasler, N. D., Camplair, P. S., & Leininger, B. E. (1990). A practical guide to family intervention following adult traumatic brain injury. In J. S. Kreutzer & P. Wehman (Eds.), *Community integration following traumatic brain injury* (pp. 249–284). Baltimore: Paul H. Brookes.

Laatsch, L. K., Thulborne, R. R., Krisky, C. M., Shobat, D. M., & Sweeney, J. A. (2004). Investigating the neurobiological basis of cognitive rehabilitation therapy with fMRI. *Brain Injury*, *18*, 957–974.

Lambooy, N., vander Zwan, A., & Fossen, A. (1965). End-results after long term unconsciousness due to head injury. *Psychiatrica Neurologica Neurochirugica Amsterdam*, *68*, 431–442.

Langfitt, T. W., & Zimmerman, R. A. (1985). Imaging and in vivo biochemistry of the brain in head injury. In D. P. Becker & J. T. Povlishock (Eds.), *Cen-tral nervous system trauma status report* (pp. 53–63). Washington, DC: National Institutes of Neurological and Communicative Disorder and Health.

Langlois, J. A., Rutland-Brown, W., & Thomas, K. E. (2004). *Traumatic brain injury in the United States*. Centers for Disease Control and Prevention. Atlanta, GA: National Center for Prevention and Control.

Langlois, J. A., Rutland-Brown, W., & Wald, M. M. (2006). The epidemiology and impact of traumatic brain injury. *Journal of Head Trauma Rehabilitation, 21,* 375–378.

Lashley, K. S. (1938). Factors limiting recovery after central nervous system lesions. *Journal of Nervous and Mental Disease, 88,* 833–855.

Lashley, K. S. (1963). *Brain mechanisms and intelligence.* New York: Dover.

Lawson, M., & Rice, D. (1989). Effects of training use of executive strategies on a verbal memory problem resulting from closed head injury. *Journal of Clinical and Experimental Neuropsychology, 11,* 842–854.

Lazarus, R. S., & Folkman, S. (1984). *Stress, appraisal, and coping.* New York: Springer.

Lehr, E. (1990). *Psychosocial management of traumatic brain injuries in children and adolescents.* Rockville, MD: Aspen.

Lehr, E., & Savage, R. C. (1990). Community and school integration from a developmental perspective. In J. S. Kreutzer & P. Wehman (Eds.), *Community integration following traumatic brain injury* (pp. 301–312). Baltimore: Brookes.

Lengfelder, A., & Gollwitzer, P. M. (2001). Reflective and reflexive action control in patients with frontal brain lesions. *Neuropsychology, 15,* 80–100.

Levin, H. S. (1985). Neurobehavioral recovery. In D. P. Becker & J. T. Povlishock (Eds.), *Central nervous system trauma status report, 1985* (pp. 65–78). Bethesda, MD: National Institutes of Health.

Levin, H. S. (1987). Neurobehavioral sequelae of head injury. In P. R. Cooper (Ed.), *Head injury* (2nd ed., pp. 442–463). Baltimore: Williams and Wilkins.

Levin, H. S., Benton, A. L., & Grossman, R. G. (1982). *Neurobehavioral consequences of closed head injury.* New York: Oxford University Press.

Levin, H. S., Goldstein, F. C, High, W. M., Jr., & Williams, D. (1988). Automatic and effortful processing after severe closed head injury. *Brain and Cognition, 7,* 283–297.

Levin, H. S., & Grossman, R. G. (1978). Behavioral sequelae of closed head injury: A quantitative study. *Archives of Neurology, 35,* 720–727.

Levin, H. S., Grossman, R. G., & Kelly, P. J. (1976). Aphasic disorder in patients with closed head injury. *Journal of Neurology, Neurosurgery and Psychiatry, 39,* 1062–1070.

Levin, H. S., Grossman, R. G., & Kelly, P. J. (1977). Impairment of facial recognition after closed head injuries of varying severity. *Cortex, 13,* 119–130.

Levin, H. S., Grossman, R. G., Rose, J. E., & Teasdale, G. (1979). Long-term neuropsychological outcome of closed head injury. *Journal of Neurosurgery, 50,* 412–422.

Levin, H. S., O'Donnell, V. M., & Grossman, R. G. (1979). The Galveston Orientation and Amnesia Test: A practical scale to assess cognition after head injury. *Journal of Nervous and Mental Disease, 167,* 675–684.

Levin, W. (1991). Computer applications in cognitive rehabilitation. In J. S. Kreutzer & P. H. Wehman (Eds.), *Cognitive rehabilitation for persons with traumatic brain injury* (pp. 163–179). Bisbee, AZ: Imaginart.

Levine, B., Cabeza, R., McIntosh, A. R., Black, S. E., Grady, C. L., & Stuss, D. T. (2002). Functional reorganization of memory systems following traumatic brain injury. *Journal of Neurology, Neurosurgery and Psychiatry, 73,* 173–181.

Levine, B., Robertson, I. H., Clare, L., Carter, G., Hong, J., Wilson, B. A., et al. (2000). Rehabilitation of executive functioning: An experimental clinical validation of Goal Management Training. *Journal of the International Neuropsychological Society, 6,* 299–312.

Levinson, D. J., Darrow, C. H., Klein, E. B., Levinson, M. H., & McKee, B. (1978). *The seasons of a man's life.* New York: Alfred A. Knopf.

Lewelt, W., Jenkins, L. W., & Miller, J. D. (1980). Autoregulation of cerebral blood flow after experimental fluid percussion injury. *Journal of Neurosurgery, 53,* 500–511.

Lewis, B., & Schutz, L. (1984, September). *Treatment of a working professional with a severe head injury.* Paper presented at New Frontiers in Cognitive Rehabilitation: An Advanced Conference, Princeton, NJ.

Lezak, M. (1976). Recovery of memory and learning functions following traumatic brain injury. *Cortex, 15,* 63–72.

Lezak, M. (1978). Living with the characterologically altered brain-injured patient. *Journal of Clinical Psychology, 39,* 592–615.

Lezak, M. (1982). The problem of assessing executive functions. *International Journal of Psychology, 17,* 281–297.

Lezak, M. (1983). *Neuropsychological assessment* (2nd ed.). New York: Oxford University Press.

Lezak, M. (1987). Relationships between personality disorders, social disturbances, and physical disability following traumatic brain injury. *Journal of Head Trauma Rehabilitation, 2,* 57–69.

Lezak, M. (1987). Making neuropsychological assessment relevant to head injury. In H. S. Levin, J. Grafman, & H. M. Eisenberg (Eds.), *Neurobehavioral recovery from head injury* (pp. 116–128). New York: Oxford University Press.

Lezak, M. (1988). Brain damage is a family affair. *Journal of Clinical and Experimental Neuropsychology, 10,* 111–123.

Lezak, M. (1995). *Neuropsychological assessment* (3rd ed.). New York: Oxford University Press.

Lezak, M., Howieson, D., & Loring, R. (2004). *Neuropsychological assessment* (4th ed.). New York: Oxford University Press.

Lezak, M., & O'Brien, K. P. (1990). Chronic emotional, social and physical changes after traumatic brain injury. In E. D. Bigler (Ed.), *Traumatic brain injury* (pp. 365–380). Austin, TX: Pro-Ed.

L'Hermitte, F. (1986). Human anatomy and the frontal lobes: Part II. Patient behavior in complex social situations: The environmental dependency syndrome. *Annals of Neurology, 19*(4), 335–343.

Lindgren, S. O. (1966). Experimental studies of mechanical effects in head injury. *Acta Chirurgica Scandinavica* (Suppl. 132), 1.

Lishman, W. A. (1968). Brain damage in relation to psychiatric disability after head injury. *British Journal of Psychiatry, 114*, 373–410.

Lishman, W. A. (1973). The psychiatric sequelae of head injury: A review. *Psychological Medicine, 3*, 304–318.

Lishman, W. A. (1978). *Organic psychiatry: The psychological consequences of cerebral disorder.* Oxford, England: Blackwell Scientific.

Lishman, W. A. (1987). *Organic psychiatry: The psychological consequences of cerebral disorder* (2nd ed.). Oxford, England: Blackwell Science.

Liu, K., Chan, C., Lee, T., Li, L., & Hui-Chan, C. (2002). Self-regulatory learning and generalization for people with brain injury. *Brain Injury, 16*, 817–824.

Livingston, M. G. (1990). Effects on the family system. In M. Rosenthal, E. R. Griffith, M. R. Bond, & J. D. Miller (Eds.), *Rehabilitation of the adult and child with traumatic head injury* (2nd ed., pp. 225–235). Philadelphia: Davis.

Locke, E. A., & Latham, G. P. (2002). Building a practically useful theory of goal setting and task motivation: A 35-year odyssey. *American Psychologist, 57*, 705–717.

Long, C. J. (1998). Neuropsychological tests: A look at our past and the impact that ecological issues may have on our future. In R. Sbordone & C. Long (Eds.), *Ecological validity of neuropsychological testing* (pp. 1–14). Boca Raton, FL: St. Lucie Press.

Long, C. J., & Williams, J. M. (1988). Neuropsychological assessment and treatment of head trauma patients. In H. A. Whitaker (Ed.), *Neuropsychological studies of nonfocal brain damage* (pp. 132–161). New York: Springer-Verlag.

Luna, G. K., Maier, R. V., Sowder. L., Copass, M. K., & Oneskovich, M. R. (1984). The influence of ethanol intoxication on outcome of injured motorcyclists. *Journal of Trauma, 24*, 695–700.

Luria, A. R. (1948/1963). *Restoration of function after brain injury.* New York: Pergamon.

Luria, A. R. (1966). *Human brain and psychological processes.* New York: Harper and Row.

Luria, A. R. (1973). *The working brain.* New York: Basic Books.

Luria, A. R. (1979). *The making of mind: A personal account of Soviet psychology.* Cambridge, MA: Harvard University Press.

Luria, A. R. (1980). *Higher cortical functions in man.* New York: Basic Books.

Lux, W. E. (1996). Pharmacological strategies in the management of cognition and behavior following traumatic brain injury. In B. P. Uzzell & H. H. Stonnington (Eds.), *Recovery after traumatic brain injury* (pp. 99–112). Mahwah, NJ: Erlbaum.

Lynch, W. J. (1982). Emotional consequences of brain injury. In L. E. Trexler (Ed.), *Cognitive rehabilitation: Conceptualization and intervention* (pp. 63–76). New York: Plenum Press.

Lynch, W. J. (1982). The use of electronic games in cognitive rehabilitation. In L. E. Trexler (Ed.), *Cognitive rehabilitation: Conceptualization and intervention* (pp. 263–274). New York: Plenum Press.

MacNiven, E. (1994). Factors affecting head injury rehabilitation outcome: Premorbid and clinical parameters. In M. A. Finlayson & S. H. Garner (Eds.), *Brain injury rehabilitation: Clinical considerations* (pp. 57–82). Baltimore: Williams and Wilkins.

Maestu, F., Campo, P. Capilla, A., Simos, P. G., Paul, M., Fernandez, S., et al. (2005). Prefrontal brain magnetic activity: Effects of memory task demands. *Neuropsychology, 19*, 301–308.

Mailhan, L., Azouvi, P., Dazord, A. (2005). Life satisfaction and disability after severe traumatic brain injury. *Brain Injury, 19*, 227–238.

Malec, J. (1985). Personality factors associated with severe traumatic disability. *Rehabilitation Psychology, 30*, 165–172.

Malec, J. (1996). Cognitive rehabilitation. In R. W. Evans (Ed.), *Neurology and trauma* (pp. 231–248). Philadelphia: Saunders.

Malec, J. F. (2001). Impact of comprehensive day treatment on societal participation for persons with acquired brain injury. *Archives of Physical Medicine & Rehabilitation, 82*, 885–895.

Malec, J. (2005, June). *Personality, depression, and outcome after traumatic brain injury*. Paper presented at the 12th Annual Brain Injury Conference, Mayo Clinic, Rochester, MN.

Malec, J. F., & Basford, J. S. (1996). Post-acute brain injury rehabilitation. *Archives of Physical Medicine and Rehabilitation, 77*, 198–207.

Malec, J. F., Smigielski, J. S., DePompolo, R. W., & Thompson, J. M. (1993). Outcome evaluation and prediction in a comprehensive-integrated post-acute outpatient brain injury programme. *Brain Injury, 7*, 15–29.

Malec, J. F., Testa, J. A., Rush, B. K., Brown, A. W., & Moessner, A. M. (2007). Self-assessment of impairment, impaired self-awareness, and depression after traumatic brain injury. *Journal of Head Trauma Rehabilitation, 22*, 156–166.

Manchester, D., Priestly, N., & Jackson, H. (2004). The assessment of executive functions: Coming out of the office. *Brain Injury, 18*, 1067–1081.

Mandleberg, I. A. (1975). Cognitive recovery after severe head injury: 2. Wechsler Adult Intelligence Scale during post-traumatic amnesia. *Journal of Neurology, Neurosurgery and Psychiatry, 38*, 1121–1126.

Mandleberg, I. A., & Brooks, D. N. (1975). Cognitive recovery after severe head injury: 1. Serial testing on the Wechsler Adult Intelligence Scale. *Journal of Neurology, Neurosurgery and Psychiatry, 39*, 1001–1007.

Manly, T. (2003). Rehabilitation of attention disorders. In B. A. Wilson (Ed.), *Neuropsychological rehabilitation: Theory and practice* (pp. 23–52). Lisse, The Netherlands: Swets and Zeitlinger.

Manly, T., Heutink, J., Davison, B., Gaynord, B., Greenfield, E., Parr, A., et al. (2004). An electronic knot in the handkerchief: "Content free cuing" and the maintenance of attentive control. *Neuropsychological Rehabilitation*, *14*, 89-116.

Marceil, J. C. (1977). Implicit dimensions of idiography and nomothesis: A reformulation. *American Psychologist*, *32*, 1046-1055.

Marin, R. S., & Chakravorty, S. (2005). Disorders of diminished motivation. In J. M. Silver, T. W. McAllister, & S. C. Yudofsky (Eds.), *Traumatic brain injury* (pp. 337-352). Washington, DC: American Psychiatric Publishing.

Marion, D., Darby, J., & Yonas, H. (1991). Acute regional cerebral blood flow changes caused by severe head injury. *Journal of Neurosurgery*, *74*, 407-414.

Markus, H. (1977). Self-schemata and processing information about the self. *Journal of Personality and Social Psychology*, *35*, 63-78.

Marshall, L. F. (1987). Neurobehavioral outcome: The neurosurgeon's perspective. In H. S. Levin, J. Grafman, & H. M. Eisenberg (Eds.), *Neurobehavioral recovery from head injury* (pp. 206-212). New York: Oxford University Press.

Martinelli, M. F., Zasler, N. D., & Tiernan, P. J. (2005). Skill acquisition and automatic process development after brain injury. *Brain Injury Professional*, *2*, 10-17.

Maruishi, M., Miyatani, M., Nakao, T., & Muranaka, H. (2007). Compensatory cortical activation during performance of an attention task by patients with diffuse axonal injury: A functional magnetic resonance imaging study. *Journal of Neurology, Neurosurgery and Psychiatry*, *78*, 168-173.

Mateer, C. A. (2005). Fundamentals of cognitive rehabilitation. In P. W. Halligan & D. T. Wade (Eds.), *The effectiveness of rehabilitation for cognitive deficits* (pp. 21-29). New York: Oxford University Press.

Mateer, C. A., & Raskin, S. (1999). Cognitive rehabilitation. In M. Rosenthal, E. R. Griffith, J. S. Kreutzer, & B. Pentland (Eds.), *Rehabilitation of the adult and child with traumatic brain injury* (3rd ed., pp. 254-269). Philadelphia: Davis.

Mauss-Clum, N., & Ryan, M. (1981). Brain injury and the family. *Journal of Neurosurgical Nursing*, *13*, 165-169.

Max, J. E. (2005). Children and adolescents. In J. M. Silver, T. W. McAllister, & S. C. Yudofsky (Eds.), *Textbook of traumatic brain injury* (pp. 477-494). Washington, DC: American Psychiatric Publishing.

Mayer, N. (1989). Acute care to rehabilitation: Concepts in transition. In P. Bach-y-Rita (Ed.), *Traumatic brain injury* (pp. 135-146). New York: Demos.

Mazziotta, J. C., & Phelps, M. E. (1986). Positron emission tomography. In M. E. Phelps, J. C. Mazziotta, & H. R. Schelbert (Eds.), *Positron emission tomography and autoradiography: Principles and applications for the brain and heart* (pp. 493-579). New York: Raven Press.

McCall, R. J. (1975). *The varieties of abnormality.* Springfield, IL: Charles C. Thomas.

McCord, W., & McCord, J. (1964). *The psychopath.* New York: Van Nostrand Reinhold.

McGlynn, S. M., & Schacter, D. L. (1989). Unawareness of deficits in neuropsychological syndromes. *Journal of Clinical and Experimental Neuropsychology, 11*, 143–205.

McGrath, J. (2004). Beyond restoration to transformation: Positive outcomes in the rehabilitation of acquired brain injury *Clinical Rehabilitation, 18*, 767–775.

McGrath, J. C., & Linley, P. A. (2006). Post-traumatic growth in acquired brain injury: A preliminary small scale study. *Brain Injury, 20*, 767–773.

McGuinness, D., & Pribram, K. (1980). The neuropsychology of attention: Emotional and motivational controls. In M. C. Wittrock (Ed.), *The brain and psychology* (pp. 95–139). London: Academic Press.

McKinlay, W. W., Brooks, D. N., Bond, M. R., Martinage, D. P., & Marshall, M. M. (1981). The short-term outcome of severe blunt head trauma as reported by the relatives of the injured person. *Journal of Neurology, Neurosurgery and Psychiatry, 44*, 527–533.

McKinlay, W. W., & Watkiss, A. J. (1999). Cognitive and behavioral effects of brain injury. In M. Rosenthal, E. R. Griffith, J. S. Kreutzer, & B. Pentland (Eds.), *Rehabilitation of the adult and child with traumatic brain injury* (3rd ed., pp. 74–86). Philadelphia: Davis.

McLean, A., Dikmen, S., Temkin, N., Wyler, A. R., & Gale, J. L. (1984). Psychosocial functioning at one month after head injury. *Neurosurgery, 14*, 393–399.

McMahon, B. T., & Frasier, R. T. (1998). Vocational rehabilitation. In K. B. Fralish & M. J. McMorrow (Eds.), *Innovations in head injury rehabilitation* (Chap. 12). White Plains, NY: Ahab Press.

McMordie, W. R., Barker, S. L., & Paolo, T. M. (1990). Return to work after head injury. *Brain Injury, 4*, 57–69.

McNeny, R. (1999). Activities of daily living. In M. Rosenthal, E. R. Griffith, J. S. Kreutzer, & B. Pentland (Eds.), *Rehabilitation of the adult and child with traumatic brain injury* (3rd ed., pp. 242–253). Philadelphia: Davis.

McQueen, J., & Posey, J. (1975). Changes in intracranial pressure and brain hydration during acute ethanolism. *Surgical Neurology, 4*, 375–379.

Meichenbaum, D. (1977). *Cognitive-behavior modification: An integrative approach.* New York: Plenum Press.

Meichenbaum, D. (1993). The "potential" contributions of cognitive behavior modification to the rehabilitation of individuals with traumatic brain injury. *Seminars in Speech and Language, 14*, 18–30.

Meier, M. J., Strauman, S., & Thompson, W. G. (1987). Individual differences in neuropsychological recovery: An overview. In M. J. Meier, A. L. Benton, & L. Diller (Eds.), *Neuropsychological rehabilitation* (pp. 71–110). New York: Guilford.

Mesulam, M.-M. (1985). Patterns in behavioral neurology: Association areas, the limbic system and hemispheric specialization. In M.-M. Mesulam (Ed.), *Principles of behavioral neurology* (pp. 1–70). Philadelphia: Davis.

Mesulam, M.-M. (1986). Frontal cortex and behavior. *Annals of Neurology, 19,* 320–324.

Mesulam, M.-M. (2000). Behavioral neuroanatomy: Large-scale networks, association cortex, frontal syndromes, the limbic system and hemispheric specialization. In M.-M. Mesulam (Ed.), *Principles of behavioral and cognitive neurology* (pp. 1–120). New York: Oxford University Press.

Mesulam, M.-M. (2002). The human frontal lobes: Transcending the default mode through contingent encoding. In D. Stuss & R. Knight (Eds.), *Principles of frontal lobe function* (pp. 8–30). New York: Oxford University Press.

Miller, B. L., Benson, D. F., & Johnson, J. K. (2003). Frontal lobes: Clinical and anatomic issues. In T. E. Feinberg & M. J. Farah (Eds.), *Behavioral neurology and neuropsychology* (2nd ed., pp. 385–392). New York: McGraw-Hill.

Miller, E. (1984). *Recovery and management of neuropsychological impairments*. New York: Wiley.

Miller, E. K., & Cohen, J. D. (2001). An integrative theory of prefrontal function. *Annual Review of Neuroscience, 24,* 167–202.

Miller, G., Galanter, E., & Pribram, K. (1960). *Plans and the structure of behavior*. New York: Holt, Rinehart and Winston.

Miller, J. D., Sweet, R. C., Narayan, R., & Becker, D. P. (1978). Early insults to the injured brain. *Journal of the American Medical Association, 240,* 439–442.

Miller, J. D., & Teasdale, G. M. (1985). Clinical trials for assessing treatment for severe head injury. In D. P. Becker & J. T. Povlishock (Eds.), *Central nervous system trauma status report* (pp. 17–32). Washington, DC: National Institutes of Neurological and Communicative Disorder and Health.

Millis, S. R., Rosenthal, M., Novack, T. A., Sherer, M., Todd, N. G., Kreutzer, J. S., et al. (2001). Long-term neuropsychological outcome after traumatic brain injury. *Journal of Head Trauma Rehabilitation, 16,* 343–355.

Millon, T. (1968). *Modern psychopathology*. Philadelphia: Saunders.

Milner, G. (1977). Marijuana and driving hazards. *Medical Journal of Australia, 1,* 208–211.

Morris, G. F., & Marshall, L. F. (1998). Traumatic central nervous system injury. In J. Corey-Bloom & R. B. David (Eds.), *Adult neurology* (pp. 251–267). St. Louis, MO: Mosby.

Morris, J., & Bleiberg, J. (1986). Neuropsychological rehabilitation and traditional psychotherapy. *International Journal of Clinical Neuropsychology, 8,* 133–134.

Multi-Society Task Force on PVS. (1994). Medical aspect of the persistent vegetative state: Second of two parts. *New England Journal of Medicine, 330*(22), 1572–1579.

Muraven, M., Baumeister, R. F., & Tice, D. M. (1999). Longitudinal improvement in self-regulation through practice: Building self-control through repeated exercise. *Journal of Social Psychology, 139,* 446–457.

Najenson, T., Grosswasser, Z., Mendelson, L, & Hackett, P. (1989). Rehabilitation outcome of brain-damaged patients after severe head injury. *International Rehabilitation Medicine, 2*, 17–22.

Najenson, T., Mendleson, L., Schechter, I., David, C., Mintz, N., & Grosswasser, Z. (1974). Rehabilitation after severe head injury. *Scandinavian Journal of Rehabilitation Medicine, 6*, 5–14.

National Center for Injury Prevention and Control. (1999). *Traumatic brain injury in the United States: A report to Congress.* Atlanta, GA: Centers for Disease Control and Prevention.

National Head Injury Foundation. (1982). *The silent epidemic.* Framingham, MA: Author.

National Institute of Health. (1998). *Consensus statement.* Washington, DC: Author.

Neisser, U. (1967). *Cognitive psychology.* Englewood Cliffs, NJ: Prentice-Hall.

Nelson, V. S. (1992). Pediatric head injury. In S. Berrol (Ed.), *Physical medicine and rehabilitation clinics of North America: Traumatic brain injury* (pp. 461–474). Philadelphia: Saunders.

Newcombe, F. (1969). *Missile wounds of the brain.* Oxford, England: Oxford University Press.

Newcombe, F. (1987). Psychometric and behavioral evidence: Scope, limitations, and ecological validity. In H. S. Levin, J. Grafman, & H. M. Eisenberg (Eds.), *Neurobehavioral recovery from head injury* (pp. 129–145). New York: Oxford University Press.

Nimgade, A., & Costello, M. C. (2003). Return to work for a company president with a traumatic brain injury. *Journal of Head Trauma Rehabilitation, 18*, 464–467.

Nochi, M. (1997). Dealing with the "Void": Traumatic brain injury as a story. *Disability and Society, 12*, 533–555.

Nochi, M. (1998). Struggling with the labeled self: People with traumatic brain injuries in social settings. *Qualitative Health Research, 8*, 665–681.

Nochi, M. (1998). "Loss of self" in the narratives of people with traumatic brain injuries: A qualitative analysis. *Social Science and Medicine, 46*, 869–878.

Nochi, M. (2000). Reconstructing self-narratives in coping with traumatic brain injury. *Social Science and Medicine, 51*, 1795–1804.

Norman, D. A. (1988). *The psychology of everyday things.* New York: Basic Books.

Norman, D. A., & Shallice, T. (1986). Attention to action: Willed and automatic control of behavior. In R. J. Davidson, G. E. Schwartz, & D. Shapiro (Eds.), *Consciousness and self-regulation* (Vol. 4, pp. 1–18). New York: Plenum Press.

Oddy, M. (1984). Head injury and social adjustment. In N. Brooks (Ed.), *Closed head injury: Psychological, social and family consequences* (pp. 108–122). Oxford, England: Oxford University Press.

Oddy, M. (1993). Head injury during childhood. *Neuropsychological Rehabilitation, 3*, 301–320.

Oddy, M., & Cogan, J. (2004). Case study of a severe memory impairment after ACA aneurysm. *Neuropsychological Rehabilitation, 14*, 481–486.

Oddy, M., Coughlan, A., Tyerman, A. D., & Jenkins, D. (1985). Social adjustment after closed head injury: A further follow-up several years after injury. *Journal of Neurology, Neurosurgery and Psychiatry, 48*, 464–468.

Oddy, M., Humphrey, M., & Utley, D. (1978). Subjective impairment and social recovery after closed head injury. *Journal of Neurology, Neurosurgery and Psychiatry, 41*, 611–616.

Oddy, M., Humphrey, M., & Utley, D. (1978). Stresses upon the relatives of head-injured patients. *British Journal of Psychiatry, 133*, 507–513.

Olver, J. H., Ponsford, J. L., & Curtin, C. A. (1996). Outcome following traumatic brain injury: A comparison between 2 and 5 years after injury. *Brain Injury, 10*, 841–848.

Ommaya, A. K., & Gennarelli, T. A. (1974). Cerebral concussion and traumatic unconsciousness: Correlation of experimental and clinical observations on blunt head injuries. *Brain, 97*, 633–654.

Ommaya, A. K., Grubb, R. L., & Naumann, R. A. (1970). Coup and contre-coup cerebral contusions: An experimental analysis. *Neurology, 20*, 388–389.

Ommaya, A. K., Grubb, R. L., & Naumann, R. A. (1971). Coup and contre-coup injuries: Observations on the mechanics of visible brain injuries in the rhesus monkey. *Journal of Neurosurgery, 35*, 503–516.

Orosz, E. (1979). Factors influencing the outcome of coma in severely injured patients. *Acta Neurochirugica, 28*, 137–139.

Osborne, C. L. (1998). *Over my head.* Kansas City, MO: Andrews McMeel.

O'Shanick, G. J., & O'Shanick, A. M. (2005). Personality disorders. In J. M. Silver, T. W. McAllister, & S. C. Yudofsky, (Eds.), *Textbook of traumatic brain injury* (pp. 245–258). Washington, DC: American Psychiatric Publishing.

Overgaard, J., Hvnd-Hansen, O., Land, A. M., Petersen, K. K., Christensen, S., Haase, J., et al. (1973). Prognosis after head injury based on early clinical examination. *Lancet, ii*, 631–635.

Ownsworth, T., & Fleming, J. (2005). The relative importance of metacognitive skills, emotional status, and executive function in psychosocial adjustment following acquired brain injury. *Journal of Head Trauma Rehabilitation, 20*, 315–332.

Pagni, C. A. (1973). The prognosis of head injured patients in a state of coma with decerebrated posture: Analysis of 471 cases. *Journal of Neurosurgical Sciences, 17*, 289–295.

Panikoff, L. B. (1983). Recovery trends of functional skills in the head-injured adult. *American Journal of Occupational Therapy, 37*, 735–743.

Panting, A., & Merry, P. (1972). The long-term rehabilitation of severe head injuries with particular reference to the need for social and medical support for the patient's family. *Rehabilitation, 38*, 33–38.

Parente, R. (1994). Effect of monetary incentive on performance after traumatic brain injury. *Neurorehabilitation, 4*, 198–203.

Park, J. W., Moscovitch, M., & Robertson, I. H. (1999). Divided attention impairments after traumatic brain injury. *Neuropsychologia, 37,* 1119–1133.

Partridge, W. M. (1985). Cerebral vascular permeability status in brain injury. In D. P. Becker & J. T. Povlishock (Eds.), *Central nervous system trauma status report* (pp. 503–512). Washington, DC: National Institutes of Neurological and Communicative Disorder and Health.

Pashler, H. E. (1998). *The psychology of attention.* Cambridge, MA: MIT Press.

Passingham, R. (1995). *The frontal lobes and voluntary action.* New York: Oxford University Press.

Paterson, D. (1980). Is your brain really necessary? *World Medicine, 5/3,* 21–24.

Pazzaglia, P., Frank, G., Frank, F., & Gaist, G. (1975). Clinical course and prognosis of acute post-traumatic coma. *Journal of Neurology, Neurosurgery and Psychiatry, 38,* 149–154.

Pelham, M. F., & Lovell, M. R. (2005). Issues in neuropsychological assessment. In J. Silver, T. McAllister, & S. Yudofsky (Eds.), *Textbook of traumatic brain injury,* (pp. 159–174). Washington, DC: American Psychiatric Press.

Peters, L. C., Stambrook, M., Moore, A. D., & Esses, L. (1990). Psychosocial sequelae of closed head injury: Effects on the marital relationship. *Brain Injury. 4,* 39–47.

Peterson, B. S., Skudlarski, P., Anderson, A. W., Zhang, H., Gatenby, J. C., Lacadie, C. M., et al. (1998). A functional magnetic resonance imaging study of tic suppression in Tourette's syndrome. *Archives of General Psychiatry, 55,* 326–333.

Piasetsky, E. (1982). The relevance of brain-behavior relationships for rehabilitation. In L. E. Trexler (Ed.), *Cognitive rehabilitation: Conceptualization and intervention* (pp. 115–130). New York: Plenum Press.

Piasetsky, E., Ben-Yishay, Y., Weinberg, J., & Diller, L. (1982). The systematic remediation of specific disorders: Selected applications of methods derived in a clinical research setting. In L. E. Trexler (Ed.), *Cognitive rehabilitation: Conceptualization and intervention* (pp. 205–222). New York: Plenum Press.

Pickelsimer, E. E., Selassie, A. W., Sample., P. L., Heinemann, A., Gu, J., & Veldheer, L. (2007). Unmet service needs of persons with traumatic brain injury. *The Journal of Head Trauma Rehabilitation, 22,* 1–13.

Picton, T. W., Alain, C., & McIntosh, A. R. (2002). The theatre of the mind: Physiological studies of the human frontal lobes. In D. T. Stuss & R. Knight (Eds.), *Principles of frontal lobe function* (pp. 109–126). New York: Oxford University Press.

Pilz, P. (1983). Axonal injury in head injury. *Acta Neurochirugica, 32,* 119–126.

Plum, F., & Posner, J. (1980). *The diagnosis of stupor and coma.* Philadelphia: Davis.

Pollack, I. W. (2005). Psychotherapy. In J. M. Silver, T. W. McAllister, & S. C. Yudofsky, (Eds.), *Textbook of traumatic brain injury* (pp. 641–654). Washington, DC: American Psychiatric Publishing.

Ponsford, J. L., & Kinsella, G. (1988). Evaluation of a remedial programme for attentional deficits following closed head injury. *Journal of Clinical and Experimental Neuropsychology, 10*, 693–708.

Ponsford, J. L., Olver, J. H., & Curran, C. (1996). Outcome following traumatic brain injury: An Australian study. In B. P. Uzzell & H. H. Stonnington (Eds.), *Recovery after traumatic brain injury* (pp. 219–234). Mahwah, NJ: Erlbaum.

Poppelreuter, W. (1917). *Disturbances of lower and higher visual capacities caused by occipital damage.* Oxford, UK: Clarendon Press.

Porch, B. E., Collins, M. J., & Wertz, R. T. (1974, April). *Statistical and clinical procedures for predicting recovery from aphasia.* Paper presented at the Clinical Aphasiology Conference, Albuquerque, NM.

Posner, M. I., & DiGirolamo, G. J. (1998). Executive attention: Conflict, target detection, and cognitive control. In R. Parasuraman (Ed.), *The attentive brain* (pp. 401–424). Cambridge, MA: MIT Press.

Posner, M. I., & Fan, J. (2007). Attention as an organ system. In J. Pomerantz (Ed.), *Neurobiology of perception and communication: From synapse to society. De Lange Conference IV* (pp. 31–61). London: Cambridge University Press.

Posner, M. I., & Petersen, S. E. (1990). The attentional system of the human brain. *Annual Review of Neuroscience, 13*, 25–42.

Povlishock, J. T. (1989). Structural aspects of brain injury. In P. Bach-y-Rita (Ed.), *Traumatic brain injury* (pp. 87–96). New York: Demos.

Povlishock, J. T., Becker, D. P., Sullivan, H. G., & Miller, J. D. (1978). Vascular permeability alterations to horseradish peroxidase in experimental brain injury. *Brain Research, 153*, 223–239.

Povlishock, J., Kontos, H. A., & Ellis, E. F. (1989). Physiological effects of traumatic brain injury. In D. P. Becker & S. K. Gudeman (Eds.), *Textbook of head injury* (pp. 451–465). Philadelphia: Saunders.

Povlishock, J. T., & Valadka, A. B. (1994). Pathobiology of traumatic brain injury. In M. A. Finlayson & S. H. Garner (Eds.), *Brain injury rehabilitation: Clinical considerations* (pp. 11–33). Baltimore: Williams and Wilkins.

Pribram, K. H. (1960). The intrinsic systems of the forebrain. In J. Field, H. W. Magoun, & V. E. Hall (Eds.), *Handbook of physiology* (Vol. 2, pp. 1323–1344). Washington, DC: American Physiological Society.

Pribram, K. H. (1971). *Languages of the brain.* Englewood Cliffs, NJ: Prentice-Hall.

Pribram, K. H. (1973). The primate frontal cortex: Executive of the brain. In K. H. Pribram & A. R. Luria (Eds.), *Psychophysiology of the frontal lobes* (pp. 293–314). New York: Academic Press.

Pribram K. H. (1976). Self-consciousness and intentionality. In G. Schwartz & D. Shapiro (Eds.), *Consciousness and self-regulation* (pp. 51–100). New York: Plenum Press.

Pribram, K. H. (1986). Non-locality and localization in the primate forebrain. In S. Filskov & T. Boll (Eds.), *Handbook of clinical neuropsychology* (Vol. 2, pp. 606–651). New York: John Wiley.

Pribram, K. H., & McGuinness, D. (1975). Arousal, activation, and effort in the control of attention. *Psychological Review, 82,* 116–149.

Price, D., & Murray, A. (1972). The influence of hypoxia and hypotension on recovery from head injury. *Injury, 3,* 218–223.

Prigatano, G. (1987). Psychiatric aspects of head injury: Problem areas and suggested guidelines for research. In H. S. Levin, J. Grafman, & H. M. Eisenberg (Eds.), *Neurobehavioral recovery from head injury* (pp. 215–231). New York: Oxford University Press.

Prigatano, G. (1990). Recovery and cognitive retraining after cognitive brain injury. In E. D. Bigler (Ed.), *Traumatic brain injury* (pp. 297–311). Austin, TX: Pro-Ed.

Prigatano, G. (1991). Disturbances of self-awareness of deficit after traumatic brain injury. In G. P. Prigatano & D. L. Schacter (Eds.), *Awareness of deficit after brain injury* (pp. 111–126). New York: Oxford University Press.

Prigatano, G. (1994). The problem of lost normality in brain injury. *Journal of Head Trauma Rehabilitation, 10,* 87–95.

Prigatano, G. (1999a). *Principles of neuropsychological rehabilitation.* New York: Oxford University Press.

Prigatano, G. (1999b). Motivation and awareness in cognitive rehabilitation. In D. T. Stuss, G. Winocur, & I. H. Robertson (Eds.), *Cognitive neurorehabilitation* (pp. 240–251). New York: Cambridge University Press.

Prigatano, G. (2005). Disturbances of self-awareness and rehabilitation of patients with traumatic brain injury. *Journal of Head Trauma Rehabilitation, 20,* 19–29.

Prigatano, G., & Ben-Yishay, Y. (1999). Psychotherapy and psychotherapeutic interventions in brain injury rehabilitation. In M. Rosenthal, E. R. Griffith, J. S. Kreutzer, & B. Pentland (Eds.), *Rehabilitation of the adult and child with traumatic brain injury* (3rd ed., pp. 271–283). Philadelphia: Davis.

Prigatano, G., Fordyce, D. J., Zeiner, H. K., Roueche, J. R., Pepping, M., & Wood, B. C. (1986). *Neuropsychological rehabilitation after brain injury.* Baltimore: The Johns Hopkins University Press.

Prigatano, G., Glisky, E., & Klonoff, P. (1996). Cognitive rehabilitation after traumatic brain injury. In P. W. Corrigan & S. C. Yudofsky (Eds.), *Cognitive rehabilitation for neuropsychiatric disorders* (pp. 223–242). Washington, DC: American Psychiatric Press.

Prigatano, G., & Johnson, S. C. (2003). The three vectors of consciousness and their disturbances after brain injury. *Neuropsychological Rehabilitation, 13,* 13–29.

Prigatano, G., Klonoff, P., O'Brien, K., Altman, I., & Amin, K. (1994). Productivity after neuropsychologically oriented milieu rehabilitation. *Journal of Head Trauma Rehabilitation, 9,* 91–102.

Prigatano, G. P., O'Brien, K. P., & Klonoff, P. S. (1993). Neuropsychological rehabilitation of young adults who suffer brain injury in childhood: Clinical observations. *Neuropsychological Rehabilitation, 3*, 411–421.

Prigatano, G., & Schacter, D. (1991). Introduction. In G. Prigatano & D. Schacter (Eds.), *Awareness of deficit after brain injury* (pp. 3–16). New York: Oxford University Press.

Quartz, S. R., & Sejnowski, T. J. (2002). *Liars, lovers, heroes: What the new brain science reveals about how we become who we are*. New York: Harper-Collins.

Rabbitt, P. (1998). Introduction: Methodology and models in the study of executive functions. In P. Rabbitt (Ed.), *Methodology of frontal and executive function* (pp. 1–38). London: Psychology Press.

Raizata, R., & Poldrack, R. (2006). Challenge-driven attention: Interacting frontal and brainstem systems. *Frontiers in Human Neuroscience, 1*(3), 1–8.

Ramachandran, V. S., & Blakeslee, S. (1998). *Phantoms in the brain*. New York: Quill.

Raskin, S. A., & Mateer, C. A. (2000). *Neuropsychological management of mild traumatic brain injury*. New York: Oxford University Press.

Rath, J. F., Simon, D., Langenbahn, D. M., Sherr, R. L., & Diller, L. (2003). Group treatment of problem-solving deficits in outpatients with traumatic brain injury: A randomized outcome study. *Neuropsychological Rehabilitation, 13*, 441–459.

Raz, A. (2004). Anatomy of attentional networks. *The Anatomical Record, 28*, 21–36.

Reason, J. (1990). *Human error*. New York: Cambridge University Press.

Reitan, R. M. (1988). Integration of neuropsychological theory, assessment and clinical applications. *The Clinical Neuropsychologist, 2*, 331–349.

Reitan, R., & Wolfson, D. (1986). *Traumatic brain injury* (Vol. I). Tucson, AZ: Neuropsychology Press.

Retzlaff, P. D., & Gibertini, M. (1994). Neuropsychometric issues and problems. In R. D. Vanderploeg (Ed.), *Clinician's guide to neuropsychological assessment* (pp. 185–209). Hillsdale, NJ: Erlbaum.

Richards, L., & Chiarello, D. (1997). Activation with selection: Parallel right-hemisphere roles in language and intentional movement. *Brain and Language, 58*, 151–178.

Rivers, K. O., Schutz, L., & Lobato. (2007, November). *Prevalence of traumatic brain injury in a college population*. Paper presented at the American Speech-Language-Hearing Association Annual Convention, Boston.

Roberts, A. H. (1969). *Brain damage in boxers*. London: Pittman Medical Publishing.

Roberts, A. H. (1979). *Severe accidental head injury*. New York: Macmillan Press.

Robertson, I. H., Stuss, D. T., & Winocur, G. (1999). Epilogue: The future of cognitive rehabilitation. In D. T. Stuss, H. Winocur, & I. H. Robertson (Eds.), *Cognitive neurorehabilitation* (pp. 362–366). Cambridge, UK: Cambridge University Press.

Robertson, I. H., Tegnér, R., Tham, K., Lo, A., & Nimmo-Smith, I. (1995). Sustained attention training for unilateral neglect: Theoretical and rehabilitation implications. *Journal of Clinical and Experimental Neuropsychology, 17*(3), 416–430.

Rose, D., & Johnson, D. (1996). Brain injuries and outcome. In F. D. Rose & D. A. Johnson (Eds.), *Brain injury and after: Towards improved outcome* (pp. 1–20). New York: Wiley and Sons.

Rose, M. (1988). Medical considerations in brain injury rehabilitation. In I. Fussey & G. Giles (Eds.), *Rehabilitation of the severely brain-injured adult: A practical approach* (pp. 30–42). London: Croom Helm.

Rosenbaum, M., & Najenson, T. (1976). Changes in life patterns and symptoms of low mood reported by wives of severely brain-injured soldiers. *Journal of Consulting and Clinical Psychology, 44*, 881–888.

Rosenthal, M. (1983). Preface. In M. Rosenthal, E. R. Griffith, M. R. Bond, & J. D. Miller (Eds.), *Rehabilitation of the head injured adult* (pp. ix–xi). Philadelphia: Davis.

Rosenthal, M. (1989). Understanding and optimizing family adaptation to traumatic brain injury. In P. Bach-y-Rita (Ed.), *Traumatic brain injury* (pp. 191–202). New York: Demos.

Rosenthal, M. (1999a). Preface to the third edition. In M. Rosenthal, E. R. Griffith, J. S. Kreutzer, & B. Pentland (Eds.), *Rehabilitation of the adult and child with traumatic brain injury* (3rd ed., pp. vii–viii). Philadelphia: Davis.

Rosenthal, M. (1999). Preface to the first edition. In M. Rosenthal, E. R. Griffith, J. S. Kreutzer, & B. Pentland (Eds.), *Rehabilitation of the adult and child with traumatic brain injury* (3rd ed., pp. xi–xii). Philadelphia: Davis.

Rosenthal, M., & Bond, M. R. (1990). Behavioral and psychiatric sequelae. In M. Rosenthal, E. R. Griffith, M. R. Bond, & J. D. Miller (Eds.), *Rehabilitation of the adult and child with traumatic head injury* (2nd ed., pp. 179–192). Philadelphia: Davis.

Rosner, B. S. (1970). Brain functions. In P. H. Mussen & M. R. Rosenzweig (Eds.), *Annual review of psychology 1970* (pp. 555–593). Palo Alto, CA: Annual Reviews, Inc.

Rothbart, M. K., & Rueda, M. R. (2005). The development of effortful control. In U. Mayr, E. Awh, & S. Keele (Eds.), *Developing individuality in the human brain: A tribute to Michael I. Posner* (pp. 167–188). Washington, DC: American Psychological Association.

Rotondi, A. J., Sinkule, J., Balzer, K., Harris, J., & Moldovan, R. (2007). A qualitative needs assessment of persons who have experienced traumatic brain injury and their primary family caregivers. *Journal of Head Trauma Rehabilitation, 22,* 14–25.

Ruesch, J., & Moore, B. E. (1943). The measurement of intellectual functions in the acute stage of head injury. *Archives of Neurological Psychiatry, 50,* 165–170.

Ruff, R. M., Marshall, L. F., Klauber, M. R., Blunt, B. A., Grant, I., Foulkes, M. A., et al. (1990). Alcohol abuse and neurological outcome of the severely head injured. *Journal of Head Trauma Rehabilitation, 5,* 21–31.

Rusk, H. A., Block, J. M., & Lowman, E. W. (1969). Rehabilitation of the brain-injured patient: A report of 157 cases with follow-up of 118. In A. E. Walker, W. F. Caveness, & M. Critchley (Eds.), *The late effects of head injury.* Springfield, IL: Thomas.

Russell, D., & Sharratt, A. (1992). *Academic recovery after head injury.* Springfield, IL: Thomas.

Russell, W. R., & Nathan, P. W. (1946). Traumatic amnesia. *Brain, 69,* 280–300.

Russell, W. R., & Smith, A. (1961). Post-traumatic amnesia in closed head injuries. *Archives of Neurology, 5,* 4–17.

Salthouse, T. (2007). Implications of within-person variability in cognitive and neuropsychological functioning in the interpretation of change. *Neuropsychology, 21,* 401–411.

Sapolsky, R. (1996). *The biological basis of individuality.* Houston, TX: The Teaching Company.

Savage, R., & Wolcott, G. (1994). Overview of acquired brain injury. In R. Savage & G. Wolcott (Eds.), *Educational dimensions of acquired brain injury* (pp. 3–12). Austin, TX: Pro-Ed.

Sbordone, R. J. (1987). A conceptual model of neuropsychologically based cognitive rehabilitation. In J. M. Williams & C. J. Long (Eds.), *The rehabilitation of cognitive disabilities* (pp. 3–27). New York: Plenum Press.

Sbordone, R. J. (1990). Psychotherapeutic treatment of the client with traumatic brain injury: A conceptual model. In J. S. Kreutzer & P. Wehman (Eds.), *Community integration following traumatic brain injury* (pp. 139–153). Baltimore: Paul H. Brookes.

Sbordone, R. J. (1991). Overcoming obstacles in cognitive rehabilitation of persons with severe traumatic brain injury. In J. S. Kreutzer & P. H. Wehman (Eds.), *Cognitive rehabilitation for persons with traumatic brain injury* (pp. 105–116). Bisbee, AZ: Imaginart.

Sbordone, R. (1997). The ecological validity of neuropsychological testing. In A. M. Horton, D. Wedding, & J. Webster (Eds.), *The neuropsychology handbook: Foundations and assessment* (2nd ed., pp. 365–392). New York: Springer.

Sbordone, R. J. (1998). Ecological validity: Some critical issues for the neuropsychologist. In R. J. Sbordone & C. Long (Eds.), *Ecological valid-*

ity of neuropsychological testing (pp. 15–41). Boca Raton, FL: St. Lucie Press.

Sbordone, R. J., Liter, J. C., & Pettler-Jennings, P. (1995). Recovery of function following severe traumatic brain injury: A retrospective 10-year follow-up. *Brain Injury, 9*, 285–299.

Schacter, D. L., & Glisky, E. (1986). Memory remediation: Restoration, alleviation and the acquisition of domain-specific knowledge. In B. Uzzell & Y. Gross (Eds.), *Clinical neuropsychology of intervention* (pp. 257–282). Boston: Martinus-Nijhoff.

Scheff, T. (1990). *Microsociology: Discourse, emotion, and social structure*. Chicago: University of Chicago Press.

Scheibel, R. S., Pearson, D. A., Faria, L. P., Kotrla, K. J., Aylward, E., Bachevalier, J., et al. (2003). An fMRI study of executive functioning after severe diffuse TBI. *Brain Injury, 17*, 919–930.

Schloss, P. J., Thompson, C. K., Gajar, A. H., & Schloss, C. K. (1985). Influence of self-monitoring on heterosexual conversational behavior of head trauma youth. *Applied Research in Mental Retardation, 6*, 269–282.

Schmidt, R. A., & Lee, T. D. (1999). *Motor control and learning: A behavioral emphasis* (3rd ed.). Champaign, IL: Human Kinetics.

Schmitter-Edgecombe, M. (2006). Implications of basic science research for brain injury rehabilitation: A focus on intact learning mechanisms. *Journal of Head Trauma Rehabilitation, 21*(2), 131–141.

Schmitter-Edgecombe, M., Fahy, M., Whelan, J., & Long, C. (1995). Memory remediation after severe closed head injury: Notebook training versus supportive therapy. *Journal of Consulting and Clinical Psychology, 63*, 484–489.

Schootman, M., & Fuortes, L. (1999). Functional status following traumatic brain injuries: Population-based rural-urban differences. *Brain Injury, 13*, 995–1004.

Schulkin, J. (2000). *Roots of social sensibility and neural function*. Cambridge, MA: MIT Press.

Schulz, K. P., Tang, C. Y., Fan, J., Marks, D. J., Newcorn, J. H., Cheung, A. M., et al. (2005). Differential prefrontal cortex activation with and without childhood attention-deficit/hyperactivity disorder. *Neuropsychology, 19*, 390–402.

Schutz, L. (1989, June). *Clinical strategies for the treatment of patients who achieve exceptional recoveries following cognitive rehabilitation*. Paper presented at The Postgraduate Course on Rehabilitation of the Brain-Injured Adult and Child, Williamsburg, VA.

Schutz, L. (2005). Broad-perspective perceptual disorder of the right cerebral hemisphere. *Neuropsychology Review, 15*, 11–27.

Schutz, L. (2005). Response optimization: A central issue in recovery from traumatic brain injury [Abstract]. *Archives of Clinical Neuropsychology, 20,* 938–939.

Schutz, L. (2005). Public policy implications of advances in cognitive neurorehabilitation [Abstract]. *Archives of Clinical Neuropsychology, 20,* 940.

Schutz, L. (2005). Neurorehabilitation treatment interventions for stimulus flooding [Abstract]. *Archives of Clinical Neuropsychology, 20,* 939.

Schutz, L. (2005). Pull the thorn from her paw and she will follow you anywhere: A neurorehabilitation fable [Abstract]. *Archives of Clinical Neuropsychology, 20*(7), 874.

Schutz, L. (2005). The girl most likely to succeed, head injury and all [Abstract]. *Archives of Clinical Neuropsychology, 20*(7), 809–810.

Schutz, L. (2006). *Self-therapy for head injury: Teaching yourself to prevent head-injured moments.* Unpublished manuscript. Available at http://www.givebackorlando.com/hepusef/hepindex.html

Schutz, L. (2006a). *Self-therapy: Learning how to fix my head injury.* Government Printing Office, Washington, DC. (for distribution to members of Congress only). Available from: http://givebackorlando.com/index1a.html.

Schutz, L. (2006b). *Helping your family member to recover from a head injury.* Government Printing Office, Washington, DC. (for distribution to members of Congress only). Available: at http://givebackorlando.com/index1a.html.

Schutz, L. (2007). Cognitive variability: A primary symptom of multiple sclerosis. In A. M. Columbus (Ed.), *Advances in psychology research* (Vol. 51, pp. 15–42). Hauppage, NY: NovaScience.

Schutz, L. (2007). Exceptional adaptation in recovery from traumatic brain injury: A case series. *The Journal of Head Trauma Rehabilitation, 22,* 48–55.

Schutz, L., Barry, P., Gross, Y., & Tupper, D. (1984, April). *Can we predict (or even explain) the functional outcomes of cognitive rehabilitation treatment?* Symposium on Models and Techniques in Cognitive Rehabilitation, Indianapolis, IN.

Schutz, L., & Gorman, P. (1996). Neuropsychological correlates of driving recovery after postacute neurorehabilitation [Abstract]. *Archives of Clinical Neuropsychology, 11,* 446.

Schutz, L., Kleinschmidt, D., & Gorman, P. (1998, April). *Practical approaches to dealing with social and interpersonal problems.* Paper presented at New Directions in TBI Services, Brain Injury Association of Florida Third Annual Educational Conference for Professionals, Tampa, FL.

Schutz, L., & Langenbahn, D. (1985, June). *Facilitating the generalization of cognitive rehabilitation treatment.* Paper presented at The Postgraduate Course on Rehabilitation of the Brain-Injured Adult and Child, Williamsburg, VA.

Schutz, L., & Lewis, B. (1985, August). *Family variables and cognitive rehabilitation treatment success.* Paper presented at the American Psychological Association Annual Convention, Los Angeles.

Schutz, L., & Micucci, J. (1984, October). *Personality classification and cognitive rehabilitation treatment planning.* Paper presented at the Fifth Annual Head Trauma Conference, Braintree Hospital, Braintree, MA.

Schutz, L., Rivers, K., & Ratusnik, D. (2009). The role of external validity in evidence-based practice for rehabilitation. *Rehabilitation Psychology, 53,* 294–302.

Schutz, L., & Schutz, J. (1999, April). *Do-it-yourself cognitive remediation: A system for training the survivor, the family and other caregivers in the process of doing cognitive retraining.* Paper presented at the Fourth Annual Educational Conference for Professionals of the Brain Injury Association of Florida, Inc., Orlando, FL.

Schutz, L., & Schutz, J. (2000). Successful educational re-entry after severe traumatic brain injury: The contribution of cognitive compensation strategies. *Florida Journal of Communication Disorders, 20,* 28–36.

Schutz, L., & Schutz, J. (2004). *Understanding and overcoming students' traumatic brain injuries: An educator's manual.* Tallahassee, FL: Department of Education.

Schutz, L., & Schutz, J. (2005, October). *Cognitive remediation in the classroom: Why, how and by whom?* Poster presented at the American Psychological Association Annual Meeting, Washington, DC.

Schutz, L., & Tercero, D. (1985, June). *Prediction of the outcome of cognitive rehabilitation from data available at intake: The relationship of neuropsychological test scores and demographic variables to independent adaptive functioning at discharge.* The Postgraduate Course on Rehabilitation on the Brain-Injured Adult and Child, Williamsburg, VA.

Schutz, L., & Trainor, K. (2007). Evaluation of cognitive rehabilitation as a treatment paradigm. *Brain Injury, 21,* 545–557.

Schutz, L., & Wanlass, R. (1986, June). *A model for predicting vocational activity following comprehensive post-acute head injury rehabilitation.* Paper presented at The Postgraduate Course on Rehabilitation of the Brain-Injured Adult and Child, Williamsburg, VA.

Schwartz, J. M., & Begley, S. (2002). *The mind and the brain.* New York: Regan Books.

Seignourel, P. J., Robins, D. L., Larson, M. J., Demery, J. A., Cole, M., & Perlstein, W. M. (2005). Cognitive control in closed head injury: Context maintenance dysfunction or prepotent response inhibition deficit? *Neuropsychology, 19,* 578–590.

Seitelberger, F., & Jellinger, K. (1971). Protracted post-traumatic encephalopathy. In *International Symposium on Head Injuries.* Edinburgh: Churchill-Livingstone.

Serle, J. R. (1979). *Expression and meaning: Studies in the theory of speech acts.* Cambridge, MA: Cambridge University Press.

Shallice, T. (1972). Dual functions of consciousness. *Psychological Review, 79,* 383–393.

Shallice, T. (1982). Specific impairments of planning. *Philosophical Transactions of the Royal Society of London B, 298,* 199–209.

Shallice, T. (1988). *From neuropsychology to mental structure.* New York: Cambridge University Press.

Shallice, T. (2000). Cognitive neuropsychology and rehabilitation: Is pessimism justified? *Neuropsychological Rehabilitation, 10,* 209–217.

Shallice, T. (2002). Fractionation of the supervisory system. In D. T. Stuss & R. T. Knight (Eds.), *Principles of frontal lobe function* (pp. 261–277). New York: Oxford University Press.

Shallice, T., & Burgess, P. (1991). Deficits in strategy application following frontal lobe damage in man. *Brain, 114,* 727–741.

Shallice, T., & Burgess, P. (1996). The domain of supervisory processes and temporal organization of behavior. *Philosophical Transactions of the Royal Society of London B, 351,* 1405–1412.

Shallice, T., & Evans, E. M. (1978). The involvement of the frontal lobes in cognitive estimation. *Cortex, 14,* 294–303.

Shapiro, D. (2000). *Dynamics of character.* New York: Basic Books.

Sherer, M., Bergloff, P., Levin, E., High, W. M., Oden, K. E., & Nick, T. G. (1998). Impaired awareness and employment outcome after traumatic brain injury. *Journal of Head Trauma Rehabilitation, 13,* 52–61.

Sherr, R. L, & Langenbahn, D. M. (1992). An approach to large-scale outpatient rehabilitation. *Neuropsychology, 6,* 417–426.

Shiffrin, R. M., & Schneider, W. (1977). Controlled and automatic human information processing: II. Perceptual learning, automatic attending, and a general theory. *Psychological Review, 84,* 127–190.

Siesjo, B. K., & Wieloch, T. (1985). Brain injury: Neurochemical aspects. In D. P. Becker & J. T. Povlishock (Eds.), *Central nervous system trauma status report* (pp. 513–532). Washington, DC: National Institutes of Neurological and Communicative Disorder and Health.

Sigman, M., & Dehaene, S. (2006). Dynamics of the central bottleneck: Dual-task and task uncertainty. *PLoS Biology, 4*(7), e220. Available at http://www.plosbiology.org/article/info:doi/10.1371/journal.pbio.0040220

Silver, J. M., McAllister, T. W., & Yudofsky, S. C. (2005). Preface. In J. Silver, T. McAllister, & S. Yudofsky (Eds.), *Textbook of traumatic brain injury* (p. xix). Washington, DC: American Psychiatric Publishing.

Simon, D. (2001). Enhancing emotional control in persons with acquired brain injury [Abstract]. *Rehabilitation Psychology, 46,* 330.

Sivak, M., Hill, C., & Olson, P. (1984). Computerized video tasks as training techniques for driving related perceptual deficits of persons with brain damage: A pilot evaluation. *International Rehabilitation Research*, 7, 389–398.

Slomine, B., McCarthy, M., Ding, R., MacKenzie, E., Jaffe, K., Aitken, M., et al. (2006). Health care utilization and needs after pediatric traumatic brain injury. *Pediatrics*, *117*, 663–674.

Smith, E. (1974). Influence of site of impact on cognitive impairment persisting long after severe closed head injury. *Journal of Neurology, Neurosurgery and Psychiatry*, *37*, 719–726.

Smith, M. (1996). Acute care. In F. D. Rose & D. A. Johnson (Eds.), *Brain injury and after: Towards improved outcome* (pp. 21–48). New York: Wiley and Sons.

Smith, P., Jostmann, N., Galinsky, A., & van Dijk, W. (2008). Lacking power impairs executive functions. *Psychological Science*, *19*, 441–447.

Sohlberg, M. M. (2005). Can disabilities resulting from attentional impairments be treated effectively? In P. W. Halligan & D. T. Wade (Eds.), *Effectiveness of rehabilitation for cognitive deficits* (pp. 91–102). Oxford, England: Oxford University Press.

Sohlberg, M. M., & Mateer, C. A. (1987). Effectiveness of an attention training program. *Journal of Clinical and Experimental Neuropsychology*, *9*, 117–130.

Sohlberg, M. M., & Mateer, C. A. (1989). *Introduction to cognitive rehabilitation: Theory and practice*. New York: Guilford Press.

Sohlberg, M. M., & Mateer, C. A. (2001). *Cognitive rehabilitation: An integrative neuropsychological approach*. New York: Guilford Press.

Sohlberg, M. M., Sprunk, H., & Metzelaar, K. (1998). Efficacy of an external cuing system in an individual with severe frontal lobe damage. *Cognitive Rehabilitation*, *4*, 36–40.

Solch, O., & Schyra, B. (1972). The late results of severe cranio-cerebral injury. *Monatsschrift fur Unfallheilkunde, Versicherungs-, Versorgungs- und Verkehrsmedizin*, *75*, 141–155.

Sparedo, F. R., & Gill, D. (1989). Effects of prior alcohol use on head injury recovery. *Journal of Head Trauma Rehabilitation*, *4*, 75–82.

Spatz, H. (1950). Brain trauma in aviation. In *German aviation medicine in World War II*. Washington, DC: U.S. Air Force.

Stein, D. G. (1988). In pursuit of new strategies for understanding recovery from brain damage: Problems and perspectives. In T. Boll & B. Bryant (Eds.), *Clinical neuropsychology and brain function: Research, measurement and practice* (pp. 9–55). Washington, DC: American Psychological Association.

Stein, D. G., Brailowski, S., & Will, B. (1995). *Brain repair*. New York: Oxford University Press.

Story, T. B. (1991). Cognitive rehabilitation services in home and community settings. In J. S. Kreutzer & P. H. Wehman (Eds.), *Cognitive rehabilitation for persons with traumatic brain injury* (pp. 251–267). Bisbee, AZ: Imaginart.

Strangman, G. E. (2006, March). *Functional neuroimaging and cognition following TBI: Prediction of rehabilitation outcome and patterns of recovery*. Paper presented at the Second Federal Interagency Conference on Traumatic Brain Injury, Bethesda, MD.

Strich, S. J. (1961). Shearing of nerve fibers as a cause of brain damage due to head injury. *Lancet, ii*, 446–448.

Stuss, D. T. (1987). Contribution of frontal lobe injury to cognitive impairment after closed head injury: Methods of assessment and recent findings. In H. S. Levin, J. Grafman, & H. M. Eisenberg (Eds.), *Neurobehavioral recovery from head injury* (pp. 166–177). New York: Oxford University Press.

Stuss, D. T. (1991). Disturbance of self-awareness after frontal system damage. In G. P. Prigatano & D. L. Schacter (Eds.), *Awareness of deficit after brain injury* (pp. 63–83). New York: Oxford University Press.

Stuss, D. T., & Benson, D. F. (1986). *The frontal lobes*. New York: Raven Press.

Stuss, D. T., & Buckle, L. (1992). Traumatic brain injury: Neuropsychological deficits and evaluation at different stages of recovery and in different patient subtypes. *Journal of Head Trauma Rehabilitation*, 7, 40–54.

Stuss, D. T., & Gow, C. A. (1992). Frontal dysfunction after traumatic brain injury. *Neuropsychiatry, Neuropsychology and Behavioral Neurology*, 5, 272–282.

Stuss, D. T., & Levine, B. (2002). Adult clinical neuropsychology: Lessons from studies of the frontal lobes. *Annual Review of Psychology*, 53, 401–433.

Stuss, D. T., Mateer, C. A., & Sohlberg, M. M. (1994). Innovative approaches to frontal lobe deficits. In M. A. Finlayson & S. H. Garner (Eds.), *Brain injury rehabilitation: Clinical considerations* (pp. 212–223). Baltimore: Williams and Wilkins.

Stuss, D. T., Murphy, K. J., Binns, M. A., & Alexander, M. P. (2003). Staying on the job: The frontal lobes control performance variability. *Brain, 126*, 2363–2380.

Stuss, D. T., Stethem, L. L., Hugenholtz, H., Picton, T., Pivik, J., & Richard, M. T. (1989). Reaction time after head injury: Fatigue, divided attention, and consistency of performance. *Journal of Neurology, Neurosurgery and Psychiatry, 52*, 742–748.

Swift, T., & Wilson, S. L. (2001). Misconceptions about brain injury among the general public and non-expert health professionals: An exploratory study. *Brain Injury, 15*, 149–165.

Symonds, C. (1970). *Studies in neurology.* Oxford, England: Oxford University Press.

Szameitat, A. J., Schubert, T., Muller, K., & Von Cramon, D. Y. (2002). Localization of executive functions in dual-task performance with fMRI. *Journal of Cognitive Neuroscience, 14*, 1184–1199.

Tarter, R., & Edwards, K. (1985). Neuropsychology of alcoholism. In R. Tarter & D. Van Thiel (Eds.), *Alcohol and the brain: Chronic effects* (pp. 217–242). New York: Guilford Press.

Taylor, H. G., Yeates, K. O., Wade, S. L., Drotar, D., Stancin, T., & Minich, N. (2002). A prospective study of short- and long-term outcomes after TBI in children: Behavior and achievement. *Neuropsychology, 16,* 15–29.

Teasdale, G., & Jennett, B. (1974). Assessment of coma and impaired consciousness: A practical scale. *Lancet, 2,* 81–83.

Teasdale, T. W., & Engberg, A. W. (2001). Suicide after traumatic brain injury: A population study. *Journal of Neurology, Neurosurgery and Psychiatry, 171,* 436–440.

Telzrow, C. (1987). Management of academic and educational problems in head injury. *Journal of Learning Disabilities, 26,* 536–545.

Telzrow, C. F. (1990). Management of academic and behavioral problems in traumatic brain injury. In E. Bigler (Ed.), *Traumatic brain injury* (pp. 251–272). Austin, TX: Pro-Ed.

Teuber, H.-L. (1964). The riddle of frontal lobe function in man. In J. M. Warren & K. Akert (Eds.), *The frontal granular cortex and behavior* (pp. 410–444). New York: McGraw-Hill.

Teuber, H.-L. (1975). Recovery of function after brain injury in man. In Ciba Foundation Symposium Number 34, *Outcome of severe damage to the central nervous system* (pp. 159–190). Amsterdam: Elsevier.

Thomas, J. D., & Trexler, L. E. (1982). Behavioral and cognitive deficits in cerebrovascular accident and closed head injury: Implications for cognitive rehabilitation. In L. E. Trexler (Ed.), *Cognitive rehabilitation: Conceptualization and intervention* (pp. 27–61). New York: Plenum Press.

Thomsen, I. V. (1974). The patient with severe head injury and his family: A follow-up study of 50 patients. *Scandinavian Journal of Rehabilitation Medicine, 6,* 180–183.

Thomsen, I. V. (1984). Late outcome of very severe blunt head trauma: A 10–15 year second follow-up. *Journal of Neurology, Neurosurgery and Psychiatry, 47,* 260–268.

Thomsen, I. V. (1989). Do young patients have worse outcomes after severe blunt head trauma? *Brain Injury, 3,* 157–162.

Thomsen, I. V. (1990). Recognizing the development of behavior disorders. In R. Ll. Wood (Ed.), *Neurobehavioural sequelae of traumatic brain injury* (pp. 52–68). New York: Taylor and Francis.

Thornton, A. E., Boudreau, V. G., Griffiths, S. Y., Woodward, T. S., Kirby, T. F., & Honer, W. G. (2007). The impact of monetary reward on memory in schizophrenia spectrum disorder. *Neuropsychology, 21,* 631–645.

Thurman, D. (2001). The epidemiology and economics of head trauma. In L. Miller & R. Hayes (Eds.) *Head trauma: Basic, preclinical and clinical directions* (pp. 327–347). New York: Wiley.

Timming, R., Orrison, W. W., & Mikula, J. A. (1982). Computerized tomography and rehabilitation outcome after severe head trauma. *Archives of Physical Medicine and Rehabilitation, 63*, 154–159.

Todis, B., & Glang, A. (2008). Redefining success: Results of a qualitative study of postsecondary transition outcomes for youth with traumatic brain injury. *Journal of Head Trauma Rehabilitation, 23*(4), 252–263.

Toglia, J. P. (1991). Generalization of treatment: A multi-context approach to cognitive-perceptual impairment in adults with brain injury. *American Journal of Occupational Therapy, 46*, 505–516.

Toglia, J., & Kirk, U. (2000). Understanding self-awareness deficits following brain injury. *Neurorehabilitation, 15*, 57–70.

Trexler, L. E. (1982). Cognitive and neuropsychological aspects of affective change following traumatic brain injury. In L. E. Trexler (Ed.), *Cognitive rehabilitation: Conceptualization and intervention* (pp. 173–197). New York: Plenum Press.

Trexler, L. (1987). Neuropsychological rehabilitation in the United States. In M. J. Meier, A. L. Benton, & L. Diller (Eds.), *Neuropsychological rehabilitation* (pp. 437–460). New York: Guilford.

Trexler, L. E., & Fordyce, D. J. (1996). Psychological perspectives on rehabilitation. In R. Braddom (Ed.), *Physical medicine and rehabilitation* (pp. 66–82). Philadelphia: W. B. Saunders.

Triplett, G., Hill, C., Freeman, L., Rajan, U., & Templer, D. I. (1996). Incidence of head injury: Lasting effects among college students and working adults in the general population. *Perceptual and Motor Skills, 83*, 1344–1346.

Truelle, J. L., & Robert-Pariset, A. (1990). Questionnaire assessment of neurobehavioural problems: European head injury evaluation chart. In R. Ll. Wood (Ed.), *Neurobehavioural sequelae of traumatic brain injury* (pp. 69–86). New York: Taylor and Francis.

Tucker, D. M., & Williamson, P. A. (1984). Asymmetric neural control systems in human self-regulation. *Psychological Review, 91*, 185–215.

Tupper, D. E., & Cicerone, K. D. (1990). *The neuropsychology of everyday life: Assessment and basic competencies.* Boston: Kluwer Academic.

Turk, D., Banfield, J., Walling, B., Heatherton, T., Grafton, S., Handy, T., et al. (2004). From facial cue to dinner for two: The neurologic substrates of personal choice. *NeuroImage, 22*, 1281–1290.

Twitchell, T. E. (1951). The restoration of motor function following hemiplegia in man. *Brain, 74*, 443–480.

Tyerman, A. D. (1996). The social context. In F. D. Rose & D. A. Johnson (Eds.), *Brain injury and after: Towards improved outcome* (pp. 97–117). New York: Wiley and Sons.

Uomoto, J. M. (1992). Neuropsychological assessment and cognitive rehabilitation after brain injury. In S. Berrol (Ed.), *Physical medicine and rehabil-*

itation clinics of North America: Traumatic brain injury (pp. 291–318). Philadelphia: Saunders.

Uomoto, P. K., & Uomoto, M. J. (1999). *Impact of traumatic brain injury on the family and spouse.* Tacoma, WA: Brain Injury Association of Washington.

Urbach, J. R., & Culbert, J. P. (1991). Head-injured parents and their children: Psychosocial consequences of a traumatic syndrome. *Psychosomatics, 32,* 24–33.

Uzzell, B. P. (1986). Pathophysiology and behavioral recovery. In B. Uzzell & Y. Gross (Eds.), *Clinical neuropsychology of intervention* (pp. 3–18). Boston: Martinus-Nijhoff.

Uzzell, B. P., Dolinskas, C. A., Wiser, R. F., & Langfitt, T. W. (1987). Influence of lesions detected by computed tomography on outcome and neuropsychological recovery after severe head injury. *Neurosurgery, 20,* 396–402.

Uzzell, B. P., & Stonnington, H. H. (1996). Final thoughts: Speculations for the future. In B. P. Uzzell & H. H. Stonnington (Eds.), *Recovery after traumatic brain injury* (pp. 323–329). Mahwah, NJ: Erlbaum.

Uzzell, B. P., & Stonnington, H. H. (1996). Introduction. In B. P. Uzzell & H. H. Stonnington (Eds.), *Recovery after traumatic brain injury* (pp. 1–3). Mahwah, NJ: Erlbaum.

Vaillant, G. E. (1977). *Adaptation to life.* Boston: Little, Brown, and Company.

Vaillant, G. E. (1993). *The wisdom of the ego.* Cambridge, MA: Harvard University Press.

Vaillant, G. E. (2002). *Aging well.* Boston: Little, Brown, and Company.

van Zomeren, A. H., & Brouwer, W. H. (1994). *Clinical neuropsychology of attention.* New York: Oxford University Press.

van Zomeren, A. H., Brouwer, W. H., & Deelman, B. G. (1984). Attentional deficits: The riddles of selectivity, speech, and alertness. In D. N. Brooks (Ed.), *Closed head injury: Psychological, social, and family consequences* (pp. 74–107). Oxford, England: Oxford University Press.

van Zomeren, A. H., Brouwer, W. H., & Minderhoud, J. M. (1987). Acquired brain damage and driving: A review. *Archives of Physical Medicine and Rehabilitation, 68,* 697–705.

van Zomeren, A. H., & Spikman, J. M. (2005). Testing speed and control: The assessment of attentional impairments. In P. W. Halligan & D. T. Wade (Eds.), *Effectiveness of rehabilitation for cognitive deficits* (pp. 71–80). New York: Oxford University Press.

van Zomeren, A. H., & Vandenburg, W. (1985). Residual complaints of patients two years after severe head injury. *Journal of Neurology, Neurosurgery and Psychiatry, 48,* 21–28.

Vapalahti, M., & Troupp, H. (1971). Prognosis for patients with severe brain injuries. *British Medical Journal, 3,* 404–407.

Varney, N. R., & Menefee, L. (1993). Psychosocial and executive deficits following closed head injury: Implications for orbital frontal cortex. *Journal of Head Trauma Rehabilitation, 8,* 32–45.

Vigoroux, R. P., Baurand, C., Naquet, R., Chament, J. H., Choux, M., Benayoun, R., et al. (1971). A series of patients with cranio-cerebral injuries studied neurologically, psychometrically, electroencephalographically, and socially. In *International Symposium on Head Injuries* (p. 335). Edinburgh: Churchill-Livingstone.

Vinogradova, O. S. (2001). Hippocampus as comparator: Role of the two input and two output systems of the hippocampus in selection and registration of information. *Hippocampus*, *11*, 578–589.

von Cramon, D., & Matthes-von Cramon, G. (1990). Frontal lobe dysfunctions in patients: Therapeutical approaches. In R. Ll. Wood & I. Fussey (Eds.), *Cognitive rehabilitation in perspective* (pp. 164–179). London: Taylor & Francis.

von Cramon, D., & Matthes-von Cramon, G. (1994). Back to work with a chronic dysexecutive syndrome. *Neuropsychological Rehabilitation*, *1*, 45–64.

von Cramon, D., Matthes-von Cramon, G., & Mai, N. (1991). Problem solving deficits in brain injured patients. A therapeutic approach. *Neuropsychological Rehabilitation*, *1*, 45–64.

Votruba, K. L., Rapport, L. J., Vangel, S. J., Hanks, R. A., Lequerica, A., Whitman, R. D., et al. (2008). Impulsivity and traumatic brain injury: The relations among behavioral observation, performance measures, and rating scales. *Journal of Head Trauma Rehabilitation*, *23*, 65–73.

Wade, D. T. (2005). Applying the WHO ICF framework to the rehabilitation of patients with cognitive deficits. In P. W. Halligan & D. T. Wade (Eds.), *Effectiveness of rehabilitation for cognitive deficits* (pp. 31–42). Oxford, England: Oxford University Press.

Walker, N. W. (1997). *Best practices in assessment and programming for students with traumatic brain injuries.* Raleigh, NC: State Department of Public Instruction.

Walsh, K. (1978). *Neuropsychology, a clinical approach.* New York: Churchill, Livingstone.

Walsh, K., & Darby, D. (1999). *Neuropsychology: A clinical approach* (4th ed.). New York: Churchill, Livingstone.

Walter, G. (1953). *The living brain.* New York: Norton.

Webster, J., & Scott, R. (1983). The effects of self-instructional training on attentional deficits following head injury. *Clinical Neuropsychology*, *4*, 69–74.

Wechsler, D. (1955). *Wechsler Adult Intelligence Scale.* New York: The Psychological Corporation.

Weddell, R., Oddy, M., & Jenkins, D. (1980). Social adjustments after rehabilitation: A two-year follow-up of patients with severe head injury. *Psychosocial Medicine*, *10*, 31–34.

Wehman, P. (1991). Cognitive rehabilitation in the workplace. In J. S. Kreutzer & P. H. Wehman (Eds.), *Cognitive rehabilitation for persons with traumatic brain injury* (pp. 269–288). Bisbee, AZ: Imaginart.

Wehman, P. (1996). Traumatic brain injury: Work outcome and supported employment. In B. P. Uzzell & H. H. Stonnington (Eds.), *Recovery after traumatic brain injury* (pp. 257–271). Mahwah, NJ: Erlbaum.

Wehman, P., Kreutzer, J., Sale, P., & West, M. (1989). Cognitive impairment and remediation: Implications for employment following traumatic brain injury. *Journal of Head Trauma Rehabilitation, 4*, 66–75.

Wehman, P., Targett, P., West, M., & Kregel, J. (2005). Productive work and employment for persons with traumatic brain injury. *Journal of Head Trauma Rehabilitation, 20*, 115–127.

Wepman, J. (1962). The language disorders. In J. Garrett & E. Levine (Eds.), *Psychological practices with the physically disabled* (pp. 197–230). New York: Columbia University Press.

Whyte, J. (1986). Outcome evaluation in the remediation of attention and memory deficits. *Journal of Head Trauma Rehabilitation, 1*, 64–71.

Willer, B., Abosch, S., & Dahmer, E. (1990). Epidemiology of disability from traumatic brain injury. In R. Ll. Wood (Ed.), *Neurobehavioural sequelae of traumatic brain injury* (pp. 18–33). New York: Taylor and Francis.

Williams, J. M. (1998). A practical model of everyday assessment. In R. J. Sbordone & C. Long (Eds.), *Ecological validity of neuropsychological testing* (pp. 129–145). Boca Raton, FL: St. Lucie Press.

Wilson, B. A. (1987). *Rehabilitation of memory.* New York: Guilford Press.

Wilson, B. A. (1995). Memory rehabilitation: Compensating for memory problems. In R. Dixon & L. Backmun (Eds.), *Compensating for psychological deficits and declines: Managing losses and promoting gains.* Mahwah, NJ: Erlbaum.

Wilson, B. A. (1999). *Case studies in neuropsychological rehabilitation.* New York: Oxford University Press.

Wilson, B. A. (2000). Compensating for cognitive deficits following brain injury. *Neuropsychology Review, 10*, 233–243.

Wilson, B. A. (2002). Toward a comprehensive model of cognitive rehabilitation. *Neuropsychological Rehabilitation, 12*, 97–110.

Wilson, B. A. (2003). The theory and practice of neuropsychological rehabilitation: An overview. In B. A. Wilson (Ed.), *Neuropsychological rehabilitation: Theory and practice* (pp. 1–10). Lisse, The Netherlands: Swets and Zeitlinger.

Wilson, B. A. (2005). The clinical neuropsychologist's dilemma. *Journal of the International Neuropsychological Society, 11*, 488–493.

Wilson, B. A., Emslie, H., Quirk, K., Evans, J., & Watson, P. (2005). A randomized control trial to evaluate a paging system for people with traumatic brain injury. *Brain Injury, 19*, 891–894.

Wilson, B. A., Scott, H., Evans, J., & Emslie, H. (2003). Preliminary report of a NeuroPage service within a health care system. *NeuroRehabilitation, 18*, 3–8.

Wilson, J. T. L., Hadley, D. M., Scott, L. C., & Harper, A. (1996). Neuropsychological significance of contusional lesions identified by MRI. In B. P. Uzzell & H. H. Stonnington (Eds.), *Recovery after traumatic brain injury* (pp. 29–37). Mahwah, NJ: Erlbaum.

World Health Organization. (1980). *International classification of impairments, disabilities and handicaps.* Geneva, Switzerland: World Health Organization.

World Health Organization. (2001). *International classification of functioning and disability*, (Beta-2 draft, short version). Geneva: World Health Organization.

Wood, R. Ll. (1987). *Brain injury rehabilitation: A neurobehavioural approach.* Rockville, MD: Aspen.

Wood, R. Ll. (1990). Neurobehavioural paradigm for rehabilitation. In R. Ll. Wood (Ed.), *Neurobehavioural sequelae of traumatic brain injury* (pp. 3–17). New York: Taylor and Francis.

Wood, R. Ll., & Fussey, I. (1987). Computer-assisted cognitive retraining: A controlled study. *International Disability Studies, 9*, 149–155.

Wood, R. Ll., & Liossi, C. (2006). Neuropsychological and neurobehavioral correlates of aggression following traumatic brain injury. *Journal of Neuropsychiatry and Clinical Neuroscience, 18*, 333–341.

Wood, R. Ll., Liossi, C., & Wood, L. (2005). The impact of head injury neurobehavioral sequelae on personal relationships: Preliminary findings. *Brain Injury, 19*(10), 845–853.

Wood, R., & Rutterford, N. A. (2006). Psychosocial adjustment 17 years after severe brain injury. *Journal of Neurology, Neurosurgery and Psychiatry, 77*, 71–73.

Worthington, A. & Walker, J. (2005). Rehabilitation of everyday living skill in the context of executive disorder. In M. Oddy & A. Worthington (Eds.), *Rehabilitation of executive disorders: A guide to theory and practice* (pp. 195–210). New York: Oxford University Press.

Worthington, A., & Walker, J. (2008). Rehabilitation of everyday living skills in the context of executive disorder. In M. Oddy & A. Worthington (Eds.). *Rehabilitation of executive disorders* (pp. 195–210). New York, NY: Oxford University Press.

Wright, J. (2000). The Glasgow Outcome Scale, and the Rappaport Disability Rating Scale. *The Center for Outcome Measurement in Brain Injury.* Retrieved September 17, 2008, from http://www.tbims.org/combi/gos

Wright, P., Rogers, N., Hall, C., Wilson, B., Evans, J., Emslie, H., et al. (2001). Comparison of pocket-computer memory aids for people with brain injury. *Brain Injury, 15*, 787–800.

Ylvisaker, M. (1998). Traumatic brain injury in children and adolescents: Introduction. In M. Ylvisaker (Ed.), *Traumatic brain injury rehabilitation: Children and adolescents* (2nd ed., pp. 1–10). Boston: Butterworth-Heinemann.

Ylvisaker, M. (2005). Children with cognitive, communicative, academic and behavioral disabilities. In W. M. High, A. M. Sander, M. A. Struchen, & K. A. Hart (Eds.), *Rehabilitation for traumatic brain injury* (pp. 205–234). New York: Oxford University Press.

Ylvisaker, M., & Gioia, G. (1998). Cognitive assessment. In M. Ylvisaker (Ed.), *Traumatic brain injury rehabilitation: Children and adolescents* (2nd ed., pp. 159–179). Boston: Butterworth-Heinemann.

Ylvisaker, M., Hanks, R., & Johnson-Greene, D. (2002). Perspectives on rehabilitation of individuals with cognitive impairment after brain injury: Rationale for reconsideration of theoretical paradigms. *Journal of Head Trauma Rehabilitation. 17*, 191–209.

Ylvisaker, M., & Szekeres, S. F. (1996). Cognitive rehabilitation for children with traumatic brain injury. In P. W. Corrigan & S. C. Yudofsky (Eds.), *Cognitive rehabilitation for neuropsychiatric disorders* (pp. 263–296). Washington, DC: American Psychiatric Association.

Ylvisaker, M., & Szekeres, S. F. (1998). A framework for cognitive rehabilitation. In M. Ylvisaker (Ed.), *Traumatic brain injury rehabilitation: Children and adolescents* (2nd ed., pp. 125–159). Boston: Butterworth-Heinemann.

Ylvisaker, M., Szekeres, S. F., & Feeney, T. J. (1998). Cognitive rehabilitation: Executive functions. In M. Ylvisaker (Ed.), *Traumatic brain injury rehabilitation: Children and adolescents* (2nd ed., pp. 221–269). Boston: Butterworth-Heinemann.

Ylvisaker, M., Todis, B., Glang, A., Urbanczyk, B., Franklin, C., DePompei, R., et al. (2001). Educating students with TBI: Themes and recommendations. *Journal of Head Trauma Rehabilitation, 16*, 76–93.

Ylvisaker, M., & Urbanczyk, B. (1994). Assessment and treatment of speech, swallowing, and communication disorders following traumatic brain injury. In M. A. Finlayson & S. H. Garner (Eds.), *Brain injury rehabilitation: Clinical considerations* (pp. 157–186). Baltimore: Williams and Wilkins.

Zaidel, E. (1987). Hemispheric monitoring. In D. Ottoson (Ed.), *Duality and unity of the brain.* London: Macmillan.

Index